# TELOMERE - A COMPLEX END OF A CHROMOSOME

Edited by **Marcelo L. Larramendy**

**Telomere - A Complex End of a Chromosome**
http://dx.doi.org/10.5772/60625
Edited by Marcelo L. Larramendy

**Contributors**

Tatsuaki Tsuruyama, Gery Lamblin, Gautier Chene, Karine Le Bail-Carval, Philippe Chabert, Georges Mellier, Andrei Tchirkov, Ekta Khattar, Vinay Tergaonkar, Leandro Sastre, Rosario Perona, Laura Iarriccio, Laura Pintado-Berninches, Javier Rodriguez-Centeno, Cristina Manguan-Garcia, Elena Garcia, Blanca Lopez-Ayllon, Alejandro Bolzan, Angayarkanni Jayaraman, Muthusamy Palaniswamy, Jayaraman Angayarkanni, K G Kiran, Yutaka Takahashi, Juliana Da Silva, Vivian Francilia Silva Kahl, Kerem Teralı, Açelya Yilmazer

**Published by InTech**

Janeza Trdine 9, 51000 Rijeka, Croatia



**Publishing Process Manager** Iva Simcic

**Technical Editor** SPi Global

**Cover** InTech Design team

First published November, 2016

Printed in Croatia

Additional hard copies can be obtained from orders@intechopen.com

Telomere - A Complex End of a Chromosome , Edited by Marcelo L. Larramendy

p. cm.

Print ISBN 978-953-51-2752-9
Online ISBN 978-953-51-2753-6

For EU product safety concerns:
IN TECH d.o.o., Prolaz Marije Krucifikse Kozulić 3, 51000 Rijeka, Croatia,
info@intechopen.com or visit our website at intechopen.com.

# Meet the editor

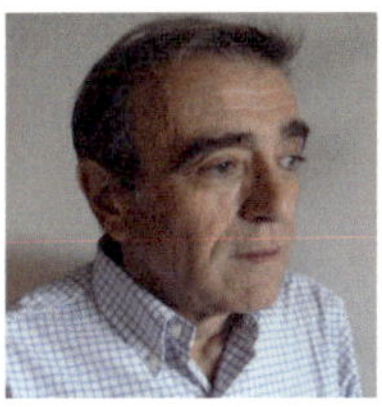

Marcelo L. Larramendy, Ph.D., serves as Professor of Molecular Cell Biology at the School of Natural Sciences and Museum (National University of La Plata, Argentina). He has been appointed as Senior Researcher of the National Scientific and Technological Research Council of Argentina. He is also Former Member of the Executive Committee of the Latin American Association of Environmental Mutagenesis, Teratogenesis and Carcinogenesis. He is author of more than 470 contributions, including scientific publications, research communications and conferences worldwide. He is recipient of several national and international awards. Prof. Larramendy is a regular Lecturer at the international A. Hollaender Courses organized by the IAEMS and is former guest scientist at the NIH, USA, and University of Helsinki, Finland. He is expert in Genetic Toxicology and is, or has been, referee for more than 30 international scientific journals. He is also member of the International Panel of Experts at the International Agency for Research on Cancer (IARC, WHO, Lyon, France) in 2015 for the evaluation of DDT, 2,4-D, and Lindane. Presently, Prof. Dr. Larramendy is Head of the Laboratory of Molecular Cytogenetics and Genotoxicology at the UNLP.

# Contents

# Preface

Historically, Hermann Muller in the 1930s was the first researcher to point out that the ends of the chromosomes had unique properties and functions as well. Muller named these chromosomal ending part “telomeres” (from the Greek words telo, meaning "end" and mere, meaning "part"), based on their terminal position. Furthermore, realizing that the ends of chromosomes were strangely resistant to X-ray-induced chromosomal damage, he hypothesized that "the terminal gene must have a special function, that of sealing the end of the chromosome, so to speak, and that "for some reason, a chromosome cannot persist indefinitely without having its ends thus sealed". Nowadays, we know that Muller was only partially correct. It is very well know and scientifically accepted that telomeres do indeed play an essential role in stabilizing the ends of chromosomes, but, on the other hand, they do not contain active genes within their DNA sequences. Instead, telomeres possess an array of highly repeated DNA sequences and specific binding proteins that form a unique, peculiar, and functional structure at the end of the chromosome. Thus, telomeres should be considered not just a simple end part of a chromosome, but instead a dynamic and functional part of them.

In addition, Barbara McClintock, a brilliant American cytogeneticist who was awarded the 1983 Nobel Prize in Physiology or Medicine, had developed reliable methods for preserving and staining maize chromosomes. McClintock observed that the broken chromosomal ends induced by clastogens were unstable. Furthermore, she noticed that these broken ends fused with any other broken ends when they contacted each other. When the replication process occurred after such contact, the cycle of breakage--fusion could, thus, be repeated. However, it was also noticed that the breakage--fusion cycle was broken when dicentric chromosomes were present, as in embryonic cells, where the broken ends of the chromosomes were somehow "healed." Nowadays, the scientific community knows that the ends were healed by the addition of a telomere, a process that is catalyzed by a specific reverse transcriptase enzyme called telomerase. Furthermore, we know that telomerase is active in germ cells, embryonic cells, and some somatic cells, but not in the endosperm cells that McClintock examined in her research work. It is worth mentioning that McClintock not only highlighted that cells do not accept the presence of unprotected chromosome ends, but also that the chromosomal broken ends are quickly fused together by the mechanism of DNA repair. Furthermore, she also observed that telomeres prevent these fusion events from occurring. Despite the magnitude and importance of these observations, 40 years of scientific research would pass by before the actual known structure of telomeres was revealed.

In the mid-1970s, Elizabeth Blackburn determined the telomere sequences for the ribosomal DNA minichromosome of the free-living ciliate protozoa Tetrahymena sp. Sequencing experiments demonstrated that the telomeres of this structure possessed 20-70 tandem copies of a simple hexanucleotide with the sequence 5'-CCCCAA-3' on one strand and 5'-TTGGGG on the complementary strand. Noteworthy, the GT-rich strand represented the 3'-end of the minichromosomes. Actually, it is well known that these tandem repeats of short GT-rich sequences are characteristic of almost all eukaryotic telomeres. They consist, generally, of a 6-8 bp sequence that is repeated hundreds or thousands of times, varying the actual repeated sequence and the number of repeats among species. In this sense, e.g., human telomeres range in size from 2-50 kb and consist of approximately 300-8,000 precise repeats of the sequence CCCTAA/TTAGGG, whereas telomeres from the budding yeast Saccharomyces cerevisiae are smaller and more heterogeneous in their composition, containing about 60-100 copies of the sequence C1-3A/TG1-3. Although such variations exist, common features of all telomeres are the orientation of the G-rich strand, which makes up the 3'-end of the chromosome, and that the terminal portion of the G-rich strand is single-stranded, generating the so-called "G-tail," with an average length of 50-100 nucleotides in yeast but up to 75-300 nucleotides in humans.

By the early 1970s, the mechanism of cellular DNA replication was clarified, and then scientists realized that this system offered an essential dilemma. Particularly, the ends of chromosomes are supposed to gradually shorten with each cycle of DNA replication. This so-called "end-replication" problem results as a direct consequence of DNA polymerase's properties. It is known that DNA polymerase requires the presence of short RNA primers to begin replication. It can then extend the primers in a 5'-to-3'-direction. Accordingly, as the replication fork progresses along the chromosome, one of the two daughter strands is synthesized continuously, whereas the other daughter strand is synthesized discontinuously in short fragments (also known as Okazaki fragments, possessing their own RNA primers), this being the so-called lagging strand. Subsequently, the RNA primers are degraded, with the gaps between the Okazaki fragments filled by the DNA enzymatic apparatus. However, a serious problem arises at the ending part of each chromosome: the DNA repair machinery is not capable of completing the gap left by the terminal RNA primer. As a consequence, the newly synthesized DNA molecule is shorter than the template (parent) DNA molecule by at least the length of one RNA primer. Without a solution to this end-replication problem, chromosomes would progressively shorten over cell-cycle divisions. We know that the "cleaver" cellular machinery must avoid such a problem, which would bring about catastrophic consequences.

By the mid-1980s, accumulating evidence started to suggest that cells are capable of solving this replication dilemma by lengthening their telomeres. Researchers from the Blackburn and Szostak laboratories were able to demonstrate not only that DNA sequences from Tetrahymena may function as telomeres for linear plasmids introduced into yeast cells, but also that the Tetrahymena telomere sequences were elongated during the process. They also demonstrated, when sequencing the new telomeres, that the elongated telomeres had repeated copies of the yeast TG1-3 repeat sequences rather than the Tetrahymena TTGGGG repeat ones. Accordingly, a new open question arose from these observations: How is it possible that yeast cells can elongate telomere sequences from another organism with copies of that organism's own telomere repeat?

Fortunately, the answer to this question was provided by the discovery of the telomerase. Carol Greider, a student in Blackburn's lab, further investigated Tetrahymena extracts able to incorporate nucleotides into a synthetic oligonucleotide that contained four copies of the Tetrahymena telomere repeat sequences. Greider purified an enzyme able to lengthen telomeres. This enzyme, later called telomerase, turned out to be a highly specialized reverse transcriptase, in other words, an enzyme able to synthesize DNA from an RNA template. The telomerase can also be classified as a ribonucleoprotein, since the RNA template is a constitutional part of the enzyme complex itself. Finally, it can also be stressed that its RNA template includes a base sequence complementary to the telomere repeat unit in the same organism.

Telomerase binds to the G-tail of the telomere through the RNA template, and it then catalyzes the extension of the G-tail. The enzyme is able to repeat this cyclic procedure many times by moving to new binding sites along the newly transcribed G-tail. In this way, in the next cycle of DNA replication, both the DNA polymerase and the DNA repair enzymes, among other enzymes, fill in the other strand. Thus, telomerase is able not only to maintain but also extend the length of telomeres.

Since the discovery of telomerase, it has become evident that this "key molecule" plays a crucial role in the regulation of the length of telomeres. Universally, telomeres are likely to shorten in cells without telomerase activity over time, and cells may stop dividing and become senescent after their telomeres shorten below a critical length. Some of the first abnormalities appear in reproductive and hematopoietic tissues. Indeed, in most animals, embryonic cells and germ cells possess telomerase activity, but many types of somatic cells do not. The exceptions include highly proliferative cells, such as those in the skin, hematopoietic tissues, and the intestinal epithelium.

Our view of the telomere has matured considerably since Blackburn and Gall provided the first information about its molecular composition. Furthermore, two new landmarks can be included in the thrilling and revolutionary history of telomeres/telomerase. The 2009 Nobel Prize in Physiology or Medicine was awarded jointly to Elizabeth H. Blackburn, Carol W. Greider, and Jack W. Szostak for the discovery of how chromosomes are protected by telomeres and the enzyme telomerase and how the enzyme impacts telomere length. A 2010 study by Mariela Jaskelioff and collaborators from Harvard Medical School showed telomere shortening to be a root cause of cellular aging.

This book, Telomere - A Complex End of a Chromosome , is organized into nine chapters containing the latest aspects of the current knowledge about the structure of telomeres and the crucial role that telomerase plays not only in maintaining chromosomal stability but also in relation to cell immortality, cell instability, and cancer biology. This book begins with two general chapters related to the structural and functional aspects of telomeres. The first chapter focuses on the structural and functional aspects of telomeric proteins and their importance in human diseases. The second chapter clearly reviews the mechanisms involved in post-transplant complications, including acute cellular rejection, chronic rejection, and chronic hepatitis of unknown cause by ageing and senescence due to telomere shortening. Then, this book includes seven chapters describing different aspects related to telomeres, telomere length, telomerase, and their relation to human health. The first reviews the current knowledge about the function of human telomeres and telomerase and their relevance in genomic instability in cancer, focusing on specific results for ovarian cancer. The second focuses on the telomerase enzyme, which maintains telomere length, as the major factor responsible for evading cell death and highlights how telomere length maintenance and telomerase expression put together are prerequisite for immortality, an essential character for cancer cells, and that understanding the mechanism of telomere and telomerase functions may pave the way for eradicating diseases like cancer. The third provides a summary of the current knowledge about telomere instability induced by anticancer drugs on mammalian cells. The fourth provides a broad evaluation of the associated mechanisms between human health and occupational exposure to different xenobiotics and telomere length, including recent findings and future perspectives. The fifth discusses the pathophysiological role of shortened telomere length in metabolic and endocrine diseases and the significance of cellular senescence. The sixth provides a review of the process by which, in a pathological context, extratelomeric effects of telomerase are related to the emergence and persistence of the cancer stem cell phenotype. Furthermore, given the common conception of cancer stemness as a major contributor to therapy resistance and tumour relapse, a more complete annotation of biological mechanisms for its regulation by telomerase will provide the opportunity to develop telomerase-targeted anticancer therapies that kill or differentiate cancer stem cells effectively. Finally, the last chapter reviews hereditary diseases caused by the presence of shortened telomeres, collectively named telomeropathies or telomere biology disorders. In these diseases, cell proliferation is impaired, which results in premature aging and dysfunction of highly proliferative tissues. Among these diseases are dyskeratosis congenita, Hoyeraal--Hreidarsson syndrome, Revesz syndrome, Coats plus syndromes, aplastic anemia, idiopathic pulmonary fibrosis, and nonalcholic, noninfectious liver disease, in which mutations present in the genes coding for the components of the telomerase and shelterin complexes and other proteins involved in telomere replication are the cause of these disease.

Many researchers have contributed to the publication of this book. Given the fast pace of new scientific publications shedding light on the matter, this book will probably be outdated very soon. We regard this as a positive and healthy fact. The editors hope that this book will continue to meet the expectations and needs of all interested in the telomere/telomerase scientific field. We now appreciate that these unusual complexes of DNA and proteins we all know as "telomeres" are dynamic and key structures that depend on telomerase and other cellular factors for continuance. Regulation of telomere activity is a dynamic area of current research, and new insights into telomeres and their role in aging and cancer, among other biological functions and pathologies, appear regularly in the scientific world. However, one fact is more than understandable in this difficult biological conundrum: the end of the telomere story is far from being totally unraveled.

**Prof. Marcelo L. Larramendy, Ph.D.**
Principal Researcher CONICET
School of Natural Sciences and Museum
National University of La Plata (UNLP)
La Plata, Argentina

Chapter 1

# Telomeres in Liver Transplantation Allografts

Tatsuaki Tsuruyama and Wulamujiang Aini

Additional information is available at the end of the chapter

http://dx.doi.org/10.5772/62196

**Abstract**

Living-donor liver transplant is a life-saving procedure for people with end-stage liver disease that has increased the number of organs available for people on the liver transplant waiting list. Patients often receive grafts from their relatives in living-donor liver transplantation. Maintenance of long-term graft function is important in liver transplant recipients. Livers from older donors have worse graft survival rates in human liver transplantation, and therefore, accurate evaluation of graft aging and senescence is expected to provide critical data for therapeutic intervention in long-term grafts. Many insults, including rejection, can contribute to post-transplant damage. Late post-transplant biopsies frequently show chronic hepatitis of unknown cause, and this can cause late graft dysfunction leading to cirrhosis. Telomere length in chronic hepatitis or cirrhosis is significantly lower than that in normal livers of the same age. Sustained cellular turnover in chronic liver disease accelerates cellular senescence or a crisis because of telomere shortening. Here, we review the mechanisms involved in post-transplant complications including acute cellular rejection, chronic rejection, and chronic hepatitis of unknown cause by ageing and senescence due to telomere shortening.

**Keywords:** Transplantation, liver, telomere

## 1. Introduction

### 1.1. Summary

Living-donor liver transplant is a life-saving procedure for people with end-stage liver disease that has increased the number of organs available for people on the liver transplant waiting list. Patients often receive grafts from their relatives in living-donor liver transplantation.

Maintenance of long-term graft function is important in liver transplant recipients. Livers from older donors have worse graft survival rates in human liver transplantation, and therefore, accurate evaluation of graft aging and senescence is expected providing critical data for therapeutic intervention in long-term grafts. Many insults, including rejection, can contribute to post-transplant damage. Late post-transplant biopsies frequently show chronic hepatitis of unknown cause, and this can cause late graft dysfunction leading to cirrhosis. Telomere length in chronic hepatitis or cirrhosis is significantly lower than that in normal livers of the same age. Sustained cellular turnover in chronic liver disease accelerates cellular senescence or a crisis because of telomere shortening. Here, we review the mechanisms involved in post-transplant complications including acute cellular rejection, chronic rejection, and chronic hepatitis of unknown cause by ageing and senescence due to telomere shortening.

### 1.2. Background

Telomeres are comprised of tandem nucleotides repeats (TTAGGG) and their functional role includes protection against the degradation of chromosomes and the maintenance of genome integrity and stability [1]. Telomere shortening relates with the etiology of liver allograft dysfunction and/or graft failure such as acute cellular rejection, chronic rejection, and chronic hepatitis of unknown cause (idiopathic post-transplant hepatitis) after liver transplantation. Older people are more sensitive to most acquired liver disorders and are more indefensibly to the consequences of liver disease. In the chronic hepatic injury and inflammation, cellular senescence functions as an essential stress-response mechanism to restrict the proliferation of damaged cells, but this benefit is at the expense of senescence-related organ dysfunction. The dual role of cell senescence in chronic liver disease will make this an intriguing but challenging area for future clinical interventions. In the setting of chronic liver disease, telomere reduction was more significant than in hepatocytes of normal livers of subjects of the same age [2-4]. In this review, we will discuss mechanism of telomere shortening involved in hepatocyte senescence after liver transplantation by examining the present-day knowledge of telomere structure. Particularly, we discuss mechanisms by which inflammation, acute stress, and oxidative stress accelerate cellular senescence.

## 2. Human telomere structure

Telomere is nucleoprotein complex at the end of chromosomes that is composed of repeated DNA sequences and interaction binding proteins [5]. Human telomeric DNA is generally in the 5–15 kb length range and contains double-stranded tandem repeats of TTAGGG, followed by single-stranded G-rich overhang [6-7]. The G-rich overhang can form a structure called t-loop [8]. T-loops have been identified by electron microscopy [9]. Moreover, the telomere fold backs on itself, so that the single-stranded G-rich overhang invades into double-stranded DNA to form a D-loop (displacement loop) [5]. The G-rich DNA sequences fold into noncanonical secondary structures called G-quadruplex. G-quadruplex is formed by stacking of several G-tetrads. The G-tetrads are formed by four guanines arranged in a plane by hydrogen bonds. These structures have been identified in human cells by using a highly specific DNA G-quadruplex antibody recently [10]. Protein complex of telomeres, known as shelterin, consists of TRF1 (telomeric repeat binding factor 1), TRF2 (telomeric repeat binding factor 2), RAP1 (repressor/activator protein 1), TIN2 (TRF1 interacting nuclear factor 2), TPP1 (TIN2-POT1 organizing protein), and POT1 (protection of telomere 1) [5, 11-12]. TRF1 and TRF2 directly bind the telomeric double-strand DNA, while POT1 binds the single-stranded overhang. TIN2 and TPP1 interact with POT1. RAP1 has no obvious effect on protection or length regulation of human telomeres [13]. Additionally, telomere-associated complex has recently been identified in mammalian cells. This complex, called CST, consists of Conserved Telomere Component 1 (CTC1), STN1 and TEN1 [14-15].

### 2.1. Telomere length regulation

Telomere length is determined by the degree of DNA elongation by telomerase, DNA erosion by incomplete DNA replication, and double-strand breaks caused by DNA damage [16]. Telomerase is a ribonucleoprotein enzyme that synthesizes new telomeric DNA to compensate for replication-associated telomere reduction [17]. Telomerase is composed of the telomerase reverse transcriptase (TERT) and a telomerase RNA component (TERC) that serves as the template for telomere extension [18]. Overexpression of human TERT (hTERT) can lead to rapid telomere elongation while hTERT knockdown or inhibition results in telomere shortening [19]. Telomere binding proteins, such as TRF2, participate in telomere length regulation in humans [20]. Human Pot1 (hPot1) as well participate in telomere length regulation by disrupting the DNA binding activity. Knocking down the expression of hPot1 in cells causes apoptosis or senescence [21]. Moreover, STN1, a part of CST complex, plays critical role in regulating telomere lengths and replicative potential of normal human fibroblasts. STN1 knockdown cells displayed a greater increase in telomere erosion and entered cellular senescence as a consequence of telomere dysfunction [22].

### 2.2. Functions of human telomeres

Human telomeres protect chromosome ends from degradation and DNA double-strand break repair [23-24]. The protective function of telomeres presumably depends on their state, whether they have "capping" or "uncapping" structures. Telomeres achieve their "capping" function by a combination of their higher-order DNA structure and binding proteins. The t-loop and G-quadruplex provide the possible cap status for telomere protection. Telomere loss leads to the disruption of telomere structures, inducing gradual telomere uncapping [25-31]. Binding proteins prevent telomeres from being recognized by the cell as a DNA break and repaired by nonhomologous end joining (NHEJ) or homologous recombination (HR)-mediated repair [5]. TRF1and TRF2 have a negative regulating function for telomere length and participate in telomere end protection [32]. TIN2 has a role of maintenance of telomere cohesion [33]. TPP1 is essential for both telomere end protection and length regulation, through repressing DNA damage signaling and modulating telomerase-dependent telomere elongation [34-35]. Protection from a DNA damage response (DDR) or unwanted DNA repair, referred to as "capped" [8, 31]. Uncapped telomeres are recognized by the DDR proteins and chromosome ends, which are referred to as telomere dysfunction-induced foci (TIFs) [36]. It has been identified that cell proliferation in vitro is accompanied by telomere shortening [1]. If telomere shortening reaches a limit and DDR foci accumulation reaches 4 or 5 foci, widespread end-to-end fusion of chromosomes and cell death would occur [37].

## 3. Age-related disease and telomere shortening

Telomere length decreases with age [38-39]. Telomere length, when shorter than the average telomere length, is associated with increased incidence of age-related diseases and/or decreased life span in humans [40-41]. Telomere length is a risk marker for cardiovascular disease [42-43]. The degree of telomere shortening correlated with the severity of heart disease [44]. Chromosomal instability in ulcerative colitis is associated with telomere shortening [45]. Liver cirrhosis correlated with hepatocyte-specific telomere shortening [3]. Type 2 diabetes was associated with reduced telomere length [46-47]. Short telomere lengths are predictors for the development of diabetic nephropathy [48]. Short telomeres are a risk factor for the development of idiopathic pulmonary fibrosis [49]. Moreover, telomere shortening has been involved in the dramatic age-related changes in the immune system as well, and this is one of the main factors believed to influence morbidity and mortality [50]. Telomere shortening promotes genome instability, leading to cancer initiation [51]. Short telomeres are likely to be recognized as double-strand breaks, resulting in induction of DNA damage repair by nonhomologous end joining pathway, leading to end-to-end chromosomal fusions. When cells with fused chromosomes enter mitotic cycles, these chromosomal fusions are likely to break and result in chromosomal abnormalities. Repeated breakage–fusion–bridge cycles cause accumulation of chromosomal instability that leads to final malignant transformation [52-53]. Telomerase activity are well correlated with development of cancer besides telomere shortening. Telomerase activity has been detected in many kinds of human cancers [54]. In addition, obesity and smoking as well as hypertension and lower socioeconomic status are associated with leucocyte telomere reduction [38, 55-57]. Telomeres in liver cells, compared to cells of other major organs, shorten most rapidly with age. The telomere shortening in hepatocytes is especially rapid in infants, and then the rate of shortening slows from adolescence to middle age, while no significant decrease is evident in adults in their forties up to centenarians [58-60].

## 4. Liver allograft rejection

### 4.1. Acute cellular rejection

The diagnosis of acute cellular rejection is determined by portal mixed cellular infiltration, bile duct inflammation or damage, and portal or central veins' endotheliitis [61]. The portal inflammatory cells include lymphocytes, neutrophils, and eosinophils predominantly. Bile duct damage is composed of variation in nuclear size, eosinophilic degeneration, vacuolation of the cytoplasm, and lymphocytic infiltration into the bile duct epithelium. However, acute cellular rejection represents an immune-mediated injury directed toward the bile ducts or vascular endothelium, rather than toward hepatocytes [62]. Sustained cellular turnover in chronic liver disease accelerates cellular senescence [2-4, 63-65]. In liver transplantation, aged donors have worse prognosis [66]. Graft survival for hepatic allografts from aged donors was significantly lower than for allografts from younger donors, suggesting there is an inability of older grafts to expand to meet the functional demands of recipients [67]. Elder donor tissue has reduced ability to withstand stress and repair. Preexisting aging presumably decreases repair and survival capacity, and post-transplant stress (e.g., rejection) further disrupts this capacity and causes graft failure [68]. Many occurrences including rejection contribute to post-transplant damage. Greater rate of telomere decline with episodes of acute rejection lead to greater telomere reduction during the post-transplant period. Accordingly, the frequency of post-transplant events (e.g., rejection) should be diminished preventing additional cell turnover.

### 4.2. Chronic rejection

Clinically, chronic rejection is characterized by progressive jaundice, unresponsive to immunosuppression, and, histologically, by obliterative vasculopathy, affecting large and medium-sized muscular arteries. Moreover, chronic rejection is characterized by the loss of small bile ducts [69-71]. Although the incidence of chronic rejection has decreased from 15–20% to 2–3% due to effective immunosuppression and early assessment of liver biopsies [69-70, 72-74], it is still an important cause of liver allograft failure. Our previous study showed that accelerated telomere intensity decline occurred in hepatocytes in chronic rejection within a year of transplantation. This accelerated telomere intensity decline might be a general process occurring in all grafts, since observed soon after liver transplantation. This observed decline may be due to premature aging following the acute stress observed in organ transplants and the high rate of cell turnover that occurs in graft regeneration immediately after transplantation [75]. Our previous data suggest that accelerated graft aging during the early post-transplantation term is inevitable even in tolerated grafts. The limit of proliferative life span by telomere shortening might be determined early after post-transplantation. Chronic rejection patients have one or more episodes of acute cellular rejection within a year of transplantation, and thus it is possible that acute cellular rejection induces a further early telomere intensity decline in hepatocytes [62, 76]. Care in organ preservation and preconditioning of the graft are important to achieve a better prognosis, which in turn is likely a consequence of the prevention of telomere erosion caused by various stressors immediately after transplantation. We have previously reported hepatocyte telomere signal intensity significantly lower than the predicted age-dependent decline observed in chronic rejection, as revealed by quantitative fluorescence in situ hybridization [77].

## 5. Idiopathic post-transplant hepatitis

Some groups have also called chronic hepatitis of unknown cause, such as idiopathic post-transplant hepatitis, *de novo* autoimmune hepatitis. This condition is commonly associated with positive autoantibodies, such as antinuclear antibody and elevation of IgG levels, and biochemically and histopathologically resembles autoimmune hepatitis in patients who did not receive transplants [78-79]. Increasing evidence suggests that late acute rejection, *de novo* autoimmune hepatitis, and idiopathic post-transplant hepatitis are part of an overlapping spectrum of immune-mediated late allograft damage occurring in long-term post-transplant patients [62]. Together with idiopathic post-transplant hepatitis, immune-mediated late allograft damage can cause late graft dysfunction leading to cirrhosis. Telomere length observed in chronic hepatitis or cirrhosis is significantly lower than that in normal livers of the same age. Sustained cellular turnover in chronic liver disease accelerates cellular senescence or a severe damage because of telomere shortening. We initially hypothesized that idiopathic post-transplant hepatitis may show more progressive telomere shortening due to higher cell turnover [3-4]. Cellular senescence in the explanted livers of young children was reported to be associated with hepatocyte damage rather than to a corresponding age-dependent phenomenon [80]. However, we observed no significant telomere reduction in hepatocytes taken from patients with idiopathic post-transplant hepatitis at late biopsy. Telomere shortening does not necessarily reflect the long-term graft status in idiopathic post-transplant hepatitis, which differs clinically and histologically. Telomere length in hepatocytes already shortened during the early post-transplant period. Increasing number of senescent cells associated with telomere shortening confirmed in a mouse model of ischemia–reperfusion injury [81]. Therefore, hepatocyte damage related to ischemia–reperfusion injury is likely to be a major factor in the accelerated telomere decline observed in the early post-transplant period. On the other hand, from the standpoint of telomere shortening in the early post-transplantation phase, telomere decline is considered a risk factor for late dysfunction of the graft. This finding is clinically significant in follow-up examinations of high-risk allografts.

## 6. Tolerance

Tolerance is a condition in which an allograft functions normally and lacks histological evidence of rejection in the absence of immunosuppression [82]. Tolerated grafts are suitable study materials for evaluating the biological organ age of grafts unaffected by inflammation and immunosuppression. We have previously reported a significant reduction in hepatocyte telomere signal intensity compared to the predicted age-dependent decline in the tolerated liver allograft, using quantitative fluorescence in situ hybridization [80,21]. Recently it has been demonstrated that measurement of relative average telomere lengths can be accomplished by real-time polymerase chain reaction (PCR) using a carefully designed pair of oligonucleotide primers [83]. In a larger number of cases, we performed quantitative real-time PCR, and confirmed accelerated telomere shortening relative to the chronological graft age in tolerated grafts. It is possible that a significant proportion of liver transplantation recipients are tolerant [84-86]. Accelerated telomere intensity decline occurred in hepatocytes in tolerated graft within a year of transplantation. The results of the previous study have suggested that even tolerated grafts might undergo a lowering of renewal capacity and a decrease in function as the recipients become older [2]. According to our previous study, the allograft could be older than the predicted age of the allograft even in tolerated grafts, and the telomere length shortened based on the graft age.

## 7. Oxidative stress after living-donor liver transplantation

Ischemia and reperfusion during transplantation produce a transient increase of reactive oxygen species in the organ, which are potent inducers of DNA breaks. In a rat model, both allogeneic and syngeneic transplants were characterized by shortened telomeres during ischemia at transplantation [87]. Oxidative stress accelerates telomere shortening [88-89]. Low ambient oxygen conditions can extend the life span of cells in culture [90]. In cell culture protected from oxidative stress through low ambient oxygen tension, the addition of antioxidants, or overexpression of antioxidant enzymes delays telomere shortening [91-93]. Further data have demonstrated the important interaction between telomere-induced senescence and oxidative stress. Senescence leads to the development of oxidative stress that reinforces the senescent state of the cell and causes further oxidative stress. The telomere decline is probably due to premature aging of the graft that might occur during ischemia–reperfusion injury or graft regeneration immediately after transplantation [81]. Thus, telomere shortening in grafts could reflect not only the proliferative history of a cell, but also the accumulation of oxidative damage during the early post-transplant period [94]. Telomere reduction is presumably accelerated by the transplantation process, in both young and old tissues, modification of peri- or post-transplantation environmental stress may probably reverse aging-dependent factors.

## 8. Telomere length in other organ transplants

Telomere length is associated with kidney function [95]. Ischemia–reperfusion during kidney transplantation is associated with rapid telomere shortening [96]. Cellular senescence in zero hour biopsies predicts outcome in renal transplantation [97]. Telomere length assessed in biopsy specimens collected in the peri-transplant period predicts long-term kidney allograft function. Complications of kidney transplantation, like delayed graft function, acute rejection, and chronic allograft dysfunction are linked with the telomere length and thus, graft ageing [98]. Moreover, telomere length is a predictive marker of transplant outcome [99]. Rapid telomere reduction in the first year after hematopoietic stem cell transplantation were identified in recipients of bone marrow grafts [100-101]. Short telomeres are associated with the presence of chronic graft versus host disease and receiving graft from a female donor [102].

## 9. Conclusions and future directions

Studies of age-related disease have mostly focused on telomere length, because excessive telomere shortening leads to diseases such as cardiovascular disease, ulcerative colitis, liver cirrhosis, diabetes, and idiopathic pulmonary fibrosis. Mechanisms of complications (e.g., rejection) of organ transplantation and consequent graft failure related with ageing and senescence are due to telomere shortening. Therefore, studying of telomere length is essential in the field of organ transplantation. Telomere length was negatively associated with patient age, male sex, acute rejection, and fatty liver, and was positively associated with time from transplantation [103]. Our previous study confirmed that accelerated telomere decline in hepatocytes in the first year post-liver-transplantation is presumably due to premature ageing following the acute stress of transplantation and the high rate of cell division that occurs during graft regeneration immediately after transplantation [77]. Accelerated telomere shortening and hepatocyte senescence identified even tolerated human liver allogarfts [104]. The main problem of older donor tissue is its lower ability to endure stress and repair. Preexisting aging may reduce repair and survival capacity, and post-transplant stress such as rejection exhausts further this capacity, leading to graft failure [68]. Ischemia and reperfusion during transplantation lead to a temporary increase of reactive oxygen species in the organ, which are predominant inducers of DNA breaks. Oxidative DNA damage advances telomere shortening [94]. Furthermore, sustained cellular turnover in chronic liver disease accelerates cellular senescence [2-4, 65-66]. The confluence of acute stress, oxidative stress, ageing, and senescence suggests possible mechanisms leading to graft failure. Avoidance of factors associated with oxidative stress and telomere dysfunction is recommended in association with current liver transplantation techniques. Telomeres in grafted livers may elongate somewhat longer if the grafts are immunologically well controlled [105]. Taken together, telomere length is one of the available indicators for evaluation of liver allograft status (Fig.1).

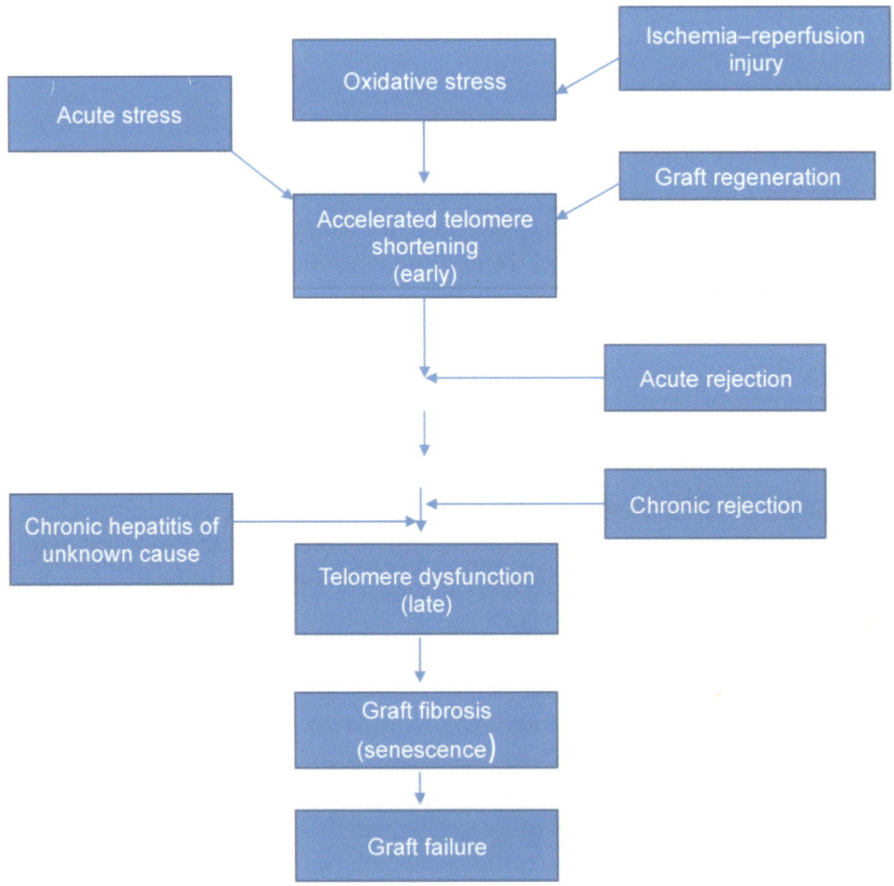


**Figure 1.** Allograft failure and telomere dysfunction

http://dx.doi.org/10.5772/62196

## Author details

Tatsuaki Tsuruyama* and Wulamujiang Aini

*Address all correspondence to: tsuruyam@kuhp.kyoto-u.ac.jp

Department of Pathology, Center for anatomical and Pathological Research, Graduate School of Medicine, Kyoto University, Kyoto, Kyoto Prefecture, Japan

The authors have declared no conflicts of interest.

## References

[1] Harley CB, Futcher AB, Greider CW. Telomeres shorten during ageing of human fibroblasts. *Nature*. 1990; 345: 458-460.

[2] Aikata H, Takaishi H, Kawakami Y, et al. Telomere reduction in human liver tissues with age and chronic inflammation. *Exp Cell Res*. 2000; 256: 578-582.

[3] Wiemann SU, Satyanarayana A, Tsahuridu M, et al. Hepatocyte telomere shortening and senescence are general markers of human liver cirrhosis. *Faseb J*. 2002; 16: 935-942.

[4] Nakajima T, Moriguchi M, Katagishi T, et al. Premature telomere shortening and impaired regenerative response in hepatocytes of individuals with NAFLD. *Liver Int*. 2006; 26: 23-31.

[5] Palm W, de Lange T. How shelterin protects mammalian telomeres. *Annu Rev Genet*. 2008; 42:301-334.

[6] Zhao Y, Sfeir AJ, Zou Y, et al. Telomere extension occurs at most chromosome ends and is uncoupled from fill-in in human cancer cells. *Cell*. 2009; 138:463-475.

[7] Chai W, Du Q, Shay JW, et al. Human telomeres have different overhang sizes at leading versus lagging strands. *Mol Cell*. 2006; 21: 427-435.

[8] de Lange T. T-loops and the origin of telomeres. *Nat Rev Mol Cell Biol*. 2004;5: 323-329.

[9] Griffith JD, Comeau L, Rosenfield S, et al. Mammalian telomeres end in a large duplex loop. *Cell*. 1999; 97: 503-514.

[10] Biffi G, Tannahill D, McCafferty J, Balasubramanian S. Quantitative visualization of DNA G-quadruplex structures in human cells. *Nat Chem*. 2013;5: 182-186.

[11] de Lange T. Shelterin: the protein complex that shapes and safeguards human telomeres. *Genes Dev*. 2005;19: 2100-2110.

[12] Diotti R, Loayza D. Shelterin complex and associated factors at human telomeres. *Nucleus*. 2011; 2: 119-135.

[13] Kabir SH, Hockemeyer D, and de Lange T. TALEN gene knockouts reveal no requirement for the conserved human shelterin protein Rap1 in telomere protection and length regulation. *Cell Rep*. 2014; 9: 1273-1280.

[14] Surovtseva YV, Churikov D, Boltz KA, et al. Conserved telomere maintenance component 1 interacts with STN1 and maintains chromosome ends in higher eukaryotes. *Mol Cell*. 2009; 36: 207-218.

[15] Miyake Y, Nakamura M, Nabetani A, et al. RPA-like mammalian Ctc1-Stn1-Ten1 complex binds to single-stranded DNA and protects telomeres independently of the Pot1 pathway. *Mol Cell*. 2009; 36: 193-206.

[16] Huffman KE, Levene SD, Tesmer VM, et al. Telomere shortening is proportional to the size of the G-rich telomeric 3′-overhang. *J Biol Chem*. 2000; 275:19719-19722.

[17] Greider CW, Blackburn EH. A telomeric sequence in the RNA of Tetrahymena telomerase required for telomere repeat synthesis. *Nature*. 1989;337:331-337.

[18] Nakamura TM, Morin GB, Chapman KB, et al. Telomerase catalytic subunit homologs from fission yeast and human. *Science*. 1997; 277: 955-959.

[19] Zhao Y, Abreu E, Kim J, et al. Processive and distributive extension of human telomeres by telomerase under homeostatic and nonequilibrium conditions. *Mol Cell*. 2011;42: 297-307.

[20] Mitchell TR, Glenfield K, Jeyanthan K, et al. Arginine methylation regulates telomere length and stability. *Mol Cell Biol*. 2009;29: 4918-4934.

[21] Veldman T, Etheridge KT, Counter CM. Loss of hPot1 function leads to telomere instability and a cut-like phenotype. *Curr Biol*. 2004; 14: 2264-2270.

[22] Boccardi V, Razdan N, Kaplunov J, et al. Stn1 is critical for telomere maintenance and long-term viability of somatic human cells. *Aging Cell*. 2015; 14: 372-381.

[23] Wellinger RJ, Zakian VA. Everything you ever wanted to know about Saccharomyces cerevisiae telomeres: beginning to end. *Genetics*. 2012; 191: 1073-1105.

[24] Pfeiffer V, Lingner J. Replication of telomeres and the regulation of telomerase. *Cold Spring Harb Perspect Biol*. 2013; 5: a010405. doi: 10. 1101/cshperspect.

[25] Blackburn EH. Telomere states and cell fates. *Nature*. 2000; 408: 53-56.

[26] Blackburn EH. Switching and signaling at the telomere. *Cell*. 2001; 106: 661-673.

[27] Cech TR. Beginning to understand the end of the chromosome. *Cell*. 2004; 116: 273-279.

[28] Blasco MA. Telomeres and human disease: ageing, cancer and beyond. *Nat Rev Genet*. 2005; 6: 611-622.

[29] Verdun RE, Karlseder J. Replication and protection of telomeres. *Nature*. 2007; 447: 924-931.

[30] O'Sullivan RJ, Karlseder J. Telomeres: protecting chromosomes against genome instability. *Nat Rev Mol Cell Biol*. 2010; 11: 171-181.

[31] Maizels N. Dynamic roles for G4 DNA in the biology of eukaryotic cells. *Nat Struct Mol Biol*. 2006; 13: 1055-1059.

[32] Smogorzewska A, van Steensel B, Bianchi A, et al. Control of human telomere length by TRF1 and TRF2. *Mol Cell Biol*. 2000; 20: 1659-1668.

[33] Canudas S, Houghtaling BR, Bhanot M, et al. A role for heterochromatin protein 1γ at human telomeres. *Genes Dev*. 2011;25: 1807-1819.

[34] Wan M, Qin J, Songyang Z, et al. OB fold-containing protein 1 (OBFC1), a human homolog of yeast Stn1, associates with TPP1 and is implicated in telomere length regulation. *J Biol Chem*. 2009; 284: 26725-26731.

[35] Chen LY, Redon S, Lingner J. The human CST complex is a terminator of telomerase activity. *Nature*. 2012;488:540-544.

[36] Takai H, Smogorzewska A, de Lange T. DNA damage foci at dysfunctional telomeres. *Curr Biol*. 2003; 13: 1549-1556.

[37] Kaul Z, Cesare AJ, Huschtscha LI, et al. Five dysfunctional telomeres predict onset of senescence in human cells. *EMBO Rep*. 2012; 13: 52-59.

[38] Valdes AM, Andrew T, Gardner JP, et al. Obesity, cigarette smoking, and telomere length in women. *Lancet*. 2005; 366: 662-664.

[39] Brouilette S, Singh RK, Thompson JR, et al. White cell telomere length and risk of premature myocardial infarction. *Arterioscler Thromb Vasc Biol*. 2003; 23: 842-846.

[40] Cawthon RM, Smith KR, O'Brien E, et al. Association between telomere length in blood and mortality in people aged 60 years or older. *Lancet*. 2003; 361: 393-395.

[41] Farzaneh-Far R, Cawthon RM, Na B, et al. Prognostic value of leukocyte telomere length in patients with stable coronary artery disease: data from the Heart and Soul Study. *Arterioscler Thromb Vasc Biol*. 2008; 28: 1379-1384.

[42] Mainous AG, Diaz VA. Telomere length as a risk marker for cardiovascular disease: the next big thing? *Expert Rev Mol Diagn*. 2010; 10: 969-971.

[43] De Meyer T, Rietzschel ER, De Buyzere ML, et al. Telomere length and cardiovascular aging: the means to the ends? *Ageing Res Rev*. 2011; 10: 297-303.

[44] van der Harst P, van der Steege G, de Boer RA, et al. Telomere length of circulating leukocytes is decreased in patients with chronic heart failure. *J Am Coll Cardiol.* 2007;49: 1459-1464.

[45] O'Sullivan JN, Bronner MP, Brentnall TA, et al. Chromosomal instability in ulcerative colitis is related to telomere shortening. *Nat Genet.* 2002; 32: 280-284.

[46] Zee RY, Castonguay AJ, Barton NS, et al. Mean leukocyte telomere length shortening and type 2 diabetes mellitus: a case-control study. *Transl Res.* 2010; 155: 166-169.

[47] Salpea KD, Humphries SE. Telomere length in atherosclerosis and diabetes. Atherosclerosis. 2010;209: 35-38.

[48] Fyhrquist F, Tiitu A, Saijonmaa O, et al. Telomere length and progression of diabetic nephropathy in patients with type 1 diabetes. *J Intern Med.* 2010; 267: 278-286.

[49] Alder JK, Chen JJ, Lancaster L, et al. Short telomeres are a risk factor for idiopathic pulmonary fibrosis. *Proc Natl Acad Sci U S A.* 2008; 105: 13051-13056.

[50] Effros RB. Genetic alterations in the ageing immune system: impact on infection and cancer. *Mech Ageing Dev.* 2003; 124: 71-77.

[51] DePinho RA, Polyak K. Cancer chromosomes in crisis. *Nat Genet.* 2004; 36: 932-934.

[52] Blasco MA, Lee HW, Hande MP, et al. Telomere shortening and tumor formation by mouse cells lacking telomerase RNA. *Cell.* 1997;91: 25-34.

[53] Rudolph KL, Chang S, Lee HW, et al. Longevity, stress response, and cancer in aging telomerase-deficient mice. *Cell.* 1999;96: 701-712.

[54] Shay JW, Bacchetti S. A survey of telomerase activity in human cancer. *Eur J Cancer.* 1997;33: 787-791.

[55] Nawrot TS, Staessen JA, Holvoet P, et al. Telomere length and its associations with oxidized-LDL, carotid artery distensibility and smoking. *Front Biosci (Elite Ed).* 2010; 2: 1164-1168.

[56] Cherkas LF, Hunkin JL, Kato BS, et al. The association between physical activity in leisure time and leukocyte telomere length. *Arch Intern Med.* 2008; 168: 154-158.

[57] Chen S, Lin J, Matsuguchi T, Blackburn E, et al. Short leukocyte telomere length predicts incidence and progression of carotid atherosclerosis in American Indians: the Strong Heart Family Study. *Aging* (Albany NY). 2014;6: 414-427.

[58] Takubo K, Nakamura K, Izumiyama N, et al. Telomere shortening with aging in human liver. *J Gerontol A Biol Sci Med Sci.* 2000; 55: B533-536.

[59] Takubo K, Izumiyama-Shimomura N, Honma N, et al. Telomere lengths are characteristic in each human individual. *Exp Gerontol.* 2002; 37: 523-531.

[60] Ishikawa N, Nakamura KI, Izumiyama N, et al. Telomere length dynamics in the human pituitary gland: robust preservation throughout adult life to centenarian age. *Age*. 2012; 34: 795-804.

[61] Banff schema for grading liver allograft rejection: an international consensus document. *Hepatology*. 1997; 25: 658-663.

[62] Neil DA, Hubscher SG: Current views on rejection pathology in liver transplantation. *Transpl Int*. 2010; 23: 971-983.

[63] Nakajima T, Nakashima T, Okada Y, et al. Nuclear size measurement is a simple method for the assessment of hepatocellular aging in non-alcoholic fatty liver disease: Comparison with telomere-specific quantitative FISH and p21 immunohistochemistry. *Pathol Int*. 2010; 60: 175-183.

[64] Gregg SQ, Gutiérrez V, Robinson AR, et al. A mouse model of accelerated liver aging caused by a defect in DNA repair. *Hepatology*. 2012; 55: 609-621.

[65] Aravinthan A, Scarpini C, Tachtatzis P, et al. Hepatocyte senescence predicts progression in non-alcohol-related fatty liver disease. *J Hepatol*. 2013; 58: 549-556.

[66] Feng S, Goodrich NP, Bragg-Gresham JL, et al. Characteristics associated with liver graft failure: the concept of a donor risk index. *Am J Transplant*. 2006; 6: 783-790.

[67] Moon JI, Kwon CH, Joh JW, Jung GO, Choi GS, Park JB, et al. Safety of small-for-size grafts in adult-to-adult living donor liver transplantation using the right lobe. *Liver Transpl*. 2010; 16: 864-869.

[68] Melk A, Schmidt BM, Braun H, et al. Effects of donor age and cell senescence on kidney allograft survival. *Am J Transplant*. 2009; 9: 114-123.

[69] Demetris A, Adams D, Bellamy C, Blakolmer K, Clouston A, Dhillon AP, et al. Update of the International Banff Schema for Liver Allograft Rejection: Working recommendations for the histopathologic staging and reporting of chronic rejection. An International Panel. *Hepatology*. 2000; 31: 792-799.

[70] Wiesner RH, Batts KP, Krom RA. Evolving concepts in the diagnosis, pathogenesis, and treatment of chronic hepatic allograft rejection. *Liver Transpl Surg*. 1999; 5: 388-400.

[71] Vierling JM. Immunologic mechanisms of hepatic allograft rejection. *Semin Liver Dis*. 1992; 12: 16-27.

[72] Jain A, Mazariegos G, Pokharna R, et al. The absence of chronic rejection in pediatric primary liver transplant patients who are maintained on tacrolimus-based immunosuppression: A long-term analysis. *Transplantation*. 2003; 75: 1020-1025.

[73] Blakolmer K, Jain A, Ruppert K, et al. Chronic liver allograft rejection in a population treated primarily with tacrolimus as baseline immunosuppression: Long-term fol-

low-up and evaluation of features for histopatho-logical staging. *Transplantation*. 2000; 69: 2330-2336.

[74] Sher LS, Cosenza CA, Michel J, Makowka L, Miller CM, Schwartz ME, et al. Efficacy of tacrolimus as rescue therapy for chronic rejection in orthotopic liver transplantation: A report of the U.S. Multicenter Liver Study Group. *Transplantation*. 1997; 64:258-263.

[75] Gupta S. Hepatic polyploidy and liver growth control. *Sem Cancer Biol*. 2000; 10: 161-171.

[76] Venick RS, McDiarmid SV, Farmer DG, et al. Rejection and steroid dependence: unique risk factors in the development of pediatric posttransplant de novo autoimmune hepatitis. *Am J Transpl*.2007, 7: 955-963.

[77] Aini W, Miyagawa-Hayashino A, Tsuruyama T, et al. Telomere shortening and karyotypic alterations in hepatocytes in long-term transplanted human liver allografts. *Transpl Int*. 2012; 25: 956-966.

[78] Banff Working Group. Liver biopsy interpretation for causes of late liver allograft dysfunction. *Hepatology*. 2006; 44: 489-501.

[79] Miyagawa-Hayashino A, Haga H, Egawa H, Hayashino Y, et al. Idiopathic post-transplantation hepatitis following living donor liver transplantation, and significance of autoantibody titre for outcome. *Transpl Int*. 2009; 22: 303-312.

[80] Gutierrez-Reyes G, del Carmen Garcia de Leon M, Varela-Fascinetto G, et al. Cellular senescence in livers from children with end stage liver disease. *PLoS One*. 2010; 5: e10231.

[81] Westhoff JH, Schildhorn C, Jacobi C, et al. Telomere shortening reduces regenerative capacity after acute kidney injury. *J Am Soc Nephrol*. 2010; 21: 327-336.

[82] Orlando G, Soker S, Wood K. Operational tolerance after liver transplantation. *J Hepatol*. 2009; 50: 1247-1257.

[83] Cawthon RM. Telomere length measurement by a novel monochrome multiplex quantitative PCR method. *Nucleic Acids Res*. 2009; 37:e21.

[84] Martinez-Llordella M, Puig-Pey I, Orlando G, et al. Multiparameter immune profiling of operational tolerance in liver transplantation. *Am J Transplant*. 2007; 7: 309-319.

[85] Martinez-Llordella M, Lozano JJ, Puig-Pey I, et al. Using transcriptional profiling to develop a diagnostic test of operational tolerance in liver transplant recipients. *J Clin Invest*. 2008; 118: 2845-2857.

[86] de la Garza RG, Sarobe P, Merino J, et al. Trial of complete weaning from immunosuppression for liver transplant recipients: Factors predictive of tolerance. *Liver Transpl*. 2013; 19: 937-944.

[87] Nawrot TS, Staessen JA, Gardner JP, et al. Telomere length and possible link to X chromosome. *Lancet*. 2004; 363:507-510.

[88] Houben JM, Moonen HJ, van Schooten FJ, et al. Telomere length assessment: biomarker of chronic oxidative stress? *Free Radic Biol Med*. 2008; 44: 235-246.

[89] Von Zglinicki T, Saretzki G, Docke W, et al. Mild hyperoxia shortens telomeres and inhibits proliferation of fibroblasts: a model for senescence? *Exp Cell Res*. 1995; 220: 186-193.

[90] Packer L, Fuehr K. Low oxygen concentration extends the lifespan of cultured human diploid cells. *Nature*. 1977; 267: 423-425.

[91] Passos JF, von Zglinicki T. Mitochondria, telomeres and cell senescence. *Exp Gerontol*. 2005; 40: 466-472.

[92] Von Zglinicki T, Pilger R, Sitte N. Accumulation of single-strand breaks is the major cause of telomere shortening in human fibroblasts. *Free Radic Biol Med*. 2000; 28: 64-74.

[93] Von Zglinicki T, Saretzki G, Docke W, et al. Mild hyperoxia shortens telomeres and inhibits proliferation of fibroblasts: a model for senescence? *Exp Cell Res*. 1995; 220: 186-193.

[94] Collado M, Blasco MA, Serrano M. Cellular senescence in cancer and aging. *Cell*. 2007; 130: 223-233.

[95] Bansal N, Whooley MA, Regan M, et al. Association between kidney function and telomere length: the heart and soul study. *Am J Nephrol*. 2012;36: 405-411.

[96] Chkhotua AB, Schelzig H, Wiegand P, et al. Influence of ischaemia/reperfusion and LFA-1 inhibition on telomere lengths and CDKI genes in ex vivo haemoperfusion of primate kidneys. *Transpl Int*. 2005; 17: 692-698.

[97] Koppelstaetter C, Schratzberger G, Perco P, et al. Markers of cellular senescence in zero hour biopsies predict outcome in renal transplantation. *Aging Cell*. 2008;7: 491-497.

[98] Domański L, Kłoda K, Kwiatkowska E, et al. Effect of delayed graft function, acute rejection and chronic allograft dysfunction on kidney allograft telomere length in patients after transplantation: a prospective cohort study. *BMC Nephrol*. 2015;16: 23.

[99] Peffault de Latour R, Calado RT, Busson M, et al. Age-adjusted recipient pretransplantation telomere length and treatment-related mortality after hematopoietic stem cell transplantation. *Blood*. 2012; 120: 3353-3359.

[100] Brümmendorf TH, Rufer N, Baerlocher GM, et al. Limited telomere shortening in hematopoietic stem cells after transplantation. *Ann N Y Acad Sci*. 2001; 938: 1-7.

[101] Robertson JD, Testa NG, Russell NH, et al. Accelerated telomere shortening following allogeneic transplantation is independent of the cell source and occurs within the first year post transplant. *Bone Marrow Transpl*. 2001; 27: 1283-1286.

[102] de Pauw ES, Otto SA, Wijnen JT, et al. Long-term follow-up of recipients of allogeneic bone marrow grafts reveals no progressive telomere shortening and provides no evidence for haematopoietic stem cell exhaustion. *Br J Haematol*. 2002; 116: 491-496.

[103] Uziel O, Laish I, Bulcheniko M, et al. Telomere shortening in liver transplant recipients is not influenced by underlying disease or metabolic derangements. *Ann Transpl*. 2013; 18: 567-575.

[104] Aini W, Miyagawa-Hayashino A, Ozeki M, et al. Accelerated telomere reduction and hepatocyte senescence in tolerated human liver allografts. *Transpl Immunol*. 2014; 31: 55-59.

[105] Kawano Y, Ishikawa N, Aida J, et al. Q-FISH measurement of hepatocyte telomere lengths in donor liver and graft after pediatric living-donor liver transplantation: donor age affects telomere length sustainability. *PLoS One*. 2014;9:e93749. doi: 10.1371/journal.pone.

Chapter 2

# Telomere and Telomerase in Cancer

Angayarkanni Jayaraman,
Kalarikkal Gopikrishnan Kiran and
Palaniswamy Muthusamy

Additional information is available at the end of the chapter

http://dx.doi.org/10.5772/64721

**Abstract**

The linear ends of chromosome are protected by specialized ribonucleoprotein (RNP) termed as telomere. These specialized terminal elements with tandem repeated sequence are the protective cap that alleviate end replication problem and cell senescence. The telomere length maintenance is essential to avoid cell death and apoptosis. Telomere shortening has been related to chronic stress due to several factors, which include not only psychological stress but also diseases such as cardiovascular diseases and cancer. Telomerase enzyme which maintains telomere length is the major factor responsible for evading cell death. Telomere length maintenance and telomerase expression put together are the prerequisite for immortality, an essential character for cancer cells. Understanding the mechanism of telomere and telomerase functions paves way for eradicating the diseases such as cancer.

**Keywords:** telomere length, telomerase, tumor progression, tumor immortality

## 1. Introduction

Telomeres are specialized DNA structures consisting of tandem arrays of hexa-nucleotide (TTAGGG) DNA sequences that cap the end of chromosomes. These structures residing near the ends of chromosomes play a very vital role in maintaining the integrity of the whole genome and prevent the loss of genetic material. As a consequence of cell division, short stretches of DNA will be lost from telomeric region and eventually lead to cellular senescence and death. There are a lot of evidences to suggest that telomere length is a better biomarker for overall health status, compared to the currently used biomarkers for the same. Few of the phenomena regarding the telomere length are unanswered till now. Till date it is unclear about the mechanistic

regarding the telomere length are unanswered till now. Till date it is unclear about the mechanistic correlation between telomere size and life span of various species. To prevent senescence of cell, the preservation of telomere length is essential, which is maintained by telomerase enzyme. Telomerase is a reverse transcriptase enzyme which has recently emerged as an attractive target for cancer as it is a crucial factor required for the tumor immortalization of a subset of cells, including cancer stem cells. Studies have proved that 80–85% of the tumor cells express telomerase whereas somatic cells lack the expression of telomerase [1]. The important paradox is that telomerase-negative normal cells have lengthier telomeres than telomerase-positive cancer cells [2]. Thus difference in telomere length and cell kinetics between normal and cancerous cells shows that targeting telomerase is a more effective way to target cancer cells. Owing to the significant role of telomere and telomerase in tumor immortalization understanding their amassed influence on cancer is crucial for cancer therapy. In this context, this book chapter is focused on disseminating the integrated impact of telomere and telomerase on cancer progression.

## 2. Telomere construction

The basic structure of telomere is conserved among eukaryotes and consists of short tandem DNA repeats, with G-rich sequence at the three-end referred to as the G-strand and the complementary strand is called the C-strand at the five-end (**Figure 1**) [3]. The length of telomeric DNA varies from 2 to 20 kilobase pairs, depending on factors such as tissue type and human age [4]. The telomere is conspicuous owing to the presence of G-overhang which extends beyond its complementary C-rich strand to form a single-stranded overhang, termed the G-tail. It has been proposed that the 3′ G-overhang can be sequestered into a lasso-like structure known as the T-loop (**Figure 2**) [5, 6]. The single-stranded G-overhang invades the double-stranded telomeric DNA, which displaces the bound G-strand base-pairing with the C-strand. As this displaced binding takes place at a distance from the physical end of the telomere, it generates a large duplex structure called the T-loop (**Figure 2**) [3, 5].

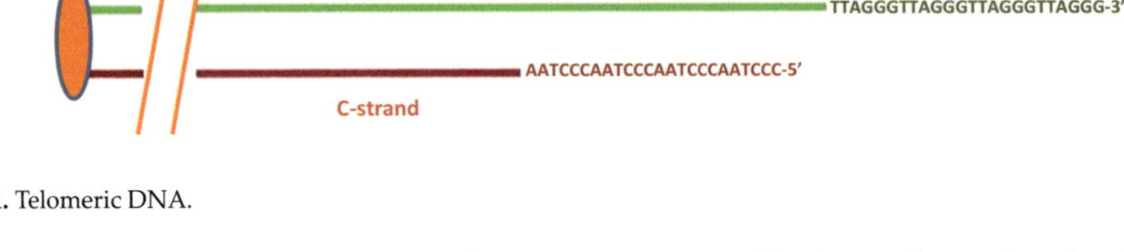


**Figure 1.** Telomeric DNA.

Telomeres can also fold into G-quadruplex DNA, an unusual DNA conformation that is based on a guanine quartet [7]. The repetitive and GC-rich nature of telomeric DNA endows it with the capability to form the higher-order DNA conformation, G-quadruplexes [8, 9]. To maintain such unusual structure of telomeres, a set of telomeric protein complex has evolved, termed shelterin. The shelterin complex consists of six individual proteins, telomeric repeat binding factor 1 (TRF1), TRF2, repressor/activator protein 1 (RAP1), TIN2 (TRF1 interacting protein 2),

http://dx.doi.org/10.5772/64721

TPP1 (TINT1/PIP1/PTOP 1), and protection of telomeres 1 (POT1) [6, 10]. The proteins TRF1 and TRF2 attach to double-stranded telomeric repeats facilitating the anchoring of the complex along the length of telomeres [11–14], whereas POT1 binds to the single-stranded overhang. TPP1 and TIN2 act as bridging proteins between the above DNA-binding modules and are crucial for chromosome end protection and telomere length regulation. TRF1 and TRF2 with the help of TIN2 [15] bind with POT1 via TPP1 [16–19]. TIN2 also connects TRF1 to TRF2, and this interaction contributes to the stabilization of TRF2 on telomeres [17–19]. Besides this shelterin complex, other proteins like TEN1 and Pinx1, which are not telomere specific, are also present at telomeres and carry out important functions in recruitment of telomerase [20].

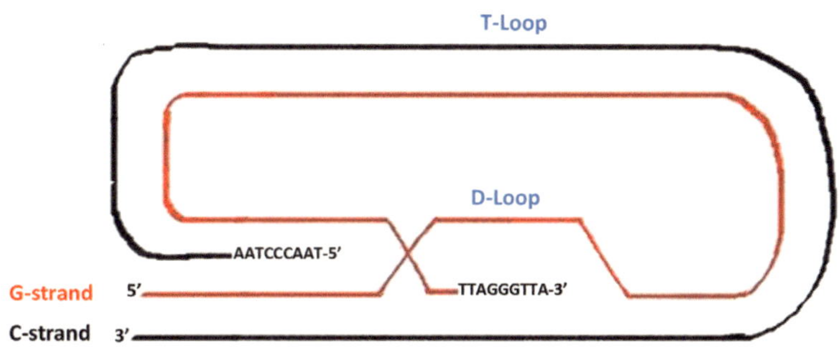


**Figure 2.** T-loop formation.

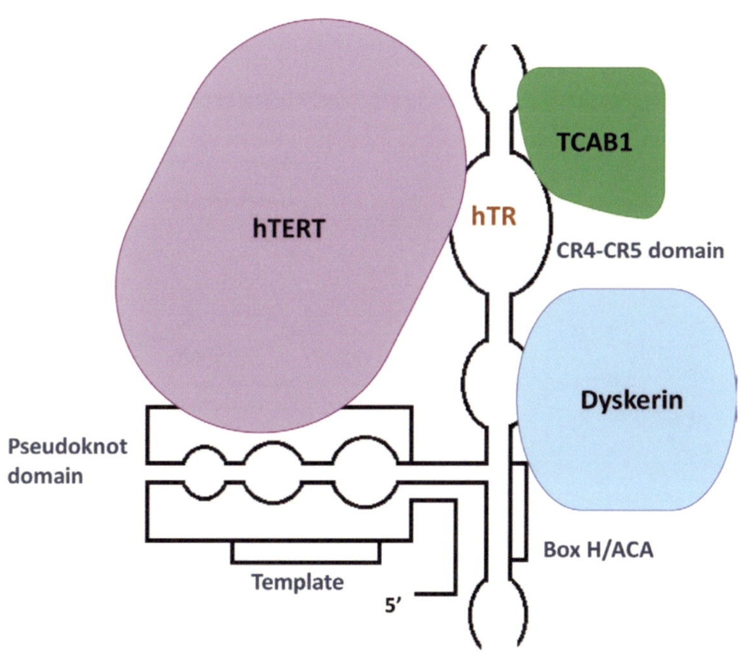


**Figure 3.** Telomere-telomerase assembly.

## 3. Telomere: a knight cap

During the evolvement of linear genome, the natural ends of linear chromosomes resemble DNA breaks and tend to induce DNA damage response (DDR). These natural linear ends are protected by the sequestration of the ribonucleoprotein (RNP) sequence, telomeres which mask the ends from continuous exposure to the DNA damage response (DDR). Telomeres serve as protective caps, preventing the chromosomal ends from being recognized as double-strand breaks by the DNA damage repair system and the activation of the p53 or p16INK4a pathway and the start of senescence or apoptosis. If the telomere cap is removed, genome instability is induced. Telomeres with its tightly regulated complexes consisting of repetitive G-rich DNA and specialized proteins accomplish the task of not only concealing the linear chromosome ends from detection and undesired repair, but also protect from checkpoints, homologous recombination, end-to-end fusions, or other events that normally promote repair of intra-chromosomal DNA breaks acts [21]. Telomeric proteins and their interacting factors create an environment at chromosome ends that inhibits DNA repair at that point; however, the repair machinery is also essential for proper telomere function.

The closed configuration of the T-loop of telomeric region provides a protective cap that defines the natural end of the chromosome and masks the telomere from the DDR machinery (**Figure 2**) [6]. In particular, T-loops could provide an architectural solution to the repression of the ataxia telangiectasia mutated (ATM) kinase pathway, which relies on a sensor (the MRN (Mre11/Rad50/Nbs1) complex) with DNA end-binding activity. In addition, T-loops could prevent the Ku70/80 heterodimer, a DNA repair factor that binds to DNA ends, from loading onto the telomere terminus, thereby blocking the initiation of the non-homologous end-joining (NHEJ) pathway (**Figure 4**).

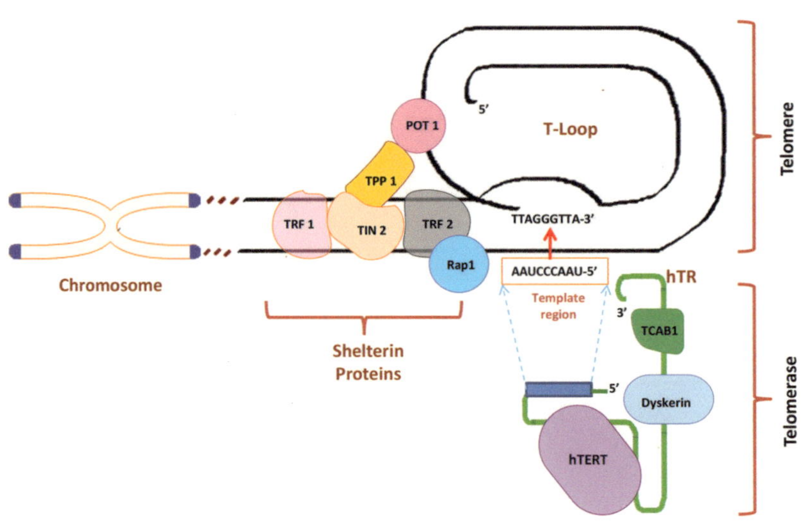


**Figure 4.** DNA damage response pathway.

Among the DNA-binding proteins, TRF1 has DNA remodeling activity [5, 22] and also shown to promote efficient replication of telomeres [23, 24]. On the contrary, TRF2 engages in chromosome end protection by inducing topological changes in telomeric DNA [25], T-loop assembly [26, 27] and by suppression of ATM dependent DDR and NHEJ (**Figure 4**) [28, 29]. Besides that, TRF2 plays a critical role in chromatin assembly, which was demonstrated by the observation that overexpression of TRF2 resulted in aberrant nucleosome spacing and decreased abundance of the core histones H3 and H4 at chromosome ends [30]. TRF2 lacking cells are reported to be growth arrested because of up-regulation of p53 and also show other hallmarks of ATM signaling, including the phosphorylation of ATM and Chk2 [31, 32]. Among the two DDR, the ATM kinase pathway at telomeres is repressed by TRF2 subunit, whereas POT1 is responsible for protection of telomere by suppression of ATR (ATM Rad3-related protein)-dependant DDR pathways [28, 33].

The high affinity of POT1 for single-stranded telomeric DNA makes it a G-strand binding component displaced from the T-loop and forms a closed configuration locking in the structure (**Figure 2**). Earlier report models suggest that POT1 and TPP1 compete with telomerase for access to the overhang [33]. Contrarily, direct interaction between TPP1 and telomerase bolsters telomerase processivity [34, 35] whereas increased loading of POT1 along the overhang block telomerase accessibility to the 3′-OH substrate. The role of RAP1 is obscure and its function has recently been elucidated. The presence of RAP1 at telomeres appears as a backup mechanism to prevent NHEJ when topology-mediated telomere protection is impaired [36]. In case of mutation in TRF2 which wraps the DNA, RAP1 has been implicated in the inhibition of NHEJ [37, 38].

Thus physically taken together, the shelterin complex and G-overhang of telomere are the protective cap that have an immensely complex role in convergence of end protection and telomere length maintenance mechanisms.

## 4. Telomerase activity

With each cell division, telomere length is reduced by ~50 to 200 bp [39] primarily because the lagging strand of DNA synthesis is unable to replicate the extreme 3′ end of the chromosome which is denoted as end replication problem [40, 41]. When telomeres become sufficiently short, cells enter an irreversible growth arrest called cellular senescence. In most eukaryotes, telomeres are stabilized, and the shortening telomeric DNA is replenished, by the action of the RNP reverse transcriptase telomerase. Progressive telomere loss has been experimentally demonstrated using non-immortalized cells in culture that lack detectable telomerase [42, 43].

In cells with active telomerase, such as cancer cells, the telomere length is continually being built up and shortened in a regulated way that maintains telomere length homeostasis and retains telomere functionality. Shortening of telomeres occur due to nucleolytic degradation and incomplete DNA replication. On the contrary, lengthening is primarily accomplished by the action of a specialized reverse transcriptase called telomerase [44] and occasionally by homologous recombination (HR) [45]. Telomerase uses the 3′ G-rich strand of a chromosome as primer to elongate chromosome end by reverse-transcribing the template region of its tightly associated RNA moiety and coordinative action with the DNA replication machinery [44, 46]. For lengthening activity, telomerase requires not only hTERT catalytic subunit and RNA template (hTR) but also other factors [47, 48].

The 3′ half of the hTR resembling the box H/ACA family of small nucleolar RNAs (snoRNAs) [49, 50] is essential for proper 3′-end processing, stability and nucleolar targeting *in vivo* [44]. The 5′ end of hTR not only acts as template for the telomere extension at chromosome ends [5, 51] but also serves as a pseudoknot that is likely to be important for telomerase function (5, 49). A 6 bp U-rich sequence at the 5′ end of hTR also interacts directly with hnRNPs C1 and C2 (**Figure 3**) [52]. Even though hTR is highly expressed in all tissues regardless of telomerase activity [53], in cancer cells hTR is generally expressed fivefold higher than normal cells [54]. However, the expression (mRNA) of the telomeric catalytic component hTERT which is closely associated with telomerase activity is estimated to be less than one to five copies per cell [54]. hTERT is generally repressed in normal cells and up-regulated in immortal cells, suggesting that hTERT is the primary determinant for the enzyme activity.

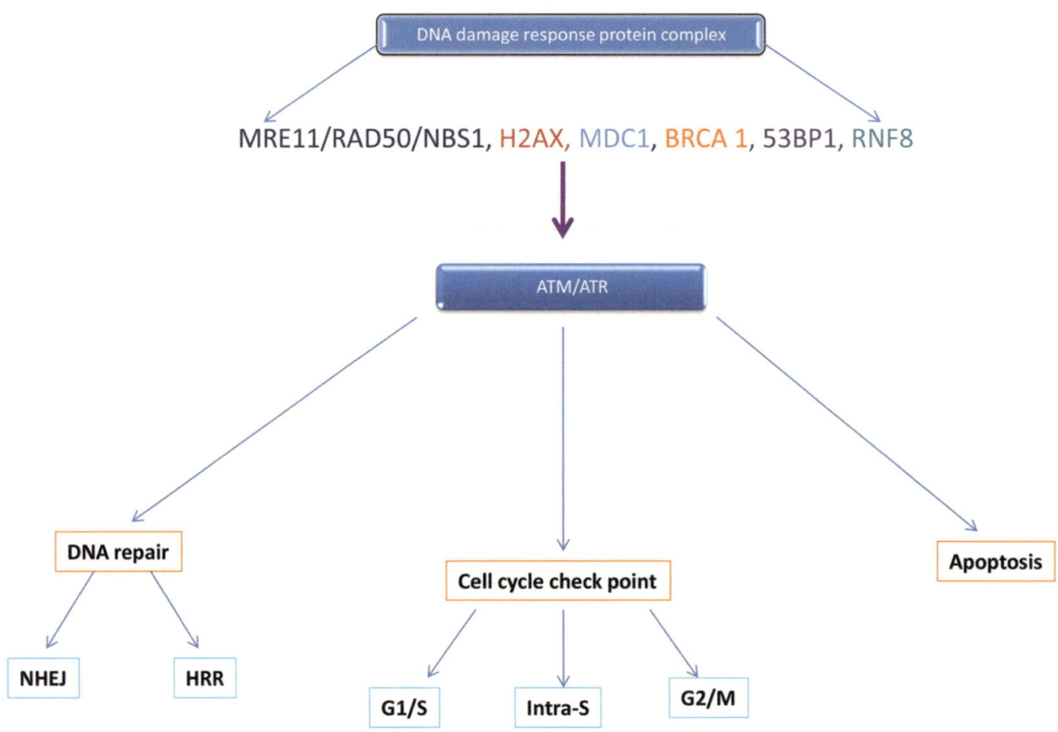


**Figure 5.** Telomerase complex.

It has been suggested that in addition to telomere elongation another aspect of telomerase RNP function is to allow even short telomeres to remain functional, which in the absence of telomerase would have caused cells to stop dividing or led to telomere–telomere fusions [55].

In other words, telomerase permits cell proliferation by stabilizing short telomeres that would be unstable in the absence of functional telomerase. In recent years, evidence has accumulated that telomerase, and in particular its catalytic subunit TERT, is involved in various non-telomere-related functions such as regulation of gene expression, growth factors and cell proliferation [56–61]. It has been reported that the telomerase has a role in modulation of Wnt/β-catenin pathway [60]. TERT has been demonstrated to bind to TBE-containing promoter elements, the specific chromatin sites of Wnt/β-catenin target genes, forming a part of the β-catenin transcriptional complex, which was facilitated by interaction with BRG1. These data endorsed the precipitous role for telomerase as a transcriptional modulator of Wnt/β-catenin signaling pathway involved in progenitor cell regulation.

In addition, various groups have shown that TERT shuttles from the nucleus and translocates to mitochondria upon exogenous stress [62–67]. Singhapol and his coworkers have demonstrated that mitochondrial telomerase localization specifically decreases mitochondrial ROS generation and cellular oxidative stress after induction of exogenous stress generated by $H_2O_2$ or irradiation in cancer cells and might thereby prevent damage to nuclear DNA [68]. Thus the presence of telomerase not only maintains telomere length imparting immortality but also play multifarious role in tumorigenesis via non-telomere-dependent mechanism which demonstrated the imperative ubiquity of telomerase in cancer cells.

## 5. Skewed expression of telomerase

Telomerase, the RNA-dependent DNA polymerase by preventing the shortening of telomeric DNA sequences, accouters unlimited proliferation. As per the telomere hypothesis of cancer cell immortalization, telomere shortening limits the life span of telomerase-negative normal cells, whereas telomerase activation in cancer cells extends their life span [4]. In normal human cells, telomerase activity is quenched during embryonic differentiation [69]. On the contrary in some tissues, like male germ cells, activated lymphocytes, and certain types of stem cell populations, the telomerase activity is induced [15, 70]. Owing to its diverse activity, the telomerase [71] which was established to be absent in most of the normal human somatic cells is recorded to be expressed in more than 90% of cancerous cells and in vitro-immortalized cells [15, 70]. A study showed that while most of the glioma tissues possess increased telomerase activity, only few (10%) anaplastic astrocytomas are reported to be telomerase positive [72–74]. In contrast to most cancerous cells, the telomerase expression is present in only 50% of glioblastoma and retinoblastoma samples, and activity is even rarely found in meningiomas and astrocytomas [75, 76].

Induction of telomerase activity in primary human keratinocytes and mammary epithelial cells has been attributed to the effect of human papillomavirus 16 E6 protein [77]. Similarly, during the menstrual cycle involving the proliferation of endometrial cells, telomerase activity is detected in normal human endometrium [78, 79]. These reports emphasis that telomerase might be the reason for tumorigenesis in hormone-dependent cancers.

It has been suggested that up-regulated expression of telomerase is contributed by the increased copy number of hTERT which was demonstrated by the report that while hTERT protein expression was strongly positive in tumor cells, the expression of hTERT in non-neoplastic mucosal cells as well as stromal elements (except lymphocytes) was weak or negative [80]. In most cases, hTERT expression is closely correlated not only with telomerase activity but also with cancer initiation and progression. In head and neck squamous cell carcinoma and human glioma cell lines, there was decrease in telomerase activity which has been correlated with overexpression of p53, E2F, p16, p21, and p15 individually [81, 82]. In malignant and nonmalignant human hematopoietic cell lines, primary leukemic cells, and normal T lymphocytes, IFN-$\alpha$ is reported to inhibit telomerase activity by suppressing hTERT transcription [83]. In addition to growth and differentiation-related regulation, telomerase activity is subject to regulation by other external and intracellular factors such as UV irradiation [84]. The telomerase having influence over several signaling pathways that determine cell proliferative or death responses when overexpressed might abrogate anti-proliferative or cell death signals. Thus cancer cells with high levels of telomerase might gain a selective growth advantage.

## 6. Telomerase as biomarker of cancer

Advent of latest cancer biomarkers has increased opportunities for improving cancer diagnostics by enhancing the quickness of detection and efficacy of treatment. In relation to the practice of new therapeutic interventions, proficient biomarkers are helpful in detection and prediction of remission or relapse of cancer at both gross and molecular levels. Telomerase activity is a hallmark of most cancer biopsies, but not generally detected in premalignant lesions and in normal tissue samples except germ cells and hematopoietic stem cells. Thus telomerase activity can be a promising biomarker for diagnosis of malignancies and a target for chemotherapy or gene therapy. Extent of telomerase activity in tumor tissues may be prognostic indicators of patient outcome. Thus, at the present time telomerase is being studied in anticipation of clinical usage. Many clinical trials for telomerase assay in cancer diagnosis are under trial. Fresh or fresh-frozen biopsies, fluids, and secretions are subject for these trials.

Other components of telomerase enzyme complex have also been utilized as biomarkers for telomerase activity. The expression of the RNA subunit of the telomerase complex (hTR) is also regarded as a diagnostic marker [85]. But the expression of hTR does not always correlate with telomerase protein expression in that particular cell type. hTR can be constitutively expressed in certain cell types in which even telomerase activity is not present [86]. Apart from this, mutation in genes of telomerase and associated proteins are considered as a diagnostic and prognostic marker for many genetic abnormalities collectively termed as telomeropathies. Early-onset melanoma tumor syndrome with multiple co-morbid cancers can be predicted from telomerase gene promoter mutation analysis. In this disorder, the mutation in promoter of telomerase gene introduces an erythroblast transformation-specific transcription factor-binding site, resulting in approximately twofold up-regulation of telomerase [87].

Introduction of telomeric repeat amplification protocol (TRAP) assay has facilitated the detection of telomerase activity in tumor biopsy samples as well as cell lines [88]. Specificity of telomerase activity in malignant phenotype further enforces the reliability of this assay. The most important advantage of TRAP assay is its low detectable limit. TRAP assay has allowed the analysis of minimal tissue samples, such as fine-needle aspirates of the breast and thyroid, cervical smears, oral washings, and urine [89, 90]. Telomerase also has been used to detect circulating tumor cells also [85]. Newly emerged technique, droplet digital TRAP assay can detect telomerase activity even in a single cell [91]. However, the positive ratios of detection of telomerase vary in sedimented cells obtained from secretion, washing, brushing samples, etc. Electrochemical telomerase assay (ECTA) is another newly emerged technique to detect telomerase activity in biological samples [92]. It is comparatively simple and rapid PCR-free method. ECTA consists of a TS primer-immobilized electrode and ferrocenyl naphthalene diimide derivative as a tetraplex binder. This method has shown a high efficiency of telomerase detection in oral cancer biopsies [93]. Taken in account of all these reports, telomerase and its functionality can be utilized as a promising diagnostic and prognostic method in cancer.

## 7. Telomeres in prognosis

Better understanding of telomere structure and its dynamics focused the research on telomeres as biomarkers for several diseases especially in early detection and prognosis of cancers. A reduced telomere length in human hematopoietic tumors predicts a reduced survival time in patients suffering from myeloid leucaemia [94], chronic lymphocytic leucaemia [95], and myelodysplastic syndromes [96]. Although telomere length in solid tumors is suggested as a potential prognostic marker, patient survival rates vary with different cancer types. For example, a short telomere length in prostate cancer correlates with short disease-free interval and shorter overall survival time [97]. Analysis of telomere length of blood cells is also considered as predictive markers for pulmonary and esophageal neoplasia as well as of lymphoma in humans [98]. It has been suggested that the reduced TL in these patients reflects the effects of increased oxidative stress which correlates with cancer risk. Advent of latest technologies to measure relative and absolute telomere lengths has paved the way to use telomere length as diagnostic and prognostic markers. Telomere restriction fragment assay, qFISH, flow FISH, qPCR assay, single telomere length analysis (STELA), and dot-blot telomere assay are the currently available assay methods for telomere length [99].

## 8. Telomerase as drug target

Telomerase enzyme has recently emerged as an attractive target for cancer as it is a crucial factor required for the tumor immortalization of a subset of cells, including cancer stem cells. Studies have shown that 80–85% of the tumor cells express telomerase, whereas somatic cells lack the expression of telomerase [1]. In the present scenario, the major concern about the chemotherapeutic approaches is the specificity of action and side effects of drugs on normal cells. Difference in telomere length and cell kinetics between normal and cancerous cells shows that targeting telomerase is an effective system to target cancer cells specifically [100]. Although telomerase is not considered as an oncogene, the expression of telomerase is the major reason for the transformation of a normal cell to cancer cell [80]. Compared to most other cancer targets, telomerase antagonists are advantageous due to the wide expression of this enzyme in cancer types [1]. Telomerase also possesses extra telomeric functions which are very crucial for tumor survival and homeostasis [101]. Studies have shown that telomerase-based cancer therapies are less likely to develop resistance against the drugs compared to drugs which target growth factor receptors or signal-transducing enzymes in cancer cells [2]. This ensures that cancer drugs based on telomerase inhibition are non-cytotoxic anticancer approach and have a broad therapeutic value.

## 9. Conclusion

Maintenance of telomere length in cancer cells is a critical factor in imparting the ability to undergo uncontrolled multiplication and thus immortality to the cells. It is imperative to discern the factors involved in telomere length preservation. Understanding the influence of telomerase and other factors in sustaining telomere length in cancer cells paves way for perceiving the theranostic role of telomere and telomerase in cancer treatment. Besides the theranostic effect, the possible side effects could be determined leading to precautionary methods to nullify the negative impact.

## Author details

Angayarkanni Jayaraman[1*], Kalarikkal Gopikrishnan Kiran[1] and Palaniswamy Muthusamy[2]

*Address all correspondence to: angaibiotech@buc.edu.in

1 Department of Microbial Biotechnology, Bharathiar University, Coimbatore, India

2 Department of Microbiology, Karpagam University, Coimbatore, India

## References

[1] Flores I, Benetti R, Blasco MA. Telomerase regulation and stem cell behaviour. Current Opinion in Cell Biology. 2006;18:254–60. doi:10.1016/j.ceb.2006.03.003

[2] Harley CB. Telomerase and cancer therapeutics. Nature Reviews Cancer. 2008;8:167–79. doi:10.1038/nrc2275

[3] Longhese MP. DNA damage response at functional and dysfunctional telomeres. Genes and Development. 2008;22:125–40. doi:10.1101/gad.1626908

[4] Mu J, Wei LX. Telomere and telomerase in oncology. Cell Research. 2002;12:1–7. doi:10.1038/sj.cr.7290104

[5] Griffith JD, Comeau L, Rosenfield S, et al. Mammalian telomeres end in a large duplex loop. Cell. 1999;97:503–14.

[6] O'Sullivan RJ, Karlseder J. Telomeres: protecting chromosomes against genome instability. Nature Reviews Molecular Cell Biology. 2010;11:171–81. doi:10.1038/nrm2848

[7] Parkinson GN, Lee MP, Neidle S. Crystal structure of parallel quadruplexes from human telomeric DNA. Nature. 2002;417:876–80. doi:10.1038/nature755

[8] Oganesian L, Bryan TM. Physiological relevance of telomeric G-quadruplex formation: a potential drug target. BioEssays: News and Reviews in Molecular, Cellular and Developmental Biology. 2007;29:155–65. doi:10.1002/bies.20523

[9] Rhodes D, Giraldo R. Telomere structure and function. Current Opinion in Structural Biology. 1995;5:311–22.

[10] Palm W, de Lange T. How shelterin protects mammalian telomeres. Annual Review of Genetics. 2008;42:301–34. doi:10.1146/annurev.genet.41.110306.130350

[11] Bilaud T, Brun C, Ancelin K, Koering CE, Laroche T, Gilson E. Telomeric localization of TRF2, a novel human telobox protein. Nature Genetics. 1997;17:236–9. doi:10.1038/ng1097-236

[12] Chong L, van Steensel B, Broccoli D, et al. A human telomeric protein. Science (New York, NY). 1995;270:1663–7.

[13] Broccoli D, Smogorzewska A, Chong L, de Lange T. Human telomeres contain two distinct Myb-related proteins, TRF1 and TRF2. Nature Genetics. 1997;17:231–5. doi:10.1038/ng1097-231

[14] Court R, Chapman L, Fairall L, Rhodes D. How the human telomeric proteins TRF1 and TRF2 recognize telomeric DNA: a view from high-resolution crystal structures. EMBO Reports. 2005;6:39–45. doi:10.1038/sj.embor.7400314

[15] Kim NW, Piatyszek MA, Prowse KR, et al. Specific association of human telomerase activity with immortal cells and cancer. Science (New York, NY). 1994;266:2011–5.

[16] Baumann P, Cech TR. POT1, the putative telomere end-binding protein in fission yeast and humans. Science (New York, NY). 2001;292:1171–5. doi:10.1126/science.1060036

[17] Houghtaling BR, Cuttonaro L, Chang W, Smith S. A dynamic molecular link between the telomere length regulator TRF1 and the chromosome end protector TRF2. Current Biology. 2004;14:1621–31. doi:10.1016/j.cub.2004.08.052

[18] Liu D, O'Connor MS, Qin J, Songyang Z. Telosome, a mammalian telomere-associated complex formed by multiple telomeric proteins. The Journal of Biological Chemistry. 2004;279:51338–42. doi:10.1074/jbc.M409293200

[19] Ye JZ, Hockemeyer D, Krutchinsky AN, et al. POT1-interacting protein PIP1: a telomere length regulator that recruits POT1 to the TIN2/TRF1 complex. Genes and Development. 2004;18:1649–54. doi:10.1101/gad.1215404

[20] Nandakumar J, Cech TR. Finding the end: recruitment of telomerase to telomeres. Nature Reviews Molecular Cell Biology. 2013;14:69–82. doi:10.1038/nrm3505

[21] Verdun RE, Karlseder J. Replication and protection of telomeres. Nature. 2007;447:924–31. doi:10.1038/nature05976

[22] Bianchi A, Smith S, Chong L, Elias P, de Lange T. TRF1 is a dimer and bends telomeric DNA. EMBO Journal. 1997;16:1785–94. doi:10.1093/emboj/16.7.1785

[23] Martinez P, Thanasoula M, Munoz P, et al. Increased telomere fragility and fusions resulting from TRF1 deficiency lead to degenerative pathologies and increased cancer in mice. Genes and Development. 2009;23:2060–75. doi:10.1101/gad.543509

[24] Sfeir A, Kosiyatrakul ST, Hockemeyer D, et al. Mammalian telomeres resemble fragile sites and require TRF1 for efficient replication. Cell. 2009;138:90–103. doi:10.1016/j.cell.2009.06.021

[25] Amiard S, Doudeau M, Pinte S, et al. A topological mechanism for TRF2-enhanced strand invasion. Nature Structural and Molecular Biology. 2007;14:147–54. doi:10.1038/nsmb1192

[26] De Lange T. Protection of mammalian telomeres. Oncogene. 2002;21:532–40. doi:10.1038/sj.onc.1205080

[27] Stansel RM, de Lange T, Griffith JD. T-loop assembly in vitro involves binding of TRF2 near the 3′ telomeric overhang. EMBO Journal. 2001;20:5532–40. doi:10.1093/emboj/20.19.5532

[28] Denchi EL, de Lange T. Protection of telomeres through independent control of ATM and ATR by TRF2 and POT1. Nature. 2007;448:1068–71. doi:10.1038/nature06065

[29] Smogorzewska A, Karlseder J, Holtgreve-Grez H, Jauch A, de Lange T. DNA ligase IV-dependent NHEJ of deprotected mammalian telomeres in G1 and G2. Current Biology. 2002;12:1635–44.

[30] Benetti R, Schoeftner S, Munoz P, Blasco MA. Role of TRF2 in the assembly of telomeric chromatin. Cell Cycle (Georgetown, TX). 2008;7:3461–8. doi:10.4161/cc.7.21.7013

[31] Celli GB, de Lange T. DNA processing is not required for ATM-mediated telomere damage response after TRF2 deletion. Nature Cell Biology. 2005;7:712–8. doi:10.1038/ncb1275

[32] Karlseder J, Broccoli D, Dai Y, Hardy S, de Lange T. p53-and ATM-dependent apoptosis induced by telomeres lacking TRF2. Science (New York, NY). 1999;283:1321–5.

[33] Loayza D, De Lange T. POT1 as a terminal transducer of TRF1 telomere length control. Nature. 2003;423:1013–8. doi:10.1038/nature01688

[34] Wang F, Podell ER, Zaug AJ, et al. The POT1-TPP1 telomere complex is a telomerase processivity factor. Nature. 2007;445:506–10. doi:10.1038/nature05454

[35] Xin H, Liu D, Wan M, et al. TPP1 is a homologue of ciliate TEBP-beta and interacts with POT1 to recruit telomerase. Nature. 2007;445:559-62. doi:10.1038/nature05469

[36] Benarroch-Popivker D, Pisano S, Mendez-Bermudez A, et al. TRF2-mediated control of telomere DNA topology as a mechanism for chromosome-end protection. Molecular Cell. 2016;61:274–86. doi:10.1016/j.molcel.2015.12.009

[37] Bae NS, Baumann P. A RAP1/TRF2 complex inhibits nonhomologous end-joining at human telomeric DNA ends. Molecular Cell. 2007;26:323–34. doi:10.1016/j.molcel.2007.03.023

[38] Sarthy J, Bae NS, Scrafford J, Baumann P. Human RAP1 inhibits non-homologous end joining at telomeres. EMBO Journal 2009;28:3390–9. doi:10.1038/emboj.2009.275

[39] Huffman KE, Levene SD, Tesmer VM, Shay JW, Wright WE. Telomere shortening is proportional to the size of the G-rich telomeric 3′-overhang. The Journal of Biological Chemistry. 2000;275:19719–22. doi:10.1074/jbc.M002843200

[40] Olovnikov AM. A theory of marginotomy: the incomplete copying of template margin in enzymic synthesis of polynucleotides and biological significance of the phenomenon. Journal of Theoretical Biology. 1973;41:181–90.

[41] Watson JD. Origin of concatemeric T7 DNA. Nature: New Biology. 1972;239:197–201.

[42] Harley CB, Futcher AB, Greider CW. Telomeres shorten during ageing of human fibroblasts. Nature. 1990;345:458–60. doi:10.1038/345458a0

[43] Vaziri H, Schachter F, Uchida I, et al. Loss of telomeric DNA during aging of normal and trisomy 21 human lymphocytes. American Journal of Human Genetics. 1993;52:661–7.

[44] Greider CW, Blackburn EH. Identification of a specific telomere terminal transferase activity in Tetrahymena extracts. Cell. 1985;43:405–13.

[45] Liu T, Chung MJ, Ullenbruch M, et al. Telomerase activity is required for bleomycin-induced pulmonary fibrosis in mice. Journal of Clinical Investigation. 2007;117:3800–9. doi:10.1172/jci32369

[46] Hug N, Lingner J. Telomere length homeostasis. Chromosoma. 2006;115:413–25. doi: 10.1007/s00412-006-0067-3

[47] Bechter OE, Eisterer W, Dlaska M, Kuhr T, Thaler J. CpG island methylation of the hTERT promoter is associated with lower telomerase activity in B-cell lymphocytic leukemia. Experimental Hematology. 2002;30:26–33.

[48] Collins K. Ciliate telomerase biochemistry. Annual Review of Biochemistry. 1999;68:187–218. doi:10.1146/annurev.biochem.68.1.187

[49] Greider CW. Telomerase activity, cell proliferation, and cancer. Proceedings of the National Academy of Sciences of the United States of America. 1998;95:90–2.

[50] Greider CW. Telomeres do D-loop-T-loop. Cell. 1999;97:419–22.

[51] Cong YS, Wen J, Bacchetti S. The human telomerase catalytic subunit hTERT: organization of the gene and characterization of the promoter. Human Molecular Genetics. 1999;8:137–42.

[52] Gu J, Andreeff M, Roth JA, Fang B. hTERT promoter induces tumor-specific Bax gene expression and cell killing in syngenic mouse tumor model and prevents systemic toxicity. Gene Therapy. 2002;9:30–7. doi:10.1038/sj.gt.3301619

[53] Avilion AA, Piatyszek MA, Gupta J, Shay JW, Bacchetti S, Greider CW. Human telomerase RNA and telomerase activity in immortal cell lines and tumor tissues. Cancer Research. 1996;56:645–50.

[54] Yi X, Tesmer VM, Savre-Train I, Shay JW, Wright WE. Both transcriptional and posttranscriptional mechanisms regulate human telomerase template RNA levels. Molecular and Cellular Biology. 1999;19:3989–97.

[55] Chan SW, Blackburn EH. New ways not to make ends meet: telomerase, DNA damage proteins and heterochromatin. Oncogene. 2002;21:553–63. doi:10.1038/sj.onc.1205082

[56] Bagheri S, Nosrati M, Li S, et al. Genes and pathways downstream of telomerase in melanoma metastasis. Proceedings of the National Academy of Sciences of the United States of America. 2006;103:11306–11. doi:10.1073/pnas.0510085103

[57] Hoffmeyer K, Raggioli A, Rudloff S, et al. Wnt/beta-catenin signaling regulates telomerase in stem cells and cancer cells. Science (New York, NY). 2012;336:1549–54. doi:10.1126/science.1218370

[58] Li S, Crothers J, Haqq CM, Blackburn EH. Cellular and gene expression responses involved in the rapid growth inhibition of human cancer cells by RNA interference-mediated depletion of telomerase RNA. Journal of Biological Chemistry. 2005;280:23709–17. doi:10.1074/jbc.M502782200

[59] Maida Y, Yasukawa M, Furuuchi M, et al. An RNA-dependent RNA polymerase formed by TERT and the RMRP RNA. Nature. 2009;461:230–5. doi:10.1038/nature08283

[60] Park JI, Venteicher AS, Hong JY, et al. Telomerase modulates Wnt signalling by association with target gene chromatin. Nature. 2009;460:66–72. doi:10.1038/nature08137

[61] Smith LL, Coller HA, Roberts JM. Telomerase modulates expression of growth-controlling genes and enhances cell proliferation. Nature Cell Biology. 2003;5:474–9. doi:10.1038/ncb985

[62] Ahmed S, Passos JF, Birket MJ, et al. Telomerase does not counteract telomere shortening but protects mitochondrial function under oxidative stress. Journal of Cell Science. 2008;121:1046–53. doi:10.1242/jcs.019372

[63] Haendeler J, Hoffmann J, Brandes RP, Zeiher AM, Dimmeler S. Hydrogen peroxide triggers nuclear export of telomerase reverse transcriptase via Src kinase family-dependent phosphorylation of tyrosine 707. Molecular and Cellular Biology. 2003;23:4598–610.

[64] Haendeler J, Drose S, Buchner N, et al. Mitochondrial telomerase reverse transcriptase binds to and protects mitochondrial DNA and function from damage. Arteriosclerosis, Thrombosis, and Vascular Biology. 2009;29:929–35. doi:10.1161/atvbaha.109.185546

[65] Indran IR, Hande MP, Pervaiz S. hTERT overexpression alleviates intracellular ROS production, improves mitochondrial function, and inhibits ROS-mediated apoptosis in cancer cells. Cancer Research. 2011;71:266–76. doi:10.1158/0008-5472.can-10-1588

[66] Santos JH, Meyer JN, Skorvaga M, Annab LA, Van Houten B. Mitochondrial hTERT exacerbates free-radical-mediated mtDNA damage. Aging Cell. 2004;3:399–411. doi:10.1111/j.1474-9728.2004.00124.x

[67] Santos JH, Meyer JN, Van Houten B. Mitochondrial localization of telomerase as a determinant for hydrogen peroxide-induced mitochondrial DNA damage and apoptosis. Human Molecular Genetics. 2006;15:1757–68. doi:10.1093/hmg/ddl098

[68] Singhapol C, Pal D, Czapiewski R, Porika M, Nelson G, Saretzki GC. Mitochondrial telomerase protects cancer cells from nuclear DNA damage and apoptosis. PloS one. 2013;8:e52989. 1-11 doi:10.1371/journal.pone.0052989

[69] Wright WE, Piatyszek MA, Rainey WE, Byrd W, Shay JW. Telomerase activity in human germline and embryonic tissues and cells. Developmental Genetics. 1996;18:173–9. doi:10.1002/(sici)1520-6408(1996)18:2<173::aid-dvg10>3.0.co;2–3

[70] Shay JW, Bacchetti S. A survey of telomerase activity in human cancer. European Journal of Cancer (Oxford, England: 1990). 1997;33:787–91. doi:10.1016/s0959-8049(97)00062-2

[71] Stewart SA, Hahn WC, O'Connor BF, et al. Telomerase contributes to tumorigenesis by a telomere length-independent mechanism. Proceedings of the National Academy of Sciences of the United States of America. 2002;99:12606–11. doi:10.1073/pnas.182407599

[72] Hiyama E, Hiyama K, Yokoyama T, et al. Rapid detection of MYCN gene amplification and telomerase expression in neuroblastoma. Clinical Cancer Research: An Official Journal of the American Association for Cancer Research. 1999;5:601–9.

[73] Poremba C, Scheel C, Hero B, et al. Telomerase activity and telomerase subunits gene expression patterns in neuroblastoma: a molecular and immunohistochemical study establishing prognostic tools for fresh-frozen and paraffin-embedded tissues. Journal of Clinical Oncology: Official Journal of the American Society of Clinical Oncology. 2000;18:2582–92.

[74] Yasui W, Tahara H, Tahara E, et al. Expression of telomerase catalytic component, telomerase reverse transcriptase, in human gastric carcinomas. Japanese Journal of Cancer Research: Gann. 1998;89:1099–103.

[75] Gupta J, Han LP, Wang P, Gallie BL, Bacchetti S. Development of retinoblastoma in the absence of telomerase activity. Journal of the National Cancer Institute.1996;88:1152–7.

[76] Langford LA, Piatyszek MA, Xu R, Schold SC, Jr., Shay JW. Telomerase activity in human brain tumours. Lancet (London, England). 1995;346:1267–8.

[77] Klingelhutz AJ, Foster SA, McDougall JK. Telomerase activation by the E6 gene product of human papillomavirus type 16. Nature. 1996;380:79–82. doi:10.1038/380079a0

[78] Kyo S, Takakura M, Kohama T, Inoue M. Telomerase activity in human endometrium. Cancer Research. 1997;57:610–4.

[79] Tanaka M, Kyo S, Takakura M, et al. Expression of telomerase activity in human endometrium is localized to epithelial glandular cells and regulated in a menstrual phase-dependent manner correlated with cell proliferation. The American Journal of Pathology. 1998;153:1985–91. doi:10.1016/s0002-9440(10)65712-4

[80] Cong Y-S, Wright WE, Shay JW. Human telomerase and its regulation. Microbiology and Molecular Biology Reviews. 2002;66:407–25. doi:10.1128/MMBR.66.3.407-425.2002

[81] Fuxe J, Akusjarvi G, Goike HM, Roos G, Collins VP, Pettersson RF. Adenovirus-mediated overexpression of p15INK4B inhibits human glioma cell growth, induces replicative senescence, and inhibits telomerase activity similarly to p16INK4A. Cell Growth and Differentiation: The Molecular Biology Journal of the American Association for Cancer Research. 2000;11:373–84.

[82] Henderson YC, Breau RL, Liu TJ, Clayman GL. Telomerase activity in head and neck tumors after introduction of wild-type p53, p21, p16, and E2F-1 genes by means of recombinant adenovirus. Head & Neck. 2000;22:347–54.

[83] Xu D, Erickson S, Szeps M, et al. Interferon alpha down-regulates telomerase reverse transcriptase and telomerase activity in human malignant and nonmalignant hematopoietic cells. Blood. 2000;96:4313–8.

[84] Hande MP, Balajee AS, Natarajan AT. Induction of telomerase activity by UV-irradiation in Chinese hamster cells. Oncogene. 1997;15:1747–52. doi:10.1038/sj.onc.1201327

[85] Xu Y, He K, Goldkorn A. Telomerase targeted therapy in cancer and cancer stem cells. Clinical Advances in Hematology and Oncology. 2011;9:442–55.

[86] Blasco MA, Rizen M, Greider CW, Hanahan D. Differential regulation of telomerase activity and telomerase RNA during multi-stage tumorigenesis. Nature Genetics. 1996;12:200–4. doi:10.1038/ng0296-200

[87] Horn S, Figl A, Rachakonda PS, et al. TERT promoter mutations in familial and sporadic melanoma. Science (New York, NY). 2013;339:959–61. doi:10.1126/science.1230062

[88] Fajkus J. Detection of telomerase activity by the TRAP assay and its variants and alternatives. Clinica Chimica Acta; International Journal of Clinical Chemistry. 2006;371:25–31. doi:10.1016/j.cca.2006.02.039

[89] Hiyama K, Ishioka S, Shay JW, et al. Telomerase activity as a novel marker of lung cancer and immune-associated lung diseases. International Journal of Molecular Medicine. 1998;1:545–9.

[90] Sugino T, Yoshida K, Bolodeoku J, et al. Telomerase activity in human breast cancer and benign breast lesions: diagnostic applications in clinical specimens, including fine needle aspirates. International Journal of Cancer. 1996;69:301–6. doi:10.1002/(sici)1097-0215(19960822)69:4<301::aid-ijc11>3.0.co;2-8

[91] Ludlow AT, Robin JD, Sayed M, et al. Quantitative telomerase enzyme activity determination using droplet digital PCR with single cell resolution. Nucleic Acids Research. 2014;42:e104-e. 1-12 doi:10.1093/nar/gku439

[92] Sato S, Kondo H, Nojima T, Takenaka S. Electrochemical telomerase assay with ferrocenylnaphthalene diimide as a tetraplex DNA-specific binder. Analytical Chemistry. 2005;77:7304–9. doi:10.1021/ac0510235

[93] Hayakawa M, Kodama M, Sato S, et al. Electrochemical telomerase assay for screening for oral cancer. British Journal of Oral and Maxillofacial Surgery. 2016;54:301–5. doi:10.1016/j.bjoms.2016.01.003

[94] Hartmann U, Brummendorf TH, Balabanov S, Thiede C, Illme T, Schaich M. Telomere length and hTERT expression in patients with acute myeloid leukemia correlates with chromosomal abnormalities. Haematologica. 2005;90:307–16.

[95] Boultwood J, Fidler C, Shepherd P, et al. Telomere length shortening is associated with disease evolution in chronic myelogenous leukemia. American Journal of Hematology. 1999;61:5–9.

[96] Ohyashiki JH, Ohyashiki K, Fujimura T, et al. Telomere shortening associated with disease evolution patterns in myelodysplastic syndromes. Cancer Research. 1994;54:3557–60.

[97] Donaldson L, Fordyce C, Gilliland F, et al. Association between outcome and telomere DNA content in prostate cancer. Journal of Urology. 1999;162:1788–92.

[98] Svenson U, Roos G. Telomere length as a biological marker in malignancy. Biochimica et Biophysica Acta. 2009;1792:317–23. doi:10.1016/j.bbadis.2009.01.017

[99] Nussey DH, Baird D, Barrett E, et al. Measuring telomere length and telomere dynamics in evolutionary biology and ecology. Methods in Ecology and Evolution/British Ecological Society. 2014;5:299–310. doi:10.1111/2041-210x.12161

[100] Zhang X, Mar V, Zhou W, Harrington L, Robinson MO. Telomere shortening and apoptosis in telomerase-inhibited human tumor cells. Genes and Development. 1999;13:2388–99.

[101] Martinez P, Blasco MA. Telomeric and extra-telomeric roles for telomerase and the telomere-binding proteins. Nature Reviews Cancer. 2011;11:161–76. doi:10.1038/nrc3025

Chapter 3

# Telomeres and Genomic Instability from Precancerous Lesions to Advanced Cancer – Understanding Through Ovarian Cancer

Gautier Chene, Gery Lamblin, Karine Le Bail-Carval, Philippe Chabert, Georges Mellier and Andrei Tchirkov

Additional information is available at the end of the chapter

http://dx.doi.org/10.5772/62259

**Abstract**

Genetic instability plays an important role in ovarian carcinogenesis. Genetic instability is one of the characteristics shared by most human cancers and seems to exist (at various levels) at all stages of the disease, from precancerous lesions to advanced cancer. It is possible that this instability is one of the first trigger events, which would facilitate the subsequent establishment of all the other cancer hallmarks. Telomere shortening appears to take place in most human preinvasive epithelial lesions: short telomeres are found in up to 88% of early precancerous conditions of the bladder, cervix, colon, esophagus, or prostate. However, little is known about ovarian carcinogenesis and telomere shortening. Recent evidence has shown that the fallopian tube may be the origin of ovarian cancer. A new tubal carcinogenic sequence has been described with precancerous lesions that could metastasize to the ovary and result in invasive ovarian cancer. In this review, we will describe the degree of telomere shortening and genomic instability (estimated by the expression of DNA damage response proteins, such as H2AX, Chk2, ATM, 53BP1, p53, and TRF2, and by array comparative genomic hybridization) in early preinvasive stages of ovarian cancer (serous tubal intraepithelial carcinoma (STIC)), ovarian high-grade serous carcinoma, and benign controls. Given that STICs have the shortest telomeres, they could be in a telomere crisis phase preceding genomic stabilization due to telomerase activation (see appended diagram). Concordant results were obtained in immunohistochemical and molecular studies. The expression of all DNA damage proteins increased from benign fallopian tubes to STICs suggesting an early activation of the DNA damage response (DDR) pathways in STICs and indicating that genomic instability may occur early in the precancerous lesions of high-grade serous ovarian cancer (HGSC). In this chapter, we propose to review current knowledge about the function of human telomeres and telomerase and their relevance in genomic instability in cancer and to focus on specific results for ovarian cancer.

**Keywords:** Telomere, genomic instability, ovarian cancer, dysplastic lesion, STIC

# 1. Introduction

## 1. 1. Telomeres, telomerases, and p53 interaction

Genomic instability is probably one of the first phases in carcinogenesis and would thus facilitate the accumulation of multiple mutations. This instability was first described in connection with the discovery of microsatellite instability with the hereditary non-polyposis colon cancer (HNPCC) or Lynch syndrome for example. In most cancers, there is another form of genomic instability, that is, the chromosomal instability (CIN), which we will describe in this review [1]. At molecular level, this instability could result in chromosome rearrangements (number and structure), duplication or segregation anomalies during mitosis, along with DNA repair system dysfunction [1–4]. The CIN may be explained by the mutator hypothesis in hereditary cancers (germline mutations in DNA repair genes as *TP53* or *BRCA* genes for instance, beginning in the precancerous lesions) and by the oncogene-induced DNA replication stress in sporadic (non-hereditary) cancers [1]. Because CIN precedes *TP53* and DNA repair genes mutations in sporadic cancer, genomic instability would be the result of activated oncogenes or antioncogenes (growth signaling pathways...) [1]. However, in both cases (sporadic and genetic cancers), CIN may be due also to telomere erosion and is likely linked to multifactorial molecular events.

Telomere dysfunction has been described to be one of the initial phases in genomic instability. Telomeres are found at the tips of the chromosomes and consist of a large number of hexamer (TTAGGG)n repeats capped with the multiprotein shelterin complex. Their main function is to protect chromosomal ends from fusion and nucleotidic degradation, which ensures chromosomal stability. Telomeres are regularly shortened during cell division due to incomplete replication of telomeric DNA. Excessive shortening (a "telomere crisis") activates DNA repair at telomeres leading to CIN and finally cell death. In tumors, telomeres are usually shortened, which makes the cell unstable, but the activation of telomerase (telomere elongation complex generally found only in stem, progenitor, and tumor cells and not in normal somatic cells) maintains the telomere length at a certain level, enabling the survival of these cells [2–4]. These unstable cells can then continue to proliferate and this results in cancer. The interaction between telomeres and p53 would thus represent one of the trigger events in carcinogenesis [5]. In physiological terms, telomere shortening represents a real "genotoxic stress" resulting in activation of the DNA damage signaling pathway (and consequently p53 tumor suppressor protein), finally leading to apoptosis or cycle arrest. When p53 is inactivated by mutations, as is the case in ovarian high-grade serous carcinoma, the telomere dysfunction is neither repaired nor signaled, resulting in genomic instability with the accompanying chromosome aberrations, which are a prelude to cancer [2–6].

DNA double-strand breaks can be the result of telomere dysfunction and are one of the most critical DNA alterations at the origin of genomic instability. One of the first response mechanisms aimed at repairing these breaks is activation of the DNA damage checkpoints. These checkpoints represent the transition state between two cell phases that may be inhibited by genotoxic lesions. There is then a slowing or complete halt in the progression from one phase to the next (checkpoint G1/S or G2/M) or during replication (checkpoint intra-S) [7].

http://dx.doi.org/10.5772/62259

The phosphorylation of ATM (a member of the phosphoinositide 3-kinase or PI3 kinase) occurs first. Then ATM phosphorylates Chk2 p53, H2AX, and 53BP1. Chk2 also phosphorylates p53 (Figure 1) [8–12]. Histone H2AX phosphorylated on residue serine 139, also called γH2AX, is a marker for cellular DNA double-strand breaks. Phosphorylation of H2AX results in the condensation of chromatin each side of the break, which makes γH2AX detectable at nuclear level by immunohistochemistry.

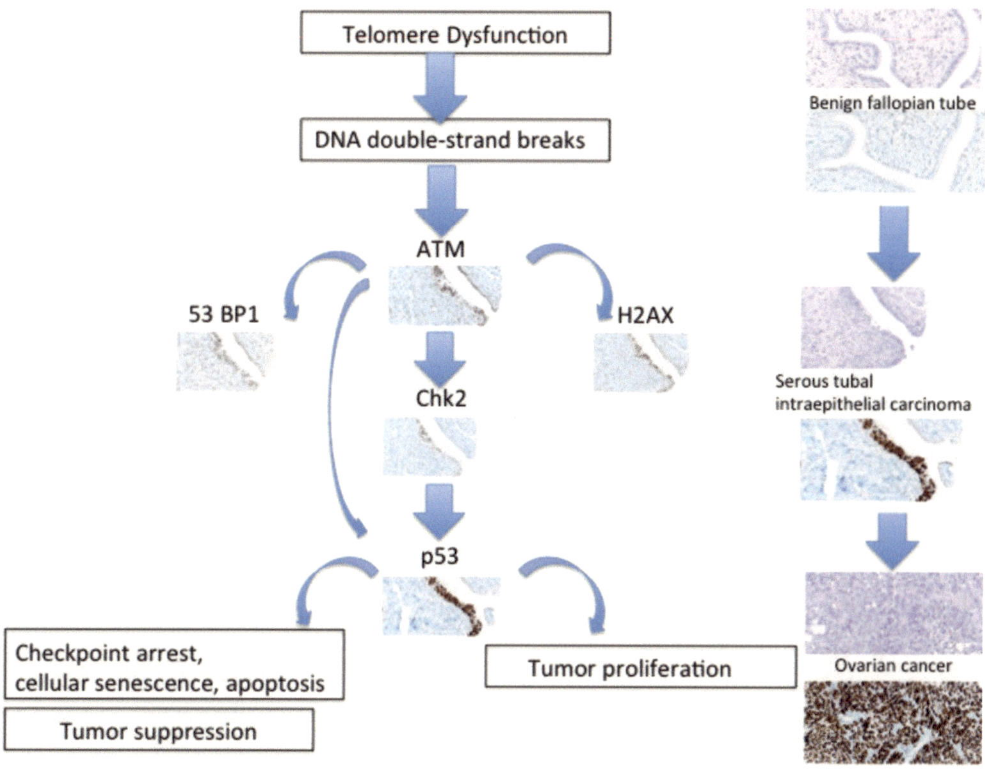


**Figure 1.** Relationship between telomeres and the DNA damage response pathway. DNA double-strand breaks may be the result of telomere dysfunction with activation of the DNA damage checkpoints. The apical kinase ATM is first activated. Then ATM activates the DNA damage mediators, H2AX and 53BP1. ATM also phosphorylates the downstream kinase Chk2, which phosphorylates p53. ATM may directly activate the effector p53. In non-cancerous situation, this pathway leads to checkpoint arrest, cellular senescence, or apoptosis. In cancerous situation, this cascade may activate tumor proliferation to invasive carcinoma. On the left side, you can see the serous carcinogenic sequence from benign fallopian tube (no p53 mutation) to serous tubal intraepithelial carcinoma (the precancerous lesion with p53 signature) and after that ovarian cancer (with also *TP 53* mutation) [15, 17].

Strong expression of γH2AX was detected in most precancerous lesions and was considered to represent an antitumor function. Experimental studies have shown that H2AX-deficient mice were at greater risk of immunodeficiency, infertility, and were also more sensitive to ionizing radiation, all of which can be explained by increased chromosomal instability related to reduced capability of the DNA repair systems. When these mice were also p53 deficient (knock-out), there was an increased risk of tumors [13, 14].

As it has been demonstrated that telomere shortening occurs early during carcinogenesis (being found in 89% of preinvasive lesions of the bladder, cervix, colon, and also the esophagus) [5], we investigated genetic instability in precancerous ovarian lesions, which has been described very recently.

## 2. Ovarian cancer: A model for greater insight into genetic instability

This review concerns high-grade serous ovarian cancer (HGSC) characterized by a higher genomic instability (see below) and very frequent *TP53* gene mutations. Germline mutations in breast cancer susceptibility 1 (BRCA 1) or BRCA 2 may lead to hereditary HGSC, whereas 90% of HGSC are sporadic (no BRCA mutations but frequent BRCA inactivation or modulation with promoter hypermethylation, loss of heterozygosity in over 50% of cases) [15].

Four hundred and eighty-nine HGSC were recently studied by the Cancer Genome Atlas Research Network [16]. *TP53* mutations were present in 96% of cases followed by mutations in *NB1, BRCA1, BCA2, RB1,* and *CDK12* genes. Homologous recombination (and the DNA damage signaling pathway) is defective in about half of the cancers analyzed [16]. Taken together, all these findings can explain why ovarian cancer may be a relevant model to explore genetic instability.

Recent histopathologic and molecular studies enabled to describe a model of tumorogenesis comprising two pathways [15]:

- Type I tumors: These are low-grade tumors for which the pathogenesis would consist of a sequence of cystadenomas/adenofibromas, then borderline tumors and finally progression towards cancer. A lesional continuum has indeed been found, that is, molecular mutations that are common to benign, borderline, and invasive lesions (BRAF and KRAS mutations in over 60% of cases, less frequently mutated PTEN (20%–46%) and β-catenin (≈30%). Note also the recent discovery of ARID1A gene mutations in endometriosis and cancers associated with endometriosis (clear cell and endometrioid cancers) [17].
- Type II tumors: These are high-grade tumors from the outset. At the molecular level, *TP53* gene mutations are found in 50%–80% of cases. These tumors show high genomic instability and are essentially represented by HGSC. This histologic subtype is the most frequent and consequently has been the subject of many studies, and a tubal carcinogenic sequence has been identified [15].

True occult intraepithelial cancerous lesions of the tube (serous tubal intraepithelial carcinoma (STIC)) have been reported unusually often in the distal portion of tubes obtained after prophylactic adnexectomy for BRCA mutation, prompting systematic and meticulous examination of these tubes [18–23]. They show epithelial stratification, nuclear atypicalities with an increase in the nucleocytoplasmic ratio, loss of nuclear polarity, nuclear pleiomorphism, and loss of ciliated cells. Immunohistochemical analysis may reveal intense and diffuse expression of *p53* (the p53 signature) and a high proliferative index (Ki67> 40%). There could be a high level of genetic instability, as demonstrated by the high positive level of γH2AX [15, 16, 18–23].

In other words, high-grade ovarian serous carcinoma could originate in the fallopian tube, and all these findings encouraged us to study STIC lesions and genomic instability.

We started by assessing the telomere length in 12 STICs, 36 non-cancerous controls, and 43 high-grade serous cancers [24, 25]. Laser microdissection of paraffin-embedded samples was used in all cases. A DNA extraction was followed by purification step. Telomere length was measured by real-time quantitative polymerase chain reaction (PCR) according to Cawthon's method [26].

STICs had the shortest telomeres (p=0.0008). Telomeres of invasive cancer were shorter than those in benign controls but longer than telomeres found in STICs. A significant correlation was also found between overexpression of p53 and H2AX proteins and shortened telomeres in STICs ($p<10^{-7}$) [24]. Kuhn *et al* [27] used fluorescence in situ hybridization technique to analyze telomere length of a series of 22 STICs in comparison with non-cancerous controls and high-grade cancers: 82% of STICs had the shortest telomeres, followed by the cancers. The controls had the longest telomeres. These findings suggest that STIC lesions are the most unstable genetically and are likely to represent one of the first steps in tubo-ovarian carcinogenesis.

We also studied these STICs by array comparative genomic hybridization (aCGH) using oligonucleotide microarrays (Agilent 180 K) [24].

The size of rearrangements in STICs was high, with an average of 2363.37 Kb (488–8161).

We found common gains at chromosomes 19q (6/12, 50%), 16p (5/12, 41.6%), 12q (5/12, 41.6%), 10q (5/12, 41.6%), 11p (4/12, 33.3%), 4p (3/12, 25%), and 8q (3/12, 25%), and common losses at chromosomes 3q (6/12, 50%), 2q (5/12, 41.6%), 11q (4/12, 33.3%), 6p (4/12, 33.3%), 22q (4/12, 33.3%), 18q (3/12, 25%), 19p (3/12, 25%), 20p (3/12, 25%), and 2 p (2/12, 16.6%) [24]. These early rearrangements could be key steps in these first phases of carcinogenesis, and the corresponding candidate genes could be involved directly in the tumor triggering process, meaning that they could represent diagnostic and/or treatment targets. More studies are required.

Finally, in another study, we investigated the level of DDR activation in STICs by immunohistochemistry (pATM, pChk2, γH2AX, 53BP1, and TRF2) [28]. We constructed a tissue microarray, including 21 benign fallopian tubes, 21 STICs, and 30 HGSCs. We demonstrated that the expression of all DDR proteins increased from benign fallopian tubes to STICs. Analysis of staining variance within cases showed that 53BP1, γH2AX, pATM, pCHK2, and TRF2 expressions were significantly higher in STICs than in HGSC [28].

Taken together, all our results have shown evidence of genomic instability in the precancerous lesions known as STICs. Of note among the frequent chromosomal breakpoints in STICs, more than half occurred at terminal bands, which is characteristic for a telomere crisis with the occurrence of telomere fusions, leading to chromosomal aberrations.

It could also be interesting to study human telomerase reverse transcriptase (hTERT) expression, which is a determinant for telomerase activity, and also the telomere architecture proteins (shelterin complex proteins TRF1, TRF2, and POT1) in STICs and HGSC [29–33]. TRF1 and TRF2 proteins are involved in negative regulation of telomere lengthening and interact with telomerase [29, 30]. POT1 appears to play a dual antagonist role, depending on cell conditions, acting as positive or negative regulator of telomere length depending on telomerase [6, 34]. In our study [28], the level of expression of TRF2 was increased in STICs in comparison with HGSC (p=0.012). It has been shown that TRF2 may shorten telomeres without telomerase inactivation [12]. TRF2 is also phosphorylated by ATM to enable DNA damage repair in response to DNA damage [12].

Telomerase would probably be activated after telomere shortening at the invasive stage and would thus counteract further telomere shortening: stabilization of telomere length at this stage would moreover represent an advantage in terms of tumor proliferation and escaping apoptosis [3].

Wang *et al* [35] investigated the relationship between telomere length and telomerase activity in 15 ovarian cancers. The authors found telomeric dysfunction in 9/15 (60%) and telomerase activation in 11/15 (73.3%) ovarian cancers. However, they did not study precancerous lesions.

Other authors demonstrated that telomerase activity was higher in ovarian carcinoma than in borderline tumors (considered as premalignant tumors) and normal ovary [36–38]. This was confirmed in cell cultures [39]. However, telomerase activity in STICs has not yet been studied.

## 3. Conclusion

Telomere shortening has been proven to be one of the potential precursors of ovarian cancer indicative of genomic instability. This could lead to significant preventive strategies such as prophylactic salpingectomy in patients with a genetic risk of ovarian cancer in order to avoid the malignant transformation of benign fallopian tube into STIC [40].

## Author details

Gautier Chene[1,2*], Gery Lamblin[1], Karine Le Bail-Carval[1], Philippe Chabert[1], Georges Mellier[1] and Andrei Tchirkov[3]

*Address all correspondence to: chenegautier@yahoo.fr

1 Department of Gynecology, Hôpital Femme Mère Enfant, HFME, Lyon CHU, Lyon, France

2 University of Claude Bernard Lyon 1, EMR 3738, Lyon, France

3 Department of Medical Cytogenetics, CHU Clermont-Ferrand & EA 4677 ERTICa, University of Auvergne, Clermont-Ferrand, France

Authors declare no conflict of interest.

## References

[1] Negrini S, Gorgoulis VG, Halazonetis TD. Genomic instability, an evolving hallmark of cancer. Nat Rev Mol Cell Biol 2010; 11: 220-8.

[2] Artandi SE, DePinho RA. Telomeres and telomerase in cancer. Carcinogenesis 2010; 31: 9-18.

[3] Svenson U, Roos G. Telomere length as a biological marker in malignancy. Bioch & Bioph Acta 2009; 1792: 317-23.

[4] Kruk PA, Godwin AK, Hamilton TC, Auersperg N. Telomeric instability and reduced proliferative potential in ovarian surface epithelial cells from women with a family history of ovarian cancer. Gynecol Oncol 1999; 73: 229-36.

[5] Artandi SE, Attardi LD. Pathways connecting telomeres and p53 in senescence, apoptosis, and cancer. BBRC 2005; 331: 881-90.

[6] Raynaud CM, Sabatier L, Philipot O, et al. Telomere length, telomeric proteins and genomic instability during the multistep carcinogenic process. Crit Rev Oncol/Hematol 2008; 66: 99-117.

[7] Gorgoulis VG, Vassiliou LVF, Karakaidos P, et al. Activation of the DNA damage checkpoint and genomic instability in human precancerous lesions. Nature 2005; 434: 907-13.

[8] Bartkova J, Horejsi Z, Koed K, et al. DNA damage response as a candidate anti-cancer barrier in early human tumorigenesis. Nature 2005; 434: 864-70.

[9] Bartek J, Lukas J, Bartkova J. DNA damage response as an anti-cancer barrier. Cell Cycle 2007; 6: 2344-47.

[10] Smith J, Tho LM, Xu N, et al. The ATM-Chk2 and ATR-Chk1 pathways in DNA damage signaling and cancer. Adv Cancer Res 2010; 108: 73-112.

[11] Perona R, Moncho-Amor V, Machado-Pinilla R, et al. Role of CHK2 in cancer development. Clin Trans Oncol 2008; 10: 538-42.

[12] Tanaka H, Mendonca MS, Bradshaw PS. DNA damage-induced phosphorylation of the human telomere-associated protein TRF2. Proc Natl Acad Sci USA 2005; 102: 15539-44.

[13] Mah LJ, El-Osta A, Karagiannis TC. γH2AX as a molecular marker of aging and disease. Epigenetics 2010; 2: 129-36.

[14] Clingen PH, Wu JYH, Miller J, Mistry N, Chin F, Wynne P, Prise KM, Hartley JA. Histone H2AX phosphorylation as a molecular pharmacological marker for DNA interstrand crosslink cancer chemotherapy. Biochem Pharmacol 2008; 76: 19-27.

[15] Chene G, Dauplat J, Robin N, et al. Tu-be or tu-be: that is the question... About serous ovarian carcinogenesis. Crit Rev Oncol/Hematol 2013; 88: 134-43.

[16] The Cancer Genome Atlas Research Network. Integrated genomic analyses of ovarian carcinoma. Nature 2011; 474: 609-15.

[17] Chene G, Ouellet V, Rahimi K, Barres V, Provencher D, Mes-Masson AM. The ARID1A pathway in ovarian clear cell and endometrioid carcinoma, contiguous endometriosis, and benign endometriosis. Int J Gynaecol Obstet 2015; 130: 27-30.

[18] Crum CP. Intercepting pelvic cancer in the distal fallopian tube: theories and realities. Mol Oncol 2009; 3: 165-70.

[19] Chene G, Lamblin G, Le Bail-Carval K, Chabert P, Bakrin N, Mellier G. Early preinvasive lesions in ovarian cancer. Biomed Res Int 2014; 2014: 639252

[20] Kindelberger D, Lee Y, Hirsch MS, Feltmate D, Medeiros F, Callahan MJ, Garner EO, Gordon RW, Birch C, Berkowitz RS, Muto MG, Crum CP. Intraepithelial carcinoma of the fimbria and pelvic serous carcinoma: evidence for a causal relationship. Am J Surg Pathol 2007; 31: 161-9.

[21] Powell CB, Kenley E, Chen LM, Crawford B, McLennan J, Zaloudek C, Komaromy M, Beattie M, Ziegler J. Risk-reducing salpingo-oophorectomy in BRCA mutation carriers: role of serial sectioning in the detection of occult malignancy. J Clin Oncol 2005; 23: 127-32.

[22] Finch A, Shaw P, Rosen B, Murphy J, Narod SA, Colgan TJ. Clinical and pathologic findings of prophylactic salpingo-oophorectomies in 159 BRCA1 and BRCA2 carriers. Gynecol Oncol 2006; 100: 58-64.

[23] Callahan MJ, Crum CP, Medeiros F, Kindelberger DW, Elvin JA, Garber JE, Feltmate CM, Berkowitz RS, Muto MG. Primary fallopian tube malignancies in BRCA-positive women undergoing surgery for ovarian cancer risk reduction. J Clin Oncol. 2007; 25: 3985-90.

[24] Chene G, Tchirkov A, Eymard-Pierre E, et al. Early telomere shortening and genomic instability in tubo-ovarian preneoplastic lesions. Clin Cancer Res 2013; 19: 2873-82.

[25] Chene G, Tchirkov A, Penault-Llorca F. Early telomere shortening and genomic instability in tubo-ovarian preneoplastic lesions-response. Clin Cancer Res 2013; 19: 5255.

[26] Cawthon RM. Telomere measurement by quantitative PCR. Nucleic Acid Res 2002; 30: 1-6.

[27] Kuhn E, Meeker A, Wang TL, Sehdev AS, Kurman RJ, Shih IM. Shortened telomeres in serous tubal intraepithelial carcinoma: an early event in ovarian high-grade serous carcinogenesis. Am J Surg Pathol 2010; 34: 829-36.

[28] Chene G, Ouellet V, Rahimi K, Barres V, Caceres K, Meunier L, Cyr L, De Laduran-taye M, Provencher D, Mes Masson AM. DNA damage signalling and apoptosis in preinvasive tubal lesions of ovarian carcinoma. Int J Gynecol Cancer 2015; 25: 761-9.

[29] Murakami J, Nagai N, Ohama K, Tahara H, Ide T. Telomerase activity in ovarian tumors. Cancer 1997; 80: 1085-92.

[30] Hu H, Zhang Y, Zou M, Yang S. Expression of TRF1, TRF2, TIN2, TERT, KU70, and BRCA1 proteins is associated with telomere shortening and may contribute to multistage carcinogenesis of gastric cancer. J Cancer Res Clin Oncol 2010; 136: 1407-14.

[31] Lantuejoul S, Soria JC, Morat L, et al. Telomere shortening and telomerase reverse transcriptase expression in preinvasive bronchial lesions. Clin Cancer Res 2005; 11: 2074-82.

[32] Oh BK, Kim YJ, Park C, Park YN. Up-regulation of telomere-binding proteins TRF1, TRF2 and TIN2 is related to telomere shortening during human multistep hepatocarcinogenesis. Am J Pathol 2005; 166: 73-80.

[33] Matsutani N, Yokozaki H, Tahara E. Expression of telomeric repeat binding factor 1 and 2 and TRF1- interacting nuclear protein 2 in human gastric carcinomas. Int J Oncol 2001; 19:507-12.

[34] Colgin LM, Baran K, Baumann P, Cech TR, Reddel RR. Human POT1 facilitates telomere elongation by telomerase. Curr Biol 2003; 13: 942-6.

[35] Wang SJ, Sakamato T, Yasuda SI, Fukasawa I, Ota Y, Hayashi M, Okura T, Zheng JH, Inaba N. The relationship between telomere length and telomerase activity in gynecologic cancers. Gynecol Oncol 2002; 84: 81-4.

[36] Sun PM, Wei LH, Luo MY, Liu G, Wang JL, Mustea A, Kongsgen D, Lichtenegger, Sehouli J. The telomerase activity and expression of hTERT gene can serve as indicators in the anti-cancer treatment of human ovarian cancer. Eur J Obstet Gynecol 2007; 130: 249-57.

[37] Kyo S, Kanaya T, Takakura M, Tanaka M, Yamashita A, Inoue H, Inoue M. Expression of human telomerase subunits in ovarian malignant, borderline and benign tumors. Int J Cancer 1999; 80: 804-9.

[38] Kyo S, Takakura M, Tanaka M, Murakami K, Saitoh R, Hirano H, Inoue M. Quantitative differences in telomerase activity among malignant, premalignant and benign ovarian lesions. Clin Cancer Res 1998; 399: 399-405.

[39] Counter CM, Hirte HW, Bacchetti S, Harley CB. Telomerase activity in human ovarian carcinoma. Proc Natl Acad Sci 1994; 91: 2900-4.

[40] Chene G, Dauplat J, Radosevic-Robin N, Cayre A, Penault-Llorca F. The fallopian tube odyssey: from the ovary to the tube. About high-grade serous ovarian carcinoma. Bull Cancer 2013; 100: 757-64.

# Chapter 4

# The Role of Telomeres and Telomere-associated Proteins as Components of Interactome in Cell-signaling Pathways

Ekta Khattar and Vinay Tergaonkar

Additional information is available at the end of the chapter

http://dx.doi.org/10.5772/62130

**Abstract**

Telomeres represent ends of all eukaryotic chromosomes and serve specialized biological role in maintaining genomic integrity by preventing end fusions and degradation. Various protein complexes associate with telomeres to either protect them from DNA damage machinery or maintain telomere length homeostasis. These protein complex subunits cross talk with a variety of cell-signaling components to either maintain telomere integrity or perform other functions, which are either dependent or independent of telomeres and/or their telomeric role. Mutations in these protein components lead to the development of various human diseases, such as age-related disorders, which occur mainly due to telomere dysfunction or cancer development due to telomerase reactivation. This chapter focuses on the structural and functional aspects of telomeric proteins and their importance in human diseases.

**Keywords:** Telomeres, shelterin, telomerase, TERT, telomere diseases, cancer

## 1. Introduction

Human telomeres consist of TTAGGG tandem repeats, which are generally 3–15 kbp in length [1]. The distal end of telomere has a 3′ single-stranded overhang, which is also termed a G-rich strand, and it forms a higher order structure (like a lariat) named t-loop [2]. In t-loop, both strands of the chromosome are joined to an earlier point in the double-stranded DNA by the 3′ strand end invading the strand pair to further form a D-loop. Formation of the D-loop completes the t-loop, thus establishing a capping structure, which protects chromosomes from degradation and recombination [3]. Figure 1A shows a schematic representation of telomere structure. The disruption of t-loop results in telomere dysfunction and induction of DNA damage response (DDR) followed by cell cycle arrest [4]. Telomeres are bound by nucleosomes and a specialized complex known as shelterin, which is composed of six core protein subunits [5]. Shelterin determines the structure of telomeres. It is implicated in the formation of t-loops and also regulates the synthesis of telomeric DNA [6]. Additional proteins capable of interacting with shelterin proteins, such as DNA damage proteins, also play a role in maintaining telomere length and chromosomal stability [7].

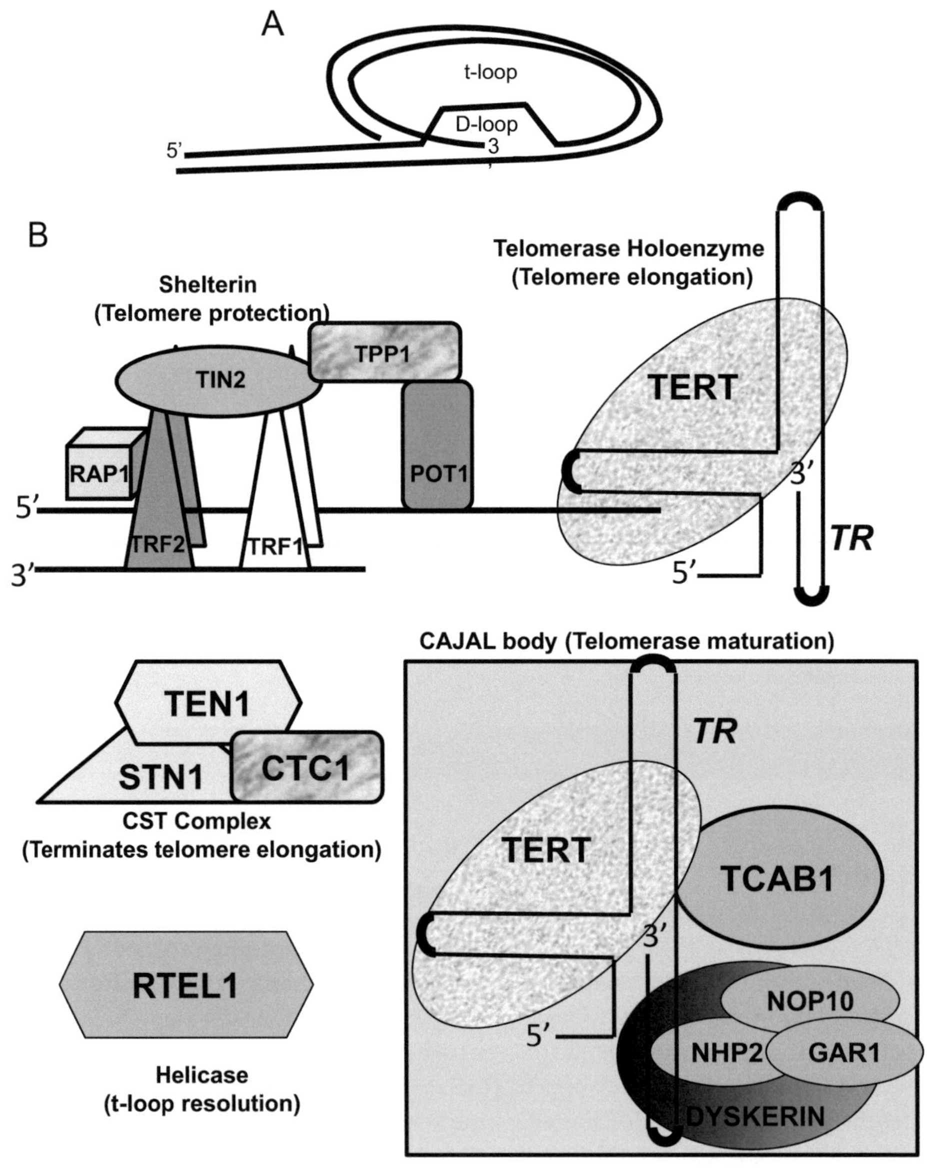


**Figure 1.** Schematic representation of telomere end structure (A) and Telomere associated protein complexes (B).

http://dx.doi.org/10.5772/62130

Telomeres shorten with replication due to two major mechanisms: (A) end-replication problem and exonuclease-mediated resection in dividing cells, and (B) damage response to reactive oxygen species in nondividing cells [8].

DNA replication involves simultaneous duplication of antiparallel DNA strands, such that replication advances in opposite directions, across a leading strand and a lagging strand. On the leading strand, daughter strand synthesis takes place continuously in the 5′–3′ direction, whereas on the lagging strand template, DNA synthesis proceeds in the 5′–3′ direction discontinuously, leading to Okazaki fragments. The leading daughter strand is completely synthesized until DNA polymerase reaches 5′ end of the leading template. However, a primer is required for DNA replication to start. At the end of replication, RNA primer occupying the 5′ end of the daughter strand is removed, and it is not possible for the overlapping strand to be replicated. Due to this, the 5′ end of each antiparallel daughter strand becomes one primer length shorter. This is referred to as the end-replication problem, which results in chromosome shortening with each subsequent cell division. Theoretically, it should result in a loss of less than 10 bp with each replication cycle; however, the rate of loss is much higher and has been calculated to be 50–200 bp per division [9]. Exonuclease activity degrading the 5′ end is another major factor, which removes the RNA primer on the lagging strand and thus also leads to the formation of 3′-end overhang structure [10]. In vitro studies have also suggested the role of oxidative stress in telomere loss [11]. Correlative and experimental studies have also suggested links between oxidative damage and telomere loss in vivo [12]. Therefore, telomere length also serves as a biological clock and marker for chronological ageing. The solution to telomere shortening is the telomerase enzyme complex, which catalyzes de novo addition of TTAGGG repeats to chromosome ends, thus preventing telomere attrition [13].

## 2. Telomere-Associated Protein Complexes (TAPs)

### 2.1. Shelterin

Shelterin, as the name suggests, provides shelter to the ends of linear chromosomes by repressing DNA damage-signaling responses, masking telomeres from DNA repair machinery, and regulating the length of telomeres [7, 14]. Shelterin is a highly specialized complex comprising six central components namely, TTAGGG repeat-binding factors TRF1 and TRF2, TRF1-interacting protein (TIN2), protection of telomeres protein (POT1), Pot1-interacting protein (TPP1), and repressor/activator protein (RAP1) [15]. All shelterin components are ubiquitously expressed and associated with telomeres throughout the cell division cycle. The complete abrogation of all shelterin subunits (except RAP1) in mice results in embryonic lethality, thereby implicating their essential roles in development [16].

**TRF1**

TRF1 was the first shelterin complex subunit to be discovered that specifically associates with double-stranded telomeric DNA, mainly as a dimer through its TRF homology domain. Recently, it has been shown that TRF1 efficiently associates with telomeric DNA in nucleosomal context and is capable of remodeling telomeric nucleosomal arrays [17]. TRF1 interacts with TIN2 in the shelterin complex as shown in Figure 1B. It also functions as a negative regulator of telomere length in telomerase-positive cells. In addition, some reports have demonstrated that it is essential for survival independent of its telomere length regulatory activity [18]. TRF1 genome-wide binding analysis revealed that it exclusively localizes at telomeres under normal conditions as well as under extreme telomere shortening unlike other shelterin members which have extra telomeric roles [19]. TRF1 has also been shown to assist Aurora-B recruitment to centromeres, thus contributing to appropriate chromosome segregation and maintenance of genomic integrity [20].

**TRF2**

TRF2 is highly similar to TRF1 in terms of protein sequence except that the N-terminal domain in TRF2 is acidic while that in TRF1 is rich in glycine and arginine residues (forming GAR domain). It possesses TRF homology domain, which mediates its dimerization. This N-terminal domain of TRF1 and TRF2 has been shown to regulate their ability to condense telomeric DNA [21]. TRF2 has been proposed to stabilize the t-loop by invasion of the upstream TTAGGG double-stranded region [22]. TRF2 has also been shown to bind at internal genomic regions, mainly at TTAGGG repeats referred to as interstitial telomeric sequences (ITSs) [23, 24]. Recent evidence suggests the role of TRF2 in the formation of novel chromosome end structures, which involve telomeres interacting with nontelomeric DNA, forming long-range chromosome loop that encompasses several megabases of chromatin and are known as interstitial telomeric loops (ITLs) [25]. Telomere-bound TRF2 is necessary to suppress the ataxia telangiectasia mutated (ATM)-dependent DNA damage response pathway [26] and the nonhomologous end joining (NHEJ) DNA repair pathway, thus playing a major role in protecting chromosome ends [9]. TRF2 also assists telomere replication by limiting resolvase activities leading to accurate repair of stalled forks [27]. It has been demonstrated that both TRF1 and TRF2 are modified post-translationally; however, the physiological relevance of these modifications is not yet completely understood [7].

**TIN2**

TIN2 (encoded by *TINF2*) associates with both TRF1 and TRF2, thus forming a bridge that connects the double-stranded telomeric DNA-binding proteins to those bound to single-stranded telomeric overhang region [28, 29]. A recent study by Frank et al demonstrates that TIN2 facilitates the recruitment of telomerase to telomeres [30]. In this study, the authors discovered a novel mutation in *TINF2* gene (which encodes TIN2 protein) and used novel functional assays to demonstrate a direct role for TIN2 in regulating telomere length through telomerase. This role is completely independent of its role in telomere protection.

**TPP1**

TPP1 interacts with TIN2 and POT1 through its carboxyl terminus and central domain, respectively [31-33]. Structurally, TPP1 possesses four domains, namely, OB (oligonucleotide/oligosaccharide-binding fold), RD (POT1 recruitment domain), S/T (serine-rich region), and TID (TIN2-interacting domain). It has been demonstrated that TPP1 recruits POT1 to telomeres [34, 35]. In addition, TPP1 has been shown to contain telomerase-interacting domain, suggest-

http://dx.doi.org/10.5772/62130

ing a role for TPP1 in the recruitment of telomerase to chromosome ends [36]. Interestingly, it has been shown that TPP1–POT1 interacts with N-terminal region of telomerase protein subunit TERT (telomerase reverse transcriptase), while TPP1 alone is also capable of interacting with C-terminal TERT residues through TPP1-OB domain [37]. TPP1-OB domain has been shown to contain a TEL patch (TPP1 glutamate (E)- and leucine (L)-rich patch), which mediates telomerase recruitment and processivity independent of its role in telomere capping [38]. In human stem cells, it has been further proven that TPP1 indeed mediates recruitment and activation of telomerase and telomere length homeostasis [39].

**POT1**

POT1 interacts with TRF1 complex via protein–protein interaction with TPP1, and this interaction is believed to affect its loading on the single-stranded TTAGGG telomeric repeat [40]. POT1 has been predicted to associate with telomeric sequences at t-loop as well as D-loop through its OB-fold domains [32]. POT1 serves a fundamental role in telomere length regulation, since it functions as a terminal transducer of telomere length control [40]. POT1–TPP1 complex has been shown to increase RAP (consecutive repeats that telomerase can add to telomere before dissociating) with minimal effect on telomerase activity [41]. Further, POT1–TPP1 has been shown to reduce the dissociation rate of telomerase from its telomeric substrate and assist in the translocation step [42].

**RAP1**

RAP1 associates with TRF2 and thus localizes to telomeres. As a component of the shelterin complex, it is dependent on TRF2 [43, 44]. RAP1 has been shown to be indispensable for telomere function in mouse and human systems [45, 46]. Further, RAP1 has been shown to possess extra telomeric roles that will be described in later part of this chapter.

### 2.2. Telomerase complex

Telomeres in human somatic cells shorten with each replication cycle due to end-replication problem consequently leading to genomic instability and cell death. Telomerase elongates telomeres and thus maintain their replicative potential. The minimal components of telomerase are a catalytic protein subunit termed as telomerase reverse transcriptase (TERT) and an RNA template known as *Terc* (*TR*) [47]. Telomerase catalyzes the addition of TTAGGG sequences to the ends of the chromosomes during each replication cycle, thus preventing telomere attrition and maintaining genomic integrity. Telomerase activity is detected predominantly in stem cells and cancer cells [48]. In normal somatic cells, telomerase activity is almost undetectable, consequently leading to shortened telomeres, which limit their life span. Furthermore, while *TR* is highly expressed in all the cell types, the levels of TERT are highly regulated at transcriptional level [49]. In somatic cells, TERT is transcriptionally turned off while stem cells display high expression of TERT, resulting in high telomerase activity. Ninety percent of cancer cells reactivate TERT expression either by mutation in *TERT* promoter or by activating oncogenic transcription factors such as NF-κB, MYC, and β-catenin that are known to activate TERT transcription [50]. This reactivation of TERT confers cancer cells with unlimited replicative potential. Distinct from its telomeric function, TERT has also been shown to cross talk with various signaling pathways and impart several additional functions to cancer cells [51].

**Terc (TR)**

Mature human *TR* is a small noncoding RNA consisting of 451 nucleotides and serves as a template for de novo telomeric repeat synthesis by telomerase. Structurally, it is subdivided into four domains namely the pseudoknot domain, the CR4-CR5 domain, the CR7, and H/ACA domain [52]. These domains perform various functions including RNA binding, dimerization, and recruitment of telomerase to telomeres. The pseudoknot domain and the CR4/5 domain along with TERT constitute the minimal requirement for reconstituted in vitro telomerase activity [53, 54]. The CR7 and H/ACA domains are required for stability and localization of telomerase [55]. H/ACA motif consists of two hairpins connected by a short single-stranded stretch, the H box, and a terminal ACA region [56] which is found in small nucleolar and small Cajal body (CB) RNAs (snoRNAs and scaRNAs). H/ACA small nucleolar ribonucleoprotein complex (H/ACA snoRNP) catalyzes pseudouridylation of small RNAs like ribosomal RNA, which may serve to stabilize their conformation [57]. The H/ACA domain of *TR* is essential for assembly into ribonucleoprotein (RNP) with four member H/ACA–RNP complex which include the core heterotrimer (Dyskerin, NHP2, and NOP10) and a fourth factor, GAR1 [56]. Dyskerin represents the catalytic subunit of H/ACA complex [57]. Major function for the association of *TR* with dyskerin is its stabilization and nuclear retention. However, no pseudouridylation of *TR* has been reported [58]. Structurally, dyskerin contains a TruB domain that functions in eukaryotic ribosomal RNA processing. The TruB domain consists of two motifs, TruB I and TruB II. In addition, it has two nuclear localization (NL) signals, N-terminal and C-terminal, and the PUA, pseudouridine synthase and archaeosine transglycosylase, domain involved in RNA modification [59]. Dyskerin and NOP10 form the stable core to which GAR1 and NHP2 subsequently bind [60]. Mutations in these proteins affect the stability of *TR* consequently affecting telomere synthesis and result in various human diseases discussed in a later section of the chapter.

Although *TR* is transcribed by RNA polymerase II, it is not polyadenylated; instead, its 3′ end is formed by exonucleolytic cleavage up to the boundary element formed by the H/ACA domain, where further cleavage is prevented by dyskerin associated with RNA [61]. The tetrameric complex of dyskerin, NOP10, NHP2, and the chaperone NAF1 associates with *TR* cotranscriptionally and is essential for its accumulation [62]. The significance of this complex formation is highlighted by a number of telomere length-associated disorders with mutations in these factors which results in reduced levels of *TR* and thus telomerase activity [63].

*TR* also harbors specialized sequence elements in the terminal loop of its 3′ hairpin namely BIO box, which stimulates *TR* stability by H/ACA RNP formation, and CAB box, which it shares with the scaRNAs. CAB box is required for trafficking *TR* to the CB, where it receives its 2,2,7-trimethyl guanosine (TMG) cap, and NAF1 is replaced by GAR1 [57, 64, 65].

**TERT**

Human TERT is a large protein consisting of 1133 amino acids and it is subdivided into four distinct domains: (a) N-terminal extension (TEN), (b) TERT RNA-binding domain (TRBD), (c) the reverse transcriptase domain (RT), and (d) the C-terminal extension (CTE) [66]. TEN domain is essential for telomerase activity and functions in proper localization and correct positioning of its catalytic site on telomeric DNA [67]. The TRBD domain functions in telomerase RNP assembly as well as RNA binding [68]. The RT domain of TERT forms the catalytic center in telomerase complex and consists of seven universally conserved RT motifs [69–71]. RT domain can be divided into two putative subdomains namely the fingers and the palm domains where fingers domain interacts with nucleic acid substrate while the palm domain contains the catalytic site [72]. CTE possesses the thumb domain and is sequentially not conserved among species [66]. CTE serves a critical role in catalytic activity and processivity of telomerase [73].

TERT interacts with chaperones HSP90 and p23 as well as with AAA$^+$ ATPases pontin and reptin [74, 75]. HSP90 and p23 interact with active telomerase; however, reptin and pontin are reported to interact with a pool of TERT, which is not assembled into active complex suggesting their role in telomerase assembly [75]. In addition, reptin and pontin are known to interact with dyskerin and are necessary for H/ACA RNP assembly, which is an essential step in TR stability [75, 76].

TERT transcription and telomerase activity is highest in the S phase of the cell cycle [77], and telomerase recruitment to telomeres has been shown to be restricted to the S phase [78, 79].

TERT interacts with two TR elements. The TRBD associates with CR4/5 region of TR and RT domain of TERT associates with pseudoknot region of TR [53, 80]. The human telomerase RNP purified from HEK293T cells overexpressing TERT and TR has been shown to be a dimeric structure, which is around 28 nm in length [81]. Although many studies have suggested the existence of multiple copies of dyskerin, NOP10, NHP2, and GAR1 with human telomerase RNP, the presence of two catalytically active TERT has been controversial since its biological significance is not clearly understood [82].

Telomerase activity in cells is limited by the levels of TERT protein (reported to be around 600 molecules/cell). All the other components of telomerase RNP are abundant [77, 83]. In normal somatic cells, TERT expression is repressed epigenetically or due to lack of activating transcription factors such as MYC, NF-κB, NFAT, RAS/RAF pathway, Ets factor steroids, and HIF [84]. Thus, transcriptional reactivation of TERT represents one of the major mechanisms responsible for activating telomerase and thus achieving replicative immortality in cancers. Recently, many cancers have been reported to harbor *TERT* promoter mutations resulting in high TERT expression and telomerase activity [85]. This is further discussed in later sections of the chapter.

### 2.3. Accessory proteins/complexes/factors for proper telomere maintenance

#### Regulator of telomere elongation helicase 1 (RTEL1)

RTEL1 is a DNA helicase, which contains N-terminal helicase domains and a C-terminal extension [86]. TRF2 recruits RTEL1 to telomeres during S phase of cell cycle to assist t-loop disassembly. RTEL1 is required for stability, protection, and elongation of telomeres [87].

RTEL1 has also been shown to interact with proliferating cell nuclear antigen (PCNA) and this interaction is important to prevent telomere fragility [87].

**CST complex**

The human CST complex consisting of CTC1, STN1, and TEN1 proteins plays a role in telomere protection and DNA metabolism [88]. Each telomerase RNP is believed to add 50–60 nucleotides to most telomeres following a single initiation event [89]. The CST complex has been proposed to set the upper limit of telomere elongation by binding to telomeric single-stranded DNA (ssDNA) and displacing telomerase, once telomeric overhang has reached certain length [90]. Study reported by Chen et al showed that CST competes with POT1–TPP1 for telomeric DNA [90]. It terminates telomerase activity through primer sequestration and physical association with the POT1–TPP1 subunits, which functions as a telomerase processivity factor [91]. CST–telomeric-DNA binding increases during late S/G2 phase following telomerase activity, concurrently with telomerase turn-off. Attenuation of CST enables excessive telomerase activity, fostering telomere elongation. It is suggested that through binding of the telomerase-extended telomere, CST limits telomerase activity at individual telomeres to approximately one binding and extension event per cell cycle.

**Telomerase Cajal body protein 1 (TCAB1)**

TCAB1 (encoded by gene *WDR79*) contains a proline-rich region and WD40 motif and is localized in CBs. CBs have been shown to accumulate telomerase as well as associate with telomeres [78]. TCAB1 has been demonstrated to be a component of active telomerase and is necessary for the telomerase holoenzyme to accumulate in CB and thus regulate telomere elongation [92]. TCAB1 interacts with CAB box motif of *TR* and functions in telomerase assembly by driving telomerase to CB. Subsequent report by Stern et al showed that TCAB1 and CB are required for telomerase recruitment to telomeres independent of each other [93].

**TERRA**

TERRA functions as a negative regulator of telomere length. It is transcribed from subtelomeric regions of telomeres that consist of UUAGGG repeats. TERRA may inhibit telomerase in cis by directly binding to telomerase [94, 95].

## 3. Cross talk of telomere-associated proteins with cellular signaling pathways

### 3.1. TAPs and DNA damage response

When the genomic DNA undergoes any damage such as single-strand DNA breaks, double-strand breaks (DSBs), nicks, or chromosome fusions, cells activate DNA repair pathway depending on the type of damage. During this process, cells seize to grow and initiate the repair, and once the repair is completed growth resumes; otherwise, they undergo apoptosis. Telomeres can also be sensed as breaks by cellular machinery. However, telomerase and shelterin complex cap the telomeres and thus maintain telomere integrity by inhibiting DNA-damage-response pathway at telomeres. Further, some of these DNA repair proteins play an essential role in telomere maintenance by directly associating with various TAPs. Recently, these TAPs have been shown to play a role in DDR at locations distinct from telomeres. TRF1, which is predominantly localized to telomeres, has been shown to interact with proteins implicated in DNA damage response such as ATM and Mre11/Rad50/Nbs1 [96]. Further, it has been shown that TRF1 is phosphorylated by Cdk1 and this form is incapable of binding to telomeres [97]. It has been shown that this phosphorylated TRF1 in a telomere-independent way facilitates end resection and homology repair (HR), activates G2/M checkpoint, and enables cell survival following double-strand break induction [98]. TRF2 is known to prevent activation of ATM-dependent DDR pathway at telomeres [26, 99, 100]. TRF2 has also been shown to localize at DNA double-strand breaks during early stages (within 2 s) of cellular response to DSBs and leaves those sites during repair processing [101]. Further reports suggested that TRF2 may also participate in HR of the extra telomeric damaged DNA [102].

It has been shown that telomerase localizes to mitochondria and protects cancer cells from nuclear DNA damage and apoptosis [103]. Further, TERT has also been shown to function in DNA damage response pathway and in regulating histone-dependent chromatin remodeling [104]. *TR* knockout mice display impaired DDR in response to damaging agents; however, the effects are evident clearly in late-generation TR null mice, which show significant telomere shortening and dysfunction [105, 106].

### 3.2. TAPs and NF-κB pathway

NF-κB transcription factors are key mediators of various cellular, inflammatory, and development pathways [107]. NF-κB family consists of five transcription factors namely RelA (p65), RelB, c-Rel, and also includes p50 and p52 (processed from p105 and p100, respectively). Rel family proteins possess REL homology domain, which harbors DNA-binding domain, dimerization, and IκB-binding domain. NF-κB family members are held inactive in cytoplasm by IκB family of proteins. Upon stimulation, IkB proteins are phosphorylated by IκB kinase (IKK) complex and thus degraded or processed to produce active dimers, which can enter the nucleus and activate the transcription response [107]. TAFs, which have been shown to modulate NF-κB signaling, independent of their role at telomeres, include shelterin complex protein RAP1 and telomerase complex protein TERT [108, 109].

A fraction of cytosolic RAP1 associates with functional IKK complex. RAP1 increases the efficiency of IKK complex in phosphorylating p65 subunit at serine 536; however, it has no effect on the degradation of IκBa inhibitory protein, thus functioning as an adaptor in the IKK complex [110]. In line with this, it was recently shown that RAP1 regulates cytokine levels followed by fine healing of corneal injury by effective modulation of NF-κB signaling [111]. Since RAP1 is also localized in cytoplasm, there are possibilities that it might function as an adaptor in various other complexes under different stimuli.

TERT has also been shown to associate with p65 in the nuclear compartment, thus directly regulating its transcriptional response. Akiyama et al demonstrated that TERT associates with p65 to mediate its translocation to nucleus in multiple myeloma cells [112]. Recently, our group showed that TERT associates with p65 to directly affect its transcriptional output [113]. We showed that *TR*-knockout mice are more resistant to inflammatory agent lipopolysaccharide (LPS), which majorly functions by activating NF-κB pathway. Ectopic expression of TERT led to increased proliferation of cancer cells as well as xenograft model, which could be abrogated by inhibiting p65. Subsequently, another group showed that TERT regulates matrix metalloproteinase (MMP) expression independently of telomerase activity via activation of NF-κB-dependent transcription [114].

### 3.3. TAPs and WNT/β-catenin pathway

WNT pathway plays a key role in development processes like cell-fate determination, progenitor cell proliferation, and cell polarity [115]. In canonical WNT pathway, WNT ligand binds to its receptor leading to stabilization of β-catenin in the cytoplasm. Stabilized β-catenin then enters nucleus to activate transcription through its interaction with TCF/Lef family members. It further recruits chromatin remodelers like BRG1 to facilitate transcription.

TERT is the only TAP shown to modulate WNT pathway independent of telomeres and telomerase catalytic activity. The first evidence demonstrating a link between TERT and WNT pathway came from Choi et al who showed that knock in of catalytically inactive TERT in hair follicle stem cells led to their proliferation [116]. Changes in gene expression as analyzed by microarray, revealed differential expression of genes involved in development/morphogenesis, signal transduction, and cytoskeleton/cell adhesion signaling pathways. Modulated gene expression pattern strongly correlated with transcriptional program of MYC and WNT, suggesting existence of a potential association of TERT with the WNT and MYC pathways. Subsequently, Park et al demonstrated the first evidence of the direct regulation of Wnt/β-catenin signaling by telomerase in mouse embryonic stem cells and *Xenopus laevis* embryos. The study reported that TERT functions as a cofactor in the β-catenin transcriptional complex through its interaction with Brg1, a chromatin-remodeling factor [117]. Ectopic expression of TERT or catalytically inactive TERT led to the activation of WNT-dependent reporters in vitro and in vivo, while chromatin immunoprecipitation assays uncovered TERT localization at WNT target gene promoters. It was shown that TERT null mice display partially penetrant homeotic transformation of vertebrae, due to the loss of 13th rib of one or both the vertebrae. Recently, another group reported that TERT forms a complex with Brg1, together with nucleostemin (NS), a nucleolar GTP-binding protein and/or its family member GNL3L and is essential for maintenance of the tumor-initiating cell phenotype in human cancer cells [118].

### 3.4. TAPs and MYC

Recently, we reported that TERT regulates MYC transcription [119]. It is well known that MYC directly regulates TERT transcription [120]. However, our study illuminated the existence of a feed-forward loop between TERT and MYC in MYC-driven cancers such as lymphomas. Using genetic and biochemical approaches, we showed that the absence of TERT delayed MYC-dependent lymphomagenesis and strikingly, this effect was not observed when the RNA component of telomerase, *TR* was removed. Using in vivo and in vitro approaches, we established that TERT stabilizes MYC and thus results in increased MYC-dependent tran-

http://dx.doi.org/10.5772/62130

scriptional output. Furthermore, we showed that this effect of TERT on MYC stability was independent of its catalytic activity. Mechanistically, we showed that TERT associates with MYC, preventing its proteasomal degradation, thus stabilizing its protein levels [119].

### 3.5. TAPs and mitochondria

Among TAPs, TERT and TIN2 have been shown to be involved in regulating mitochondrial activity. It has been shown that TERT translocates to mitochondria under certain stress conditions [121–123]. Mitochondrial TERT binds to and protects mitochondrial DNA from hydrogen peroxide-induced oxidative damage [103, 124]. Overexpression and knockdown studies involving TERT in cancer cells have shown that the role of TERT in mitochondrial pathway of apoptosis is independent of its catalytic activity [122, 125]. Interestingly, it has also been shown that TERT functions as a reverse transcriptase in mitochondria using mitochondrial tRNA as a template [126]. Furthermore, it has been shown that TERT can interact with RNA component of mitochondrial RNA-processing endoribonuclease (*RMRP*) to form a complex similar to RNA-dependent RNA polymerase (RdRP). This complex then affects gene silencing at the post-transcriptional level [126].

TIN2 has also been shown to localize to mitochondria, where it results in altered mitochondrial structure. The group showed that the reduction of TIN2 levels led to augmented mitochondrial oxidative phosphorylation and reduced aerobic glycolysis in cancer cells [127].

### 3.6. TAPs and miscellaneous associations

Apart from the above-described associations of TAPs with cellular machinery, there are various reports about many more interacting partners. TRF2 has been shown to function as a transcriptional activator by directly binding to promoter of the angiogenic tyrosine kinase platelet-derived growth factor receptor β (PDGFRβ). This study highlighted the angiogenic role of TRF2 uncoupled from its telomere-capping role [128]. Telomerase was shown to regulate rDNA transcription by directly associating with RNA polymerase I upon hyperproliferative stimuli such as during liver regeneration and Ras-induced hyperproliferation [129].

Figure 2 summarizes the role of telomere-interacting proteins in cross talk with cellular signaling pathways.

## 4. Telomeres and TAPs in human diseases: Telomeropathies

Telomeres shorten with each cell division. When telomeres become excessively short, they lose their protective role and activate a DNA damaging signal response resulting in genomic instability, cell cycle arrest, and senescence. TAPs play an essential role in maintaining telomere length, and genetic mutations affecting their activity can result in telomere dysfunction. This manifests into a wide variety of diseases collectively named as "telomeropathies" or "telomere syndromes", which exhibit impaired telomere maintenance.

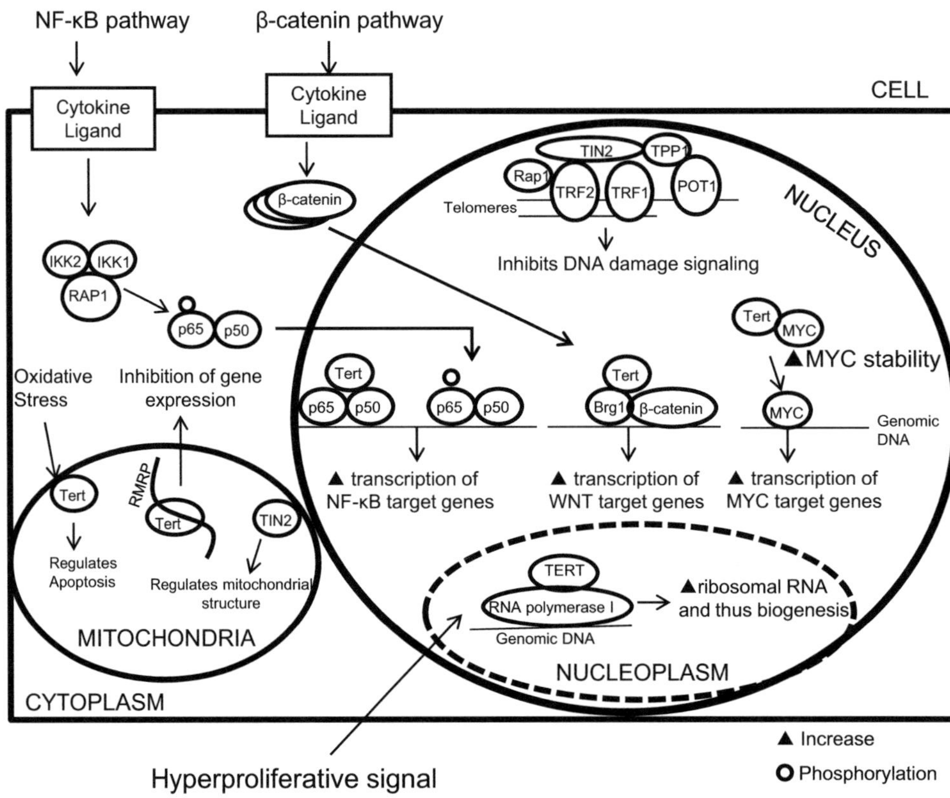


**Figure 2.** Schematic representation showing Telomere associated proteins interacting with several cell-signaling pathways.

### 4.1. Telomere-shortening syndromes

Inherited mutations, which hamper telomerase or telomere maintenance genes, result in progressive shortening of telomeres. Telomere shortening has major impact on highly proliferating tissues, such as bone marrow, where stem cells reach senescence stage and organ failure might ensue. Clinical conditions associated with shortened telomeres may be very different. This may be partly due to genetic anticipation since telomere length is inherited [63].

#### *4.1.1. Dyskeratosis congenita*

Dyskeratosis congenita (DC) arises primarily due to bone marrow failure and is associated with a diagnostic triad of oral leukoplakia, skin hyperpigmentation, nail dystrophy, and other manifestations. Dyskerin (encoded by *DKC1*), which is an essential component of telomerase enzyme in vivo, was the first gene identified as a cause of DC, and was thus named after this syndrome. DC is a heterogeneous disease showing all modes of inheritance. To date, 11 genes have been associated with DC. These include genes encoding products involved in telomere elongating enzyme, telomerase components (TERT and *TR*), telomerase stability (dyskerin,

NOP10, NHP2), telomerase recruitment (TIN2 and TPP1), telomerase trafficking (TCAB1), telomerase docking (CTC1), and telomere replication (RTEL1) [130].

Figure 3 shows schematic representation of telomere-interacting proteins with domains and positions of reported germ-line mutations, which result in various forms of DC.

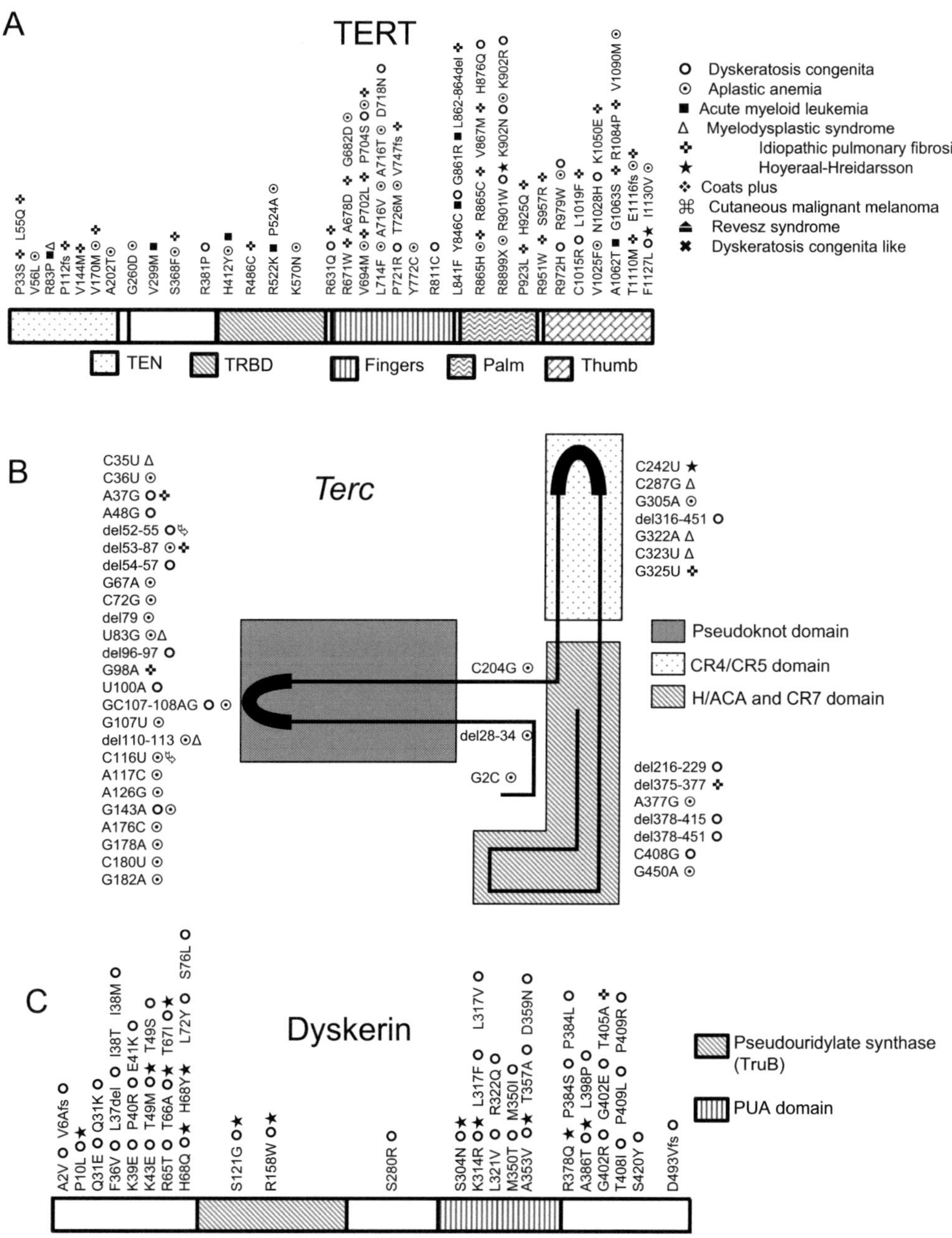

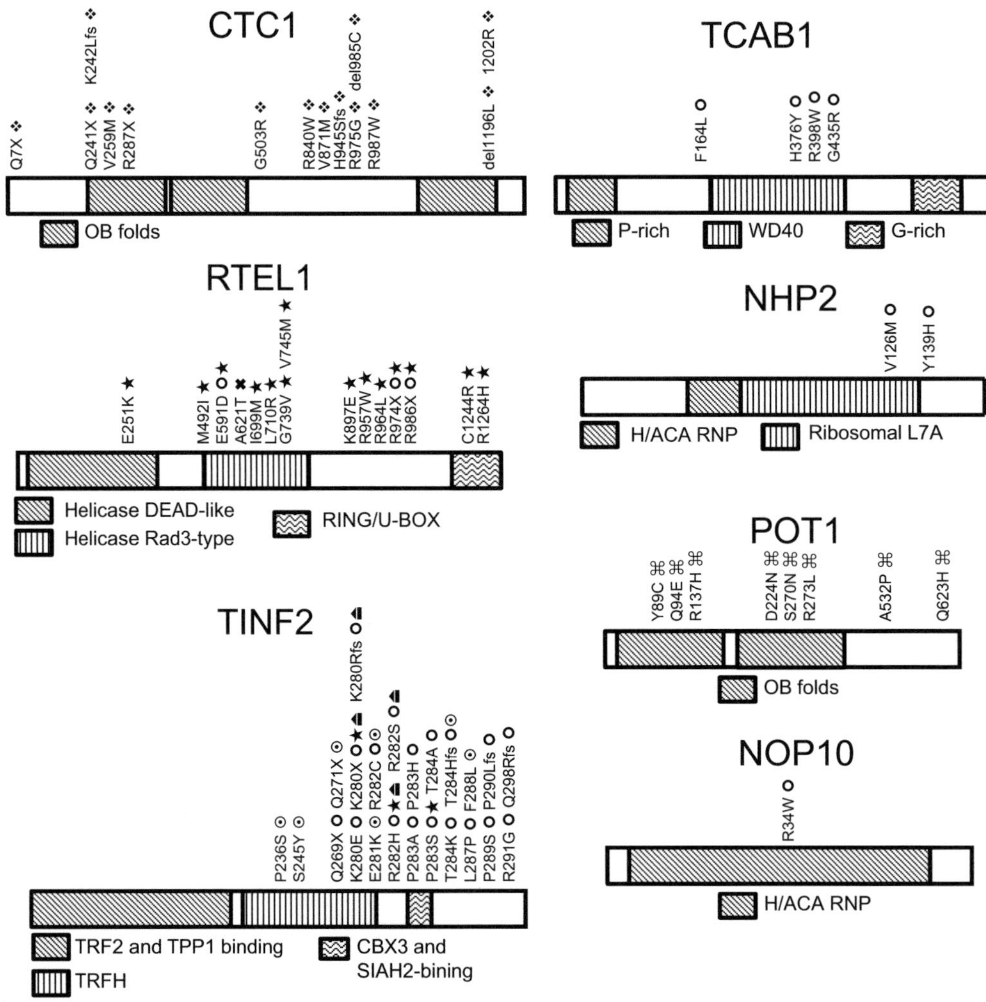


**Figure 3.** Schematic representation showing protein structure and localization of reported mutations in telomere associated proteins. The information is adapted from Espinoza et al [144].

Recently poly(A)-specific ribonuclease (*PARN*) gene mutations have been reported in a subgroup of patients with DC wherein *PARN* deficiency results in reduced stability of several key TAPs (dyskerin, TRF1, RTEL1, and *TR*) and specifically leads to telomere attrition [131]. Almost all modes of inheritance have been reported in DC, which include autosomal recessive, autosomal dominant, and X-linked. Based on functional relevance of mutated proteins and their penetrance, clinically diverse variant manifestations of DC are reported.

Calado et al reported a study of five families who were suffering from liver disease (familial liver cirrhosis) in combination with hematologic and autoimmune disorders [132]. They analyzed the mutations associated with the disease and found rare loss of function mutations in *TERT* or *TR* (3.7% vs 0.8%). Hoyeraal–Hreidarsson syndrome (HHS) is associated with intrauterine growth retardation (IUGR), microcephaly, cerebellar hypoplasia, and thrombocytopenia along with various nonspecific enteropathies. HHS patients are also found to harbor DC mucocutaneous triad in adulthood. Detailed analysis revealed mutations in *DKC1*, *TIN2* along with some cases showing autosomal recessive mutations in *TERT*, *NHP2*, *NOP10*, *TPP1*, and *RTEL1* genes [133, 134]. Revesz syndrome (RS) is associated with various disease manifestations mainly bilateral exudative retinopathy. Other symptoms reported include IUGR, intracranial calcifications, developmental delay, and nail dystrophy in different cases, which were highly overlapping with DC symptoms. It was discovered that RS patients have short telomeres and harbor germ-line mutations in *TINF2* gene [135]. Coats plus syndrome (CCS) is a rare recessive disorder that is characterized by intracranial calcifications, hematological abnormalities, and retinal vascular defects. CCS patients display shortened telomeres indicating telomere dysfunction as a major cause. Missense mutations in *CTC1* gene whose protein is a part of CST complex has been reported to occur in CCS patients [136]. HHS, RS, and CCS represent severe forms of DC.

About 10% of DC patients develop cancer at a very young age. Various DC families display an increased incidence of acute myeloid leukemia and myelodysplastic syndrome [137]. Spontaneous reversion to the functional *TR* allele in hematopoietic stem cells of haploinsufficient DC patients has been observed predisposing them to hematological disorders. The mechanism behind high cancer incidence, in spite of short telomeres that should have cancer-protecting effect, remains largely unexplained. The only proposed mechanism is genomic instability due to fusion of chromosome ends by NHEJ as has been observed in mutation carriers and in *TR*-knockout mice [138].

#### *4.1.2. Pulmonary fibrosis*

Idiopathic pulmonary fibrosis (IPF) disease is characterized by progressive lung scarring and fibrotic changes. The disease is associated with abnormal telomere maintenance and is an attenuated form where fibrosis develops with cumulative age-related changes. This disease arises from mutations in genes encoding *TERT* and *TR* leading to reduced telomerase activity and subsequently shorter telomeres, resulting in impaired growth of lung stem cells [139]. Surprisingly, short telomeres have been detected in IPF patients with intact telomerase genes, indicating that IPF may develop in people who have short telomere lengths [140]. This study also showed the development of liver cirrhosis in 3% of sporadic IPF patients, demonstrating a complication of telomere-mediated disease outside the lung even in the absence of telomerase mutations. Also, increased incidence of insulin-dependent diabetes is detected in IPF patients [141]. Short telomeres have been shown to cause insulin secretion defects and glucose intolerance in telomerase-deficient mice [142].

#### *4.1.3. Bone marrow failure*

Many bone marrow failure disease cases have been linked to telomere biology. Mutations in telomeric proteins can lead to accelerated telomere attrition in hematopoietic compartment leading to bone marrow failure. The most common gene associated with bone marrow failure is *TERT*, which generally harbors point mutations in its gene [143, 144].

## 4.2. Role of TAPs in cancer

The role of TAPs in cancer development is well known. People with long telomeres are at a greater genetic risk of developing cancers [145]. Thus, examining the role of telomere proteins in cancer holds immense prognostic, diagnostic, and therapeutic value.

### *4.2.1. Shelterin proteins and cancer*

The shelterin complex member POT1 was found to be somatically inactivated in chronic lymphocytic leukemia where it led to telomere deprotection and length extension [146]. Recently, two studies reported occurrence of rare, germ-line variants in *POT1*, making them susceptible to the development of familial melanoma [145]. In these cohorts, carrier individuals displayed significantly longer and more fragile telomeres than controls, and in some cases developed cancer in other tissues along with melanoma. Molecular and functional analysis showed that some of the variants abrogate the binding of POT1 to ssDNA, thus raising the possibility that carriers are predisposed to malignancy via telomere uncapping and a more permissive extension of chromosome ends. However, the exact biological mechanism needs further investigation. Mutation in *RAP1*, another shelterin protein member was reported in a melanoma cohort. RAP1 is involved in negative regulation of telomere length and functions by repressing homology-directed repair [147]. Mutations were reported to occur in TRF1-interacting region of RAP1. This loss of interaction with shelterin may increase the risk of cancer development.

Germ-line mutations affecting other proteins that interact with shelterin complex members and increase cancer risk have also been reported. For example, ku80, which interacts with RAP1 and PARP1, which in turn interacts with TRF2, has been found to be associated with diffuse large B-cell lymphomas.

### *4.2.2. Telomerase and cancer*

Telomerase activity is essential for immortalization. Thus, targeting telomerase activity represents an attractive approach for both cancer diagnosis and treatment [148, 149]. As described previously, TERT is the limiting factor for telomerase activity. Therefore, its reactivation mechanisms hold great significance in understanding the development of cancer and thus designing targeted therapies.

Two hot-spot mutations in the *TERT* promoter, -228 C>T and -250 C>T, were recently reported to occur at high frequency in several solid tumors, for example: melanoma, gliomas, carcinoma of bladder, urothelial cancer, thyroid and squamous cell carcinoma of the tongue, as well as in liposarcomas and hepatocellular carcinomas, which have relatively low rates of self-renewal [85, 150–153]. It was recently shown that *TERT* promoter mutations create novel binding sites for GABP, which belongs to Ets family of transcription factors [154]. These mutations have strong clinical implications with worse prognosis and poor survival, and thus may represent a novel therapeutic target [153].

*TERT* promoter mutation in skin cancers

Stem cells differentiate into normal somatic cells and as a consequence repress TERT transcription. Upon subsequent cell division, progressive telomere shortening occurs due to lack of telomerase activity. This acts as a barrier for tumor development and progression. Skin epidermal cells are highly differentiated cells, possess short telomeres, and are thus capable of undergoing limited proliferation [155]. However, in melanoma, increased telomerase activity is reported and this has been associated with high proliferation rate and early metastasis [156, 157].

High frequency of *TERT* promoter mutations has been reported in familial and sporadic melanoma (about 29–73%) [150, 151]. In primary cutaneous melanoma, *TERT* promoter mutations were found to be associated with BRAFV600E mutations, worse prognostic features, and shorter disease-free and overall survival [158, 159]. *TERT* promoter mutations have also been reported to be common in nonmelanoma skin cancer ranging from 39 to 74% in sporadic basal cell carcinoma and up to 50% mutation frequency in squamous cell carcinoma [158, 160, 161]. Various studies have assessed the association between telomere length and risk of developing skin cancer [162]. Some reports suggest no association between telomere length in peripheral blood leukocytes (PBL) and risk of nonmelanoma skin cancer [163]. On the contrary, other authors have reported that longer telomeres in PBL are protective for certain skin cancer types [162].

*TERT* promoter mutations in central nervous system (CNS) tumors

Within CNS tumors, gliomas have been shown to possess the highest frequency of *TERT* promoter mutations, while medulloblastoma and meningioma show lower frequencies [164]. Within gliomas, the percentage of cases with *TERT* promoter mutations varies depending on the histopathological type of tumor. *TERT* promoter mutations are reported in a large number of cases of glioblastoma multiforme (GBM), which is the most frequent and aggressive form of glioma, and in oligodendrogliomas, in contrast to astrocytoma and ependymoma, where only a small percentage of the tumors possess such mutations [159, 164]. Furthermore, the frequency of *TERT* promoter mutations in oligoastrocytomas, gliomas with a mixed origin, is in between that of oligodendrogliomas and astrocytomas [152]. These findings are consistent with the reported data on telomerase activity in gliomas, which is significantly higher in GBM (50–89%) and oligodendrogliomas (75–100%) than in astrocytomas (0–45%) [165–167].

Some studies also reported an association between single-nucleotide polymorphisms (SNPs) in the *TERT* gene and an increased risk of glioma development [168, 169].

*TERT* promoter mutations in other cancers

Telomerase role in bladder carcinoma (BC) has been reported. In majority of BC tumor samples, telomerase activity was detected, while it was absent in the respective normal parallel samples [170, 171]. In some reports, telomerase activity was associated with lower grade and lower stage BC [170, 172]. Other studies showed that both telomerase activity and telomerase expression are associated with more advanced and higher grade of cancers [171, 173]. Preliminary evidence obtained in cell lines suggests that BC might have *TERT* promoter mutations

[150]. *TERT* promoter mutations are also frequently detected in BC cell lines, with a prevalence ranging from 47 to 85%. These results have clearly shown that *TERT* promoter mutations represent one of the most common genetic events, perhaps the most frequent, in BC [85].

*TERT* promoter mutations also occur at high frequency in other cancer types, for example: hepatocellular carcinoma (56%), several soft tissue tumors histotypes (e.g., 93% in atypical fibroxanthoma, 79% in myxoid liposarcoma, and 76% in pleomorphic dermal sarcoma) and carcinoma of the renal pelvis (64%). Tumor histotypes with intermediate frequencies of *TERT* promoter mutations comprise laryngeal carcinoma (27%) and clear cell carcinoma of the ovary (16%) [174]. *TERT* promoter mutations are not frequently found in leukemias and colorectal cancers [174].

The high prevalence of *TERT* promoter mutations suggests the significance of telomere maintenance in cancers. Clinically, *TERT* promoter mutations represent a potential biomarker in cancer prognosis. Furthermore, *TERT* promoter mutations also serve as an attractive therapeutic target since they occur specifically in cancer cells and are absent in surrounding healthy tissues.

## 5. Conclusion

Telomeres are organized into highly specialized structures at chromosome ends. Telomerase and shelterin plays a role in telomere homeostasis. Along with telomere maintenance, telomere-associated proteins also play a significant role in various cell-signaling pathways. The significance and implication of telomerase and shelterin in human diseases have also been firmly established in various models of degenerative diseases. In cancer, telomerase dysfunction has been identified as a critical step for immortalization, although the underlying mechanisms are unclear. The recent identification of telomerase promoter mutations has stimulated research, following which numerous studies have reported similar alterations in various cancer models. In several relevant cancer types, telomerase promoter mutations seem to represent a new biomarker for prognosis with potential applications in presurgical diagnosis and in the monitoring of patients. Mechanisms regulating telomerase promoter mutations also hold immense therapeutic value since they occur specifically in cancers.

## Author details

Ekta Khattar* and Vinay Tergaonkar

*Address all correspondence to: khattare@imcb.a-star.edu.sg

Institute of Molecular and Cell Biology (IMCB), A STAR (Agency for Science, Technology and Research), Singapore, Singapore

## References

[1] Moyzis RK, Buckingham JM, Cram LS, Dani M, Deaven LL, Jones MD, Meyne J, Ratliff RL, Wu JR: A highly conserved repetitive DNA sequence, (TTAGGG)n, present at the telomeres of human chromosomes. Proceedings of the National Academy of Sciences of the United States of America 1988, 85:6622–6626.

[2] Griffith JD, Comeau L, Rosenfield S, Stansel RM, Bianchi A, Moss H, de Lange T: Mammalian telomeres end in a large duplex loop. Cell 1999, 97:503–514.

[3] Greider CW: Telomeres do D-loop-T-loop. Cell 1999, 97:419–422.

[4] d'Adda di Fagagna F, Reaper PM, Clay-Farrace L, Fiegler H, Carr P, Von Zglinicki T, Saretzki G, Carter NP, Jackson SP: A DNA damage checkpoint response in telomere-initiated senescence. Nature 2003, 426:194–198.

[5] Diotti R, Loayza D: Shelterin complex and associated factors at human telomeres. Nucleus 2011, 2:119–135.

[6] de Lange T: Shelterin: the protein complex that shapes and safeguards human telomeres. Genes & Development 2005, 19:2100–2110.

[7] Palm W, de Lange T: How shelterin protects mammalian telomeres. Annual Review of Genetics 2008, 42:301–334.

[8] Passos JF, von Zglinicki T: Mitochondria, telomeres and cell senescence. Experimental Gerontology 2005, 40:466–472.

[9] Takai H, Smogorzewska A, de Lange T: DNA damage foci at dysfunctional telomeres. Current Biology 2003, 13:1549–1556.

[10] Wai LK: Telomeres, telomerase, and tumorigenesis – a review. MedGenMed: Medscape General Medicine 2004, 6:19.

[11] Richter T, von Zglinicki T: A continuous correlation between oxidative stress and telomere shortening in fibroblasts. Experimental Gerontology 2007, 42:1039–1042.

[12] Cattan V, Mercier N, Gardner JP, Regnault V, Labat C, Maki-Jouppila J, Nzietchueng R, Benetos A, Kimura M, Aviv A, et al: Chronic oxidative stress induces a tissue-specific reduction in telomere length in CAST/Ei mice. Free Radical Biology & Medicine 2008, 44:1592–1598.

[13] Greider CW, Blackburn EH: Identification of a specific telomere terminal transferase activity in tetrahymena extracts. Cell 1985, 43:405–413.

[14] Sfeir A, de Lange T: Removal of shelterin reveals the telomere end-protection problem. Science 2012, 336:593–597.

[15] Xin H, Liu D, Songyang Z: The telosome/shelterin complex and its functions. Genome Biology 2008, 9:232.

[16] Martinez P, Blasco MA: Telomeric and extra-telomeric roles for telomerase and the telomere-binding proteins. Nature Reviews Cancer 2011, 11:161–176.

[17] Galati A, Micheli E, Alicata C, Ingegnere T, Cicconi A, Pusch MC, Giraud-Panis MJ, Gilson E, Cacchione S: TRF1 and TRF2 binding to telomeres is modulated by nucleosomal organization. Nucleic Acids Research 2015, 43:5824–5837.

[18] van Steensel B, de Lange T: Control of telomere length by the human telomeric protein TRF1. Nature 1997, 385:740–743.

[19] Garrobo I, Marion RM, Dominguez O, Pisano DG, Blasco MA: Genome-wide analysis of in vivo TRF1 binding to chromatin restricts its location exclusively to telomeric repeats. Cell Cycle 2014, 13:3742–3749.

[20] Ohishi T, Muramatsu Y, Yoshida H, Seimiya H: TRF1 ensures the centromeric function of Aurora-B and proper chromosome segregation. Molecular and Cellular Biology 2014, 34:2464–2478.

[21] Poulet A, Pisano S, Faivre-Moskalenko C, Pei B, Tauran Y, Haftek-Terreau Z, Brunet F, Le Bihan YV, Ledu MH, Montel F, et al: The N-terminal domains of TRF1 and TRF2 regulate their ability to condense telomeric DNA. Nucleic Acids Research 2012, 40:2566–2576.

[22] Doksani Y, Wu JY, de Lange T, Zhuang X: Super-resolution fluorescence imaging of telomeres reveals TRF2-dependent T-loop formation. Cell 2013, 155:345–356.

[23] Simonet T, Zaragosi LE, Philippe C, Lebrigand K, Schouteden C, Augereau A, Bauwens S, Ye J, Santagostino M, Giulotto E, et al: The human TTAGGG repeat factors 1 and 2 bind to a subset of interstitial telomeric sequences and satellite repeats. Cell Research 2011, 21:1028–1038.

[24] Yang D, Xiong Y, Kim H, He Q, Li Y, Chen R, Songyang Z: Human telomeric proteins occupy selective interstitial sites. Cell Research 2011, 21:1013–1027.

[25] Wood AM, Rendtlew Danielsen JM, Lucas CA, Rice EL, Scalzo D, Shimi T, Goldman RD, Smith ED, Le Beau MM, Kosak ST: TRF2 and lamin A/C interact to facilitate the functional organization of chromosome ends. Nature Communications 2014, 5:5467.

[26] Celli GB, de Lange T: DNA processing is not required for ATM-mediated telomere damage response after TRF2 deletion. Nature Cell Biology 2005, 7:712–718.

[27] Saint-Leger A, Koelblen M, Civitelli L, Bah A, Djerbi N, Giraud-Panis MJ, Londono-Vallejo A, Ascenzioni F, Gilson E: The basic N-terminal domain of TRF2 limits recombination endonuclease action at human telomeres. Cell Cycle 2014, 13:2469–2474.

[28] Kim SH, Kaminker P, Campisi J: TIN2, a new regulator of telomere length in human cells. Nature Genetics 1999, 23:405–412.

[29] Ye JZ, Donigian JR, van Overbeek M, Loayza D, Luo Y, Krutchinsky AN, Chait BT, de Lange T: TIN2 binds TRF1 and TRF2 simultaneously and stabilizes the TRF2 complex on telomeres. The Journal of Biological Chemistry 2004, 279:47264–47271.

[30] Frank AK, Tran DC, Qu RW, Stohr BA, Segal DJ, Xu L: The shelterin TIN2 subunit mediates recruitment of telomerase to telomeres. PLoS Genetics 2015, 11:e1005410.

[31] Hockemeyer D, Palm W, Else T, Daniels JP, Takai KK, Ye JZ, Keegan CE, de Lange T, Hammer GD: Telomere protection by mammalian Pot1 requires interaction with Tpp1. Nature Structural & Molecular Biology 2007, 14:754–761.

[32] Loayza D, Parsons H, Donigian J, Hoke K, de Lange T: DNA binding features of human POT1: a nonamer 5'-TAGGGTTAG-3' minimal binding site, sequence specificity, and internal binding to multimeric sites. The Journal of Biological Chemistry 2004, 279:13241–13248.

[33] Liu D, Safari A, O'Connor MS, Chan DW, Laegeler A, Qin J, Songyang Z: PTOP interacts with POT1 and regulates its localization to telomeres. Nature Cell Biology 2004, 6:673–680.

[34] Chen LY, Liu D, Songyang Z: Telomere maintenance through spatial control of telomeric proteins. Molecular and Cellular Biology 2007, 27:5898–5909.

[35] Kibe T, Osawa GA, Keegan CE, de Lange T: Telomere protection by TPP1 is mediated by POT1a and POT1b. Molecular and Cellular Biology 2010, 30:1059–1066.

[36] Xin H, Liu D, Wan M, Safari A, Kim H, Sun W, O'Connor MS, Songyang Z: TPP1 is a homologue of ciliate TEBP-beta and interacts with POT1 to recruit telomerase. Nature 2007, 445:559–562.

[37] Zhong FL, Batista LF, Freund A, Pech MF, Venteicher AS, Artandi SE: TPP1 OB-fold domain controls telomere maintenance by recruiting telomerase to chromosome ends. Cell 2012, 150:481–494.

[38] Nandakumar J, Bell CF, Weidenfeld I, Zaug AJ, Leinwand LA, Cech TR: The TEL patch of telomere protein TPP1 mediates telomerase recruitment and processivity. Nature 2012, 492:285–289.

[39] Sexton AN, Regalado SG, Lai CS, Cost GJ, O'Neil CM, Urnov FD, Gregory PD, Jaenisch R, Collins K, Hockemeyer D: Genetic and molecular identification of three human TPP1 functions in telomerase action: recruitment, activation, and homeostasis set point regulation. Genes & Development 2014, 28:1885–1899.

[40] Loayza D, De Lange T: POT1 as a terminal transducer of TRF1 telomere length control. Nature 2003, 423:1013–1018.

[41] Wang F, Podell ER, Zaug AJ, Yang Y, Baciu P, Cech TR, Lei M: The POT1-TPP1 telomere complex is a telomerase processivity factor. Nature 2007, 445:506–510.

[42] Latrick CM, Cech TR: POT1-TPP1 enhances telomerase processivity by slowing primer dissociation and aiding translocation. The EMBO Journal 2010, 29:924–933.

[43] Li B, Oestreich S, de Lange T: Identification of human Rap1: implications for telomere evolution. Cell 2000, 101:471–483.

[44] Takai KK, Hooper S, Blackwood S, Gandhi R, de Lange T: In vivo stoichiometry of shelterin components. The Journal of Biological Chemistry 2010, 285:1457–1467.

[45] Kabir S, Hockemeyer D, de Lange T: TALEN gene knockouts reveal no requirement for the conserved human shelterin protein Rap1 in telomere protection and length regulation. Cell Reports 2014, 9:1273–1280.

[46] Martinez P, Thanasoula M, Carlos AR, Gomez-Lopez G, Tejera AM, Schoeftner S, Dominguez O, Pisano DG, Tarsounas M, Blasco MA: Mammalian Rap1 controls telomere function and gene expression through binding to telomeric and extratelomeric sites. Nature Cell Biology 2010, 12:768–780.

[47] Gilson E, Geli V: How telomeres are replicated. Nature Reviews Molecular Cell Biology 2007, 8:825–838.

[48] Blasco MA: Telomeres and human disease: ageing, cancer and beyond. Nature Reviews Genetics 2005, 6:611–622.

[49] Liu Y, Snow BE, Hande MP, Yeung D, Erdmann NJ, Wakeham A, Itie A, Siderovski DP, Lansdorp PM, Robinson MO, et al: The telomerase reverse transcriptase is limiting and necessary for telomerase function in vivo. Current Biology: CB 2000, 10:1459–1462.

[50] Li Y, Tergaonkar V: Noncanonical functions of telomerase: implications in telomerase-targeted cancer therapies. Cancer Research 2014, 74:1639–1644.

[51] Low KC, Tergaonkar V: Telomerase: central regulator of all of the hallmarks of cancer. Trends in Biochemical Sciences 2013, 38:426–434.

[52] Theimer CA, Feigon J: Structure and function of telomerase RNA. Current Opinion in Structural Biology 2006, 16:307–318.

[53] Mitchell JR, Collins K: Human telomerase activation requires two independent interactions between telomerase RNA and telomerase reverse transcriptase. Molecular Cell 2000, 6:361–371.

[54] Autexier C, Pruzan R, Funk WD, Greider CW: Reconstitution of human telomerase activity and identification of a minimal functional region of the human telomerase RNA. The EMBO Journal 1996, 15:5928–5935.

[55] Marrone A, Dokal I: Dyskeratosis congenita: molecular insights into telomerase function, ageing and cancer. Expert Reviews in Molecular Medicine 2004, 6:1–23.

[56] Egan ED, Collins K: Biogenesis of telomerase ribonucleoproteins. RNA 2012, 18:1747–1759.

[57] Kiss T, Fayet-Lebaron E, Jady BE: Box H/ACA small ribonucleoproteins. Molecular Cell 2010, 37:597–606.

[58] Kittur N, Darzacq X, Roy S, Singer RH, Meier UT: Dynamic association and localization of human H/ACA RNP proteins. RNA 2006, 12:2057–2062.

[59] Vulliamy TJ, Marrone A, Knight SW, Walne A, Mason PJ, Dokal I: Mutations in dyskeratosis congenita: their impact on telomere length and the diversity of clinical presentation. Blood 2006, 107:2680–2685.

[60] Hamma T, Ferre-D'Amare AR: The box H/ACA ribonucleoprotein complex: interplay of RNA and protein structures in post-transcriptional RNA modification. The Journal of Biological Chemistry 2010, 285:805–809.

[61] Fu D, Collins K: Distinct biogenesis pathways for human telomerase RNA and H/ACA small nucleolar RNAs. Molecular Cell 2003, 11:1361–1372.

[62] Darzacq X, Kittur N, Roy S, Shav-Tal Y, Singer RH, Meier UT: Stepwise RNP assembly at the site of H/ACA RNA transcription in human cells. The Journal of Cell Biology 2006, 173:207–218.

[63] Armanios M, Blackburn EH: The telomere syndromes. Nature Reviews Genetics 2012, 13:693–704.

[64] Jady BE, Bertrand E, Kiss T: Human telomerase RNA and box H/ACA scaRNAs share a common Cajal body-specific localization signal. The Journal of Cell Biology 2004, 164:647–652.

[65] Girard C, Verheggen C, Neel H, Cammas A, Vagner S, Soret J, Bertrand E, Bordonne R: Characterization of a short isoform of human Tgs1 hypermethylase associating with small nucleolar ribonucleoprotein core proteins and produced by limited proteolytic processing. The Journal of Biological Chemistry 2008, 283:2060–2069.

[66] Mason M, Schuller A, Skordalakes E: Telomerase structure function. Current Opinion in Structural Biology 2011, 21:92–100.

[67] Schmidt JC, Dalby AB, Cech TR: Identification of human TERT elements necessary for telomerase recruitment to telomeres. eLife 2014, 3.

[68] Bley CJ, Qi X, Rand DP, Borges CR, Nelson RW, Chen JJ: RNA-protein binding interface in the telomerase ribonucleoprotein. Proceedings of the National Academy of Sciences of the United States of America 2011, 108:20333–20338.

[69] Nakamura TM, Morin GB, Chapman KB, Weinrich SL, Andrews WH, Lingner J, Harley CB, Cech TR: Telomerase catalytic subunit homologs from fission yeast and human. Science 1997, 277:955–959.

[70] Lingner J, Hughes TR, Shevchenko A, Mann M, Lundblad V, Cech TR: Reverse transcriptase motifs in the catalytic subunit of telomerase. Science 1997, 276:561–567.

[71] Xiong Y, Eickbush TH: Origin and evolution of retroelements based upon their reverse transcriptase sequences. The EMBO Journal 1990, 9:3353–3362.

[72] Steitz TA: DNA polymerases: structural diversity and common mechanisms. The Journal of Biological Chemistry 1999, 274:17395–17398.

[73] Huard S, Moriarty TJ, Autexier C: The C terminus of the human telomerase reverse transcriptase is a determinant of enzyme processivity. Nucleic Acids Research 2003, 31:4059–4070.

[74] Holt SE, Aisner DL, Baur J, Tesmer VM, Dy M, Ouellette M, Trager JB, Morin GB, Toft DO, Shay JW, et al: Functional requirement of p23 and Hsp90 in telomerase complexes. Genes & Development 1999, 13:817–826.

[75] Venteicher AS, Meng Z, Mason PJ, Veenstra TD, Artandi SE: Identification of ATPases pontin and reptin as telomerase components essential for holoenzyme assembly. Cell 2008, 132:945–957.

[76] King TH, Decatur WA, Bertrand E, Maxwell ES, Fournier MJ: A well-connected and conserved nucleoplasmic helicase is required for production of box C/D and H/ACA snoRNAs and localization of snoRNP proteins. Molecular and Cellular Biology 2001, 21:7731–7746.

[77] Xi L, Cech TR: Inventory of telomerase components in human cells reveals multiple subpopulations of hTR and hTERT. Nucleic Acids Research 2014, 42:8565–8577.

[78] Jady BE, Richard P, Bertrand E, Kiss T: Cell cycle-dependent recruitment of telomerase RNA and Cajal bodies to human telomeres. Molecular Biology of the Cell 2006, 17:944–954.

[79] Tomlinson RL, Ziegler TD, Supakorndej T, Terns RM, Terns MP: Cell cycle-regulated trafficking of human telomerase to telomeres. Molecular Biology of the Cell 2006, 17:955–965.

[80] Robart AR, Collins K: Human telomerase domain interactions capture DNA for TEN domain-dependent processive elongation. Molecular Cell 2011, 42:308–318.

[81] Sauerwald A, Sandin S, Cristofari G, Scheres SH, Lingner J, Rhodes D: Structure of active dimeric human telomerase. Nature Structural & Molecular Biology 2013, 20:454–460.

[82] Egan ED, Collins K: Specificity and stoichiometry of subunit interactions in the human telomerase holoenzyme assembled in vivo. Molecular and Cellular Biology 2010, 30:2775–2786.

[83] Akincilar SC, Low KC, Liu CY, Yan TD, Oji A, Ikawa M, Li S, Tergaonkar V: Quantitative assessment of telomerase components in cancer cell lines. FEBS Letters 2015, 589:974–984.

[84] Gladych M, Wojtyla A, Rubis B: Human telomerase expression regulation. Biochemistry and Cell Biology = Biochimie et biologie cellulaire 2011, 89:359–376.

[85] Vinagre J, Pinto V, Celestino R, Reis M, Populo H, Boaventura P, Melo M, Catarino T, Lima J, Lopes JM, et al: Telomerase promoter mutations in cancer: an emerging molecular biomarker? Virchows Archiv: An International Journal of Pathology 2014, 465:119–133.

[86] Faure G, Revy P, Schertzer M, Londono-Vallejo A, Callebaut I: The C-terminal extension of human RTEL1, mutated in Hoyeraal–Hreidarsson syndrome, contains harmonin-N-like domains. Proteins 2014, 82:897–903.

[87] Sarek G, Vannier JB, Panier S, Petrini JH, Boulton SJ: TRF2 recruits RTEL1 to telomeres in S phase to promote t-loop unwinding. Molecular Cell 2015, 57:622–635.

[88] Miyake Y, Nakamura M, Nabetani A, Shimamura S, Tamura M, Yonehara S, Saito M, Ishikawa F: RPA-like mammalian Ctc1-Stn1-Ten1 complex binds to single-stranded DNA and protects telomeres independently of the Pot1 pathway. Molecular Cell 2009, 36:193–206.

[89] Zhao Y, Sfeir AJ, Zou Y, Buseman CM, Chow TT, Shay JW, Wright WE: Telomere extension occurs at most chromosome ends and is uncoupled from fill-in in human cancer cells. Cell 2009, 138:463–475.

[90] Chen LY, Redon S, Lingner J: The human CST complex is a terminator of telomerase activity. Nature 2012, 488:540–544.

[91] Schmidt JC, Cech TR: Human telomerase: biogenesis, trafficking, recruitment, and activation. Genes & Development 2015, 29:1095–1105.

[92] Venteicher AS, Artandi SE: TCAB1: driving telomerase to Cajal bodies. Cell Cycle 2009, 8:1329–1331.

[93] Stern JL, Zyner KG, Pickett HA, Cohen SB, Bryan TM: Telomerase recruitment requires both TCAB1 and Cajal bodies independently. Molecular and Cellular Biology 2012, 32:2384–2395.

[94] Schoeftner S, Blasco MA: Developmentally regulated transcription of mammalian telomeres by DNA-dependent RNA polymerase II. Nature Cell Biology 2008, 10:228–236.

[95] Redon S, Reichenbach P, Lingner J: The non-coding RNA TERRA is a natural ligand and direct inhibitor of human telomerase. Nucleic Acids Research 2010, 38:5797–5806.

[96] Wu Y, Xiao S, Zhu XD: MRE11-RAD50-NBS1 and ATM function as co-mediators of TRF1 in telomere length control. Nature Structural & Molecular Biology 2007, 14:832–840.

[97] McKerlie M, Zhu XD: Cyclin B-dependent kinase 1 regulates human TRF1 to modulate the resolution of sister telomeres. Nature Communications 2011, 2:371.

[98] McKerlie M, Walker JR, Mitchell TR, Wilson FR, Zhu XD: Phosphorylated (pT371)TRF1 is recruited to sites of DNA damage to facilitate homologous recombination and checkpoint activation. Nucleic Acids Research 2013, 41:10268–10282.

[99] Karlseder J, Broccoli D, Dai Y, Hardy S, de Lange T: p53- and ATM-dependent apoptosis induced by telomeres lacking TRF2. Science 1999, 283:1321–1325.

[100] Denchi EL, de Lange T: Protection of telomeres through independent control of ATM and ATR by TRF2 and POT1. Nature 2007, 448:1068–1071.

[101] Bradshaw PS, Stavropoulos DJ, Meyn MS: Human telomeric protein TRF2 associates with genomic double-strand breaks as an early response to DNA damage. Nature Genetics 2005, 37:193–197.

[102] Fouche N, Cesare AJ, Willcox S, Ozgur S, Compton SA, Griffith JD: The basic domain of TRF2 directs binding to DNA junctions irrespective of the presence of TTAGGG repeats. The Journal of Biological Chemistry 2006, 281:37486–37495.

[103] Singhapol C, Pal D, Czapiewski R, Porika M, Nelson G, Saretzki GC: Mitochondrial telomerase protects cancer cells from nuclear DNA damage and apoptosis. PloS One 2013, 8:e52989.

[104] Masutomi K, Possemato R, Wong JM, Currier JL, Tothova Z, Manola JB, Ganesan S, Lansdorp PM, Collins K, Hahn WC: The telomerase reverse transcriptase regulates chromatin state and DNA damage responses. Proceedings of the National Academy of Sciences of the United States of America 2005, 102:8222–8227.

[105] Goytisolo FA, Samper E, Martin-Caballero J, Finnon P, Herrera E, Flores JM, Bouffler SD, Blasco MA: Short telomeres result in organismal hypersensitivity to ionizing radiation in mammals. The Journal of Experimental Medicine 2000, 192:1625–1636.

[106] Wong KK, Chang S, Weiler SR, Ganesan S, Chaudhuri J, Zhu C, Artandi SE, Rudolph KL, Gottlieb GJ, Chin L, et al: Telomere dysfunction impairs DNA repair and enhances sensitivity to ionizing radiation. Nature Genetics 2000, 26:85–88.

[107] Hayden MS, Ghosh S: Shared principles in NF-kappaB signaling. Cell 2008, 132:344–362.

[108] Ghosh AS, Tergaonkar V: Telomeres and inflammation: Rap1 joins the ends? Cell Cycle 2010, 9:3834–3835.

[109] Tergaonkar V: Catalytically inactive telomerase in oncogenesis. Oncotarget 2015, 6:14725–14726.

[110] Teo H, Ghosh S, Luesch H, Ghosh A, Wong ET, Malik N, Orth A, de Jesus P, Perry AS, Oliver JD, et al: Telomere-independent Rap1 is an IKK adaptor and regulates NF-kappaB-dependent gene expression. Nature Cell Biology 2010, 12:758–767.

[111] Poon MW, Yan L, Jiang D, Qin P, Tse HF, Wong IY, Wong DS, Tergaonkar V, Lian Q: Inhibition of RAP1 enhances corneal recovery following alkali injury. Investigative Ophthalmology & Visual Science 2015, 56:711–721.

[112] Akiyama M, Hideshima T, Hayashi T, Tai YT, Mitsiades CS, Mitsiades N, Chauhan D, Richardson P, Munshi NC, Anderson KC: Nuclear factor-kappaB p65 mediates tumor necrosis factor alpha-induced nuclear translocation of telomerase reverse transcriptase protein. Cancer Research 2003, 63:18–21.

[113] Ghosh A, Saginc G, Leow SC, Khattar E, Shin EM, Yan TD, Wong M, Zhang Z, Li G, Sung WK, et al: Telomerase directly regulates NF-kappaB-dependent transcription. Nature Cell Biology 2012, 14:1270–1281.

[114] Ding D, Xi P, Zhou J, Wang M, Cong YS: Human telomerase reverse transcriptase regulates MMP expression independently of telomerase activity via NF-kappaB-dependent transcription. FASEB Journal: official publication of the Federation of American Societies for Experimental Biology 2013, 27:4375–4383.

[115] Clevers H, Nusse R: Wnt/beta-catenin signaling and disease. Cell 2012, 149:1192–1205.

[116] Choi J, Southworth LK, Sarin KY, Venteicher AS, Ma W, Chang W, Cheung P, Jun S, Artandi MK, Shah N, et al: TERT promotes epithelial proliferation through transcriptional control of a Myc- and Wnt-related developmental program. PLoS Genetics 2008, 4:e10.

[117] Park JI, Venteicher AS, Hong JY, Choi J, Jun S, Shkreli M, Chang W, Meng Z, Cheung P, Ji H, et al: Telomerase modulates Wnt signalling by association with target gene chromatin. Nature 2009, 460:66–72.

[118] Okamoto N, Yasukawa M, Nguyen C, Kasim V, Maida Y, Possemato R, Shibata T, Ligon KL, Fukami K, Hahn WC, Masutomi K: Maintenance of tumor initiating cells of defined genetic composition by nucleostemin. Proceedings of the National Academy of Sciences of the United States of America 2011, 108:20388–20393.

[119] Koh CM, Khattar E, Leow SC, Liu CY, Muller J, Ang WX, Li Y, Franzoso G, Li S, Guccione E, Tergaonkar V: Telomerase regulates MYC-driven oncogenesis independent of its reverse transcriptase activity. The Journal of Clinical Investigation 2015, 125:2109–2122.

[120] Wu KJ, Grandori C, Amacker M, Simon-Vermot N, Polack A, Lingner J, Dalla-Favera R: Direct activation of TERT transcription by c-MYC. Nature Genetics 1999, 21:220–224.

[121] Mondello C, Bottone MG, Noriki S, Soldani C, Pellicciari C, Scovassi AI: Oxidative stress response in telomerase-immortalized fibroblasts from a centenarian. Annals of the New York Academy of Sciences 2006, 1091:94–101.

[122] Lee J, Sung YH, Cheong C, Choi YS, Jeon HK, Sun W, Hahn WC, Ishikawa F, Lee HW: TERT promotes cellular and organismal survival independently of telomerase activity. Oncogene 2008, 27:3754–3760.

[123] Santos JH, Meyer JN, Skorvaga M, Annab LA, Van Houten B: Mitochondrial hTERT exacerbates free-radical-mediated mtDNA damage. Aging Cell 2004, 3:399–411.

[124] Haendeler J, Drose S, Buchner N, Jakob S, Altschmied J, Goy C, Spyridopoulos I, Zeiher AM, Brandt U, Dimmeler S: Mitochondrial telomerase reverse transcriptase binds to and protects mitochondrial DNA and function from damage. Arteriosclerosis, Thrombosis, and Vascular Biology 2009, 29:929–935.

[125] Massard C, Zermati Y, Pauleau AL, Larochette N, Metivier D, Sabatier L, Kroemer G, Soria JC: hTERT: a novel endogenous inhibitor of the mitochondrial cell death pathway. Oncogene 2006, 25:4505–4514.

[126] Sharma NK, Reyes A, Green P, Caron MJ, Bonini MG, Gordon DM, Holt IJ, Santos JH: Human telomerase acts as a hTR-independent reverse transcriptase in mitochondria. Nucleic Acids Research 2012, 40:712–725.

[127] Chen LY, Zhang Y, Zhang Q, Li H, Luo Z, Fang H, Kim SH, Qin L, Yotnda P, Xu J, et al: Mitochondrial localization of telomeric protein TIN2 links telomere regulation to metabolic control. Molecular Cell 2012, 47:839–850.

[128] El Mai M, Wagner KD, Michiels JF, Ambrosetti D, Borderie A, Destree S, Renault V, Djerbi N, Giraud-Panis MJ, Gilson E, et al: The telomeric protein TRF2 regulates angiogenesis by binding and activating the PDGFRbeta promoter. Cell Reports 2014, 9:1047–1060.

[129] Gonzalez OG, Assfalg R, Koch S, Schelling A, Meena JK, Kraus J, Lechel A, Katz SF, Benes V, Scharffetter-Kochanek K, et al: Telomerase stimulates ribosomal DNA transcription under hyperproliferative conditions. Nature Communications 2014, 5:4599.

[130] Holohan B, Wright WE, Shay JW: Cell biology of disease: Telomeropathies: an emerging spectrum disorder. The Journal of Cell Biology 2014, 205:289–299.

[131] Tummala H, Walne A, Collopy L, Cardoso S, de la Fuente J, Lawson S, Powell J, Cooper N, Foster A, Mohammed S, et al: Poly(A)-specific ribonuclease deficiency impacts telomere biology and causes dyskeratosis congenita. The Journal of Clinical Investigation 2015, 125:2151–2160.

[132] Calado RT, Regal JA, Kleiner DE, Schrump DS, Peterson NR, Pons V, Chanock SJ, Lansdorp PM, Young NS: A spectrum of severe familial liver disorders associate with telomerase mutations. PloS One 2009, 4:e7926.

[133] Le Guen T, Jullien L, Touzot F, Schertzer M, Gaillard L, Perderiset M, Carpentier W, Nitschke P, Picard C, Couillault G, et al: Human RTEL1 deficiency causes Hoyeraal-Hreidarsson syndrome with short telomeres and genome instability. Human Molecular Genetics 2013, 22:3239–3249.

[134] Kocak H, Ballew BJ, Bisht K, Eggebeen R, Hicks BD, Suman S, O'Neil A, Giri N, Maillard I, Alter BP, et al: Hoyeraal-Hreidarsson syndrome caused by a germline mutation in the TEL patch of the telomere protein TPP1. Genes & Development 2014, 28:2090–2102.

[135] Sasa GS, Ribes-Zamora A, Nelson ND, Bertuch AA: Three novel truncating TINF2 mutations causing severe dyskeratosis congenita in early childhood. Clinical Genetics 2012, 81:470–478.

[136] Gu P, Chang S: Functional characterization of human CTC1 mutations reveals novel mechanisms responsible for the pathogenesis of the telomere disease Coats plus. Aging Cell 2013, 12:1100–1109.

[137] Alter BP, Giri N, Savage SA, Peters JA, Loud JT, Leathwood L, Carr AG, Greene MH, Rosenberg PS: Malignancies and survival patterns in the National Cancer Institute inherited bone marrow failure syndromes cohort study. British Journal of Haematology 2010, 150:179–188.

[138] Vulliamy T, Marrone A, Goldman F, Dearlove A, Bessler M, Mason PJ, Dokal I: The RNA component of telomerase is mutated in autosomal dominant dyskeratosis congenita. Nature 2001, 413:432–435.

[139] Traila D, Mladinescu OF, Oancea C, Tudorache V: Short telomeres in pulmonary fibrosis: from genetics to clinical significance. Pneumologia 2015, 64:8, 11–13.

[140] Alder JK, Chen JJ, Lancaster L, Danoff S, Su SC, Cogan JD, Vulto I, Xie M, Qi X, Tuder RM, et al: Short telomeres are a risk factor for idiopathic pulmonary fibrosis. Proceedings of the National Academy of Sciences of the United States of America 2008, 105:13051–13056.

[141] Gribbin J, Hubbard R, Smith C: Role of diabetes mellitus and gastro-oesophageal reflux in the aetiology of idiopathic pulmonary fibrosis. Respiratory Medicine 2009, 103:927–931.

[142] Guo N, Parry EM, Li LS, Kembou F, Lauder N, Hussain MA, Berggren PO, Armanios M: Short telomeres compromise beta-cell signaling and survival. PloS One 2011, 6:e17858.

[143] Yamaguchi H, Calado RT, Ly H, Kajigaya S, Baerlocher GM, Chanock SJ, Lansdorp PM, Young NS: Mutations in TERT, the gene for telomerase reverse transcriptase, in aplastic anemia. The New England Journal of Medicine 2005, 352:1413–1424.

[144] Calado RT, Regal JA, Hills M, Yewdell WT, Dalmazzo LF, Zago MA, Lansdorp PM, Hogge D, Chanock SJ, Estey EH, et al: Constitutional hypomorphic telomerase muta-

tions in patients with acute myeloid leukemia. Proceedings of the National Academy of Sciences of the United States of America 2009, 106:1187–1192.

[145] Robles-Espinoza CD, Velasco-Herrera Mdel C, Hayward NK, Adams DJ: Telomere-regulating genes and the telomere interactome in familial cancers. Molecular Cancer Research : MCR 2015, 13:211–222.

[146] Ramsay AJ, Quesada V, Foronda M, Conde L, Martinez-Trillos A, Villamor N, Rodriguez D, Kwarciak A, Garabaya C, Gallardo M, et al: POT1 mutations cause telomere dysfunction in chronic lymphocytic leukemia. Nature Genetics 2013, 45:526–530.

[147] Aoude LG, Pritchard AL, Robles-Espinoza CD, Wadt K, Harland M, Choi J, Gartside M, Quesada V, Johansson P, Palmer JM, et al: Nonsense mutations in the shelterin complex genes ACD and TERF2IP in familial melanoma. Journal of the National Cancer Institute 2015, 107.

[148] Artandi SE, DePinho RA: Telomeres and telomerase in cancer. Carcinogenesis 2010, 31:9–18.

[149] Donate LE, Blasco MA: Telomeres in cancer and ageing. Philosophical transactions of the Royal Society of London Series B, Biological Sciences 2011, 366:76–84.

[150] Huang FW, Hodis E, Xu MJ, Kryukov GV, Chin L, Garraway LA: Highly recurrent TERT promoter mutations in human melanoma. Science 2013, 339:957–959.

[151] Horn S, Figl A, Rachakonda PS, Fischer C, Sucker A, Gast A, Kadel S, Moll I, Nagore E, Hemminki K, et al: *TERT* promoter mutations in familial and sporadic melanoma. Science 2013, 339:959–961.

[152] Killela PJ, Reitman ZJ, Jiao Y, Bettegowda C, Agrawal N, Diaz LA, Jr., Friedman AH, Friedman H, Gallia GL, Giovanella BC, et al: *TERT* promoter mutations occur frequently in gliomas and a subset of tumors derived from cells with low rates of self-renewal. Proceedings of the National Academy of Sciences of the United States of America 2013, 110:6021–6026.

[153] Liu X, Wu G, Shan Y, Hartmann C, von Deimling A, Xing M: Highly prevalent *TERT* promoter mutations in bladder cancer and glioblastoma. Cell Cycle 2013, 12:1637–1638.

[154] Bell RJ, Rube HT, Kreig A, Mancini A, Fouse SD, Nagarajan RP, Choi S, Hong C, He D, Pekmezci M, et al: Cancer. The transcription factor GABP selectively binds and activates the mutant *TERT* promoter in cancer. Science 2015, 348:1036–1039.

[155] Buckingham EM, Klingelhutz AJ: The role of telomeres in the ageing of human skin. Experimental Dermatology 2011, 20:297–302.

[156] Ramirez RD, D'Atri S, Pagani E, Faraggiana T, Lacal PM, Taylor RS, Shay JW: Progressive increase in telomerase activity from benign melanocytic conditions to malignant melanoma. Neoplasia 1999, 1:42–49.

[157] Rudolph P, Schubert C, Tamm S, Heidorn K, Hauschild A, Michalska I, Majewski S, Krupp G, Jablonska S, Parwaresch R: Telomerase activity in melanocytic lesions: a potential marker of tumor biology. The American Journal of Pathology 2000, 156:1425–1432.

[158] Populo H, Boaventura P, Vinagre J, Batista R, Mendes A, Caldas R, Pardal J, Azevedo F, Honavar M, Guimaraes I, et al: *TERT* promoter mutations in skin cancer: the effects of sun exposure and X-irradiation. The Journal of Investigative Dermatology 2014, 134:2251–2257.

[159] Vinagre J, Almeida A, Populo H, Batista R, Lyra J, Pinto V, Coelho R, Celestino R, Prazeres H, Lima L, et al: Frequency of *TERT* promoter mutations in human cancers. Nature Communications 2013, 4:2185.

[160] Griewank KG, Murali R, Schilling B, Schimming T, Moller I, Moll I, Schwamborn M, Sucker A, Zimmer L, Schadendorf D, et al: *TERT* promoter mutations are frequent in cutaneous basal cell carcinoma and squamous cell carcinoma. PloS One 2013, 8:e80354.

[161] Scott GA, Laughlin TS, Rothberg PG: Mutations of the *TERT* promoter are common in basal cell carcinoma and squamous cell carcinoma. Modern Pathology: An Official Journal of the United States and Canadian Academy of Pathology, Inc 2014, 27:516–523.

[162] Anic GM, Sondak VK, Messina JL, Fenske NA, Zager JS, Cherpelis BS, Lee JH, Fulp WJ, Epling-Burnette PK, Park JY, Rollison DE: Telomere length and risk of melanoma, squamous cell carcinoma, and basal cell carcinoma. Cancer Epidemiology 2013, 37:434–439.

[163] Liang G, Qureshi AA, Guo Q, De Vivo I, Han J: No association between telomere length in peripheral blood leukocytes and the risk of nonmelanoma skin cancer. Cancer Epidemiology, Biomarkers & Prevention: a publication of the American Association for Cancer Research, cosponsored by the American Society of Preventive Oncology 2011, 20:1043–1045.

[164] Koelsche C, Sahm F, Capper D, Reuss D, Sturm D, Jones DT, Kool M, Northcott PA, Wiestler B, Bohmer K, et al: Distribution of *TERT* promoter mutations in pediatric and adult tumors of the nervous system. Acta Neuropathologica 2013, 126:907–915.

[165] Hiraga S, Ohnishi T, Izumoto S, Miyahara E, Kanemura Y, Matsumura H, Arita N: Telomerase activity and alterations in telomere length in human brain tumors. Cancer Research 1998, 58:2117–2125.

[166] Langford LA, Piatyszek MA, Xu R, Schold SC, Jr., Shay JW: Telomerase activity in human brain tumours. Lancet 1995, 346:1267–1268.

[167] Sano T, Asai A, Mishima K, Fujimaki T, Kirino T: Telomerase activity in 144 brain tumours. British Journal of Cancer 1998, 77:1633–1637.

[168] Shete S, Hosking FJ, Robertson LB, Dobbins SE, Sanson M, Malmer B, Simon M, Marie Y, Boisselier B, Delattre JY, et al: Genome-wide association study identifies five susceptibility loci for glioma. Nature Genetics 2009, 41:899–904.

[169] Zhao Y, Chen G, Song X, Chen H, Mao Y, Lu D: Fine-mapping of a region of chromosome 5p15.33 (TERT-CLPTM1L) suggests a novel locus in TERT and a CLPTM1L haplotype are associated with glioma susceptibility in a Chinese population. International Journal of Cancer: Journal international du cancer 2012, 131:1569–1576.

[170] Okumura A, Mizuno I, Nagakawa O, Fuse H: Telomerase activity is correlated with lower grade and lower stage bladder carcinomas. International journal of urology : official journal of the Japanese Urological Association 2004, 11:1082-1086.

[171] Lin Y, Miyamoto H, Fujinami K, Uemura H, Hosaka M, Iwasaki Y, Kubota Y: Telomerase activity in human bladder cancer. Clinical Cancer Research: An Official Journal of the American Association for Cancer Research 1996, 2:929–932.

[172] Morii A, Komiya A, Okumura A, Fuse H: Telomerase activity in bladder cancer tissue. Experimental and Therapeutic Medicine 2010, 1:85–88.

[173] Yang CH, Hung WC, Wang SL, Kang WY, Chen WT, Huang YC, Su YC, Chai CY: Immunoexpression and prognostic role of hTERT and cyclin D1 in urothelial carcinoma. APMIS: acta pathologica, microbiologica, et immunologica Scandinavica 2008, 116:309–316.

[174] Heidenreich B, Rachakonda PS, Hemminki K, Kumar R: *TERT* promoter mutations in cancer development. Current Opinion in Genetics & Development 2014, 24:30–37.

Chapter 5

# Molecular Diagnosis and Precision Therapeutic Approaches for Telomere Biology Disorders

Rosario Perona, Laura Iarriccio, Laura Pintado-Berninches, Javier Rodriguez-Centeno, Cristina Manguan-Garcia, Elena Garcia, Blanca Lopez-Ayllón and Leandro Sastre

Additional information is available at the end of the chapter

http://dx.doi.org/10.5772/65353

**Abstract**

Telomeres are nucleo-protein structures located at the end of chromosomes that protect them from degradation. Telomeres length is maintained by the activity of the telomerase complex. These structures are protected by a specialized protein complex named shelterin. In the absence of telomerase activity and/or protection telomeres are shortened after each round of DNA replication. When a critical size is reached, telomeres are recognized as damaged DNA by the cell p53-dependent DNA-repair system. Persistent activation of this pathway finally results in cell apoptosis or senescence.

There are a number of rare hereditary diseases caused by the presence of shortened telomeres, collectively named telomeropathies or telomere biology disorders. In these diseases, cell proliferation is impaired, which results in premature aging and dysfunction of highly proliferative tissues (bone morrow, skin and other epithelia). Among them are Dyskeratosis congenita, the Hoyeraal-Hreidarsson, Revesz and Coats plus syndromes, Aplastic anemia, Idiopathic pulmonary fibrosis and nonalcoholic, noninfectious liver disease. Mutations present in the genes coding for component of the telomerase and shelterin complexes and other proteins involved in telomere replication are the cause of these diseases. Clinical manifestations, causative mutations, diagnosis and possible therapeutic approaches to these diseases will be discussed in this chapter.

**Keywords:** telomere, telomere biology disorders, telomeropathies, pulmonary fibrosis, bone marrow failure

# 1. Introduction

Eukaryotic chromosomes are capped at their ends by specialized nucleo-protein structures, named telomeres that protect them from degradation. Human telomeres have a specific nucleotide sequence composed by thousand of repetitions of the TTAGGG hexanucleotide [1]. A protein complex, named shelterin associates to this DNA region to form the telomere-specific chromatin structure. Telomeres protects the chromosomal ends from degradation and are, therefore, essential for chromosomal and genome stability [2]. In their absence chromosomal ends are recognized as damaged DNA by the cell and can be degraded or recombined with other chromosomal ends resulting in the fusion and reorganization of chromosomes [3]. The maintenance of telomeres is, therefore, of critical importance for the genetic stability of cells and organisms.

Replication of telomeric DNA requires the contribution of a specific enzymatic machinery. DNA polymerases responsible for replication of the rest of the chromosomal DNA cannot completely synthesize telomeric DNA. DNA polymerases always require a primer molecule that cover the 5′ end of the DNA and are not able to complete the synthesis of the lagging strand of lineal DNA molecules, such as chromosomes. This end-replication problem results in the shortening of each telomere by 50-100 nucleotides at each DNA replication cycle and, therefore, at each cell division [4]. In most eukaryotic organisms, including humans, telomere length is maintained by the activity of the telomerase complex that elongates the telomeres by a replication-independent mechanism [5]. The complex is formed by a protein with reverse-transcriptase activity (TERT) and one RNA with a region of homology to the telomere DNA that is used as template for elongation [6]. Telomerase activity is, therefore, required for unlimited cell proliferation. Telomerase components and, in particular the TERT gene, are expressed to high relative levels during embryonic development allowing high cell proliferation rates. Expression of the TERT gene is, however, repressed in most human adult cells [7]. TERT expression is found only in germinal cells, in stem cells, specially in those of highly proliferative tissues such as bone marrow and epithelia and in lymphocytes [8]. The rest of the cells express very low TERT levels and their telomeres get progressively shorter after each cell division. When telomeres reach a critical size get unprotected and are recognized as damaged DNA. The ATM and ATR kinases, that regulate cellular responses to DNA damage are recruited to critically-short telomeres and activate the p53-dependent pathway that results in cell cycle arrest [3]. Prolonged arrest would finally induce apoptotic cell death or cellular senescence. Actually, most tissue-specific stem cells do not express enough TERT protein to completely replicate their telomeres at each cell division and their proliferative capacity decreases with the age of the organism [9]. With time, stem cell exhaustion impairs tissue renewal. Because of this reason, telomere shortening has been recognized as one of the hallmarks of human aging [10].

Telomere replication is also involved in the acquisition of the unlimited proliferative capacity that characterizes tumor cells [7]. Telomerase expression and activity is induced in about 85% of tumors, which allows tumor cells to completely elongate their telomeres at each cell division. In the other about 15% of tumors, telomeres length is maintained by a telomerase-independent mechanism, know as Alternative Lengthening of the Telomeres (ALT) that elongates telomeres through DNA recombination mechanisms [11].

The importance of telomere homeostasis is further enforced by the existence of a number of rare hereditary diseases that are caused by the presence of shortened telomeres, collectively named telomeropathies, short telomere syndromes or telomere biology disorders [12]. These diseases are caused by mutations in genes coding for proteins involved in telomere lengthening (telomerase complex and related proteins) or in the maintenance of telomere structure (shelterin complex). These diseases are commonly characterized by the presence of very short telomeres in the cells of the affected patients. The molecular pathology of these diseases, their diagnosis and emerging therapies will be summarized in this chapter. It is necessary to enforce the importance of telomere homeostaxis for healthy life since excessively long telomeres are also causative of disease. Recent reports have associated the presence of long telomeres to increased frequency of cancers such as melanoma or glioma [13]. Mutations in the promoter region of the TERT gene that increase gene expression are frequently found in these and other tumors [14, 15]. In addition, mutations in the coding region of genes coding for protein of the shelterin complex have been found in human tumors [16, 17].

## 2. Main body

### 2.1. Telomere structure

Telomeres have a very specialized chromatin structure that is required to protect chromosome ends from degradation and to avoid telomere-telomere fusions [2]. The general structure will be briefly summarized in this section of the chapter and is schematically shown in the upper panel of Figure 1 where the genes mutated in telomere biology disorders are indicated by asterisks. Telomere structure has been the subject of several recent excellent reviews [2, 12, 18, 19]. The nucleotide sequence of telomeres is composed for multiple repetitions of the TTAGGG hexanucleotide in humans and several other animals. The length of these regions is variable in different organisms. In humans, telomeres have and average size of 8-14 kb in peripheral blood cells in new born children [20]. The size decreases with age so that the average size in a 90-years old person is of 3-7 kb [12]. In contrast, most mice strains used in research have an average telomere length of 50-100 kb which has made more difficult the development of mouse models of telomere biology disorders [21, 22].

Telomere ends are not formed by blunt-ended double-stranded DNA, as might be expected. Instead, the 3′ strand is about 75-300 bases longer than the 5′ end strand forming an overhanging single-stranded DNA fragment (Fig 1, upper panel) [1]. The overhanging strand contains the TTAGGG sequence and is, therefore, known as the G-rich strand. The complementary strand contains the complementary CCCTAA repeats and is named the C-rich strand. The overhanging strand is not unstructured. Instead, it turns over the telomere DNA and intercalates in the neighbouring double-stranded DNA forming a loop, named the T-loop, as schematically shown in the upper panel of Figure 1 [23]. Looping results in the formation of a triple stranded DNA region known as D-loop that is required for the stability of the terminal telomeric DNA region [24].

Telomeres are further stabilized by the presence of a specific protein complex, the shelterin complex. It is composed by six different proteins: TRF1, TRF2, RAP1, TIN2, TPP1 and POT1 (upper panel of Figure 1] [2]. TRF1 (telomeric repeat binding factor 1, encoded by the TERF1 gene) binds to telomeric double-stranded DNA as a dimmer [25]. TRF2 (telomeric repeat binding factor 2, encoded by the TERF2 gene) also binds double-stranded DNA as a dimmer and associates with TRF1 [26]. The TIN2 protein (TRF1-interacting protein 2] interacts with TRF1 and TRF2 [27] and recruits the POT1(Protection of telomeres protein 1]/TPP1(POT1-interacting protein 1] heterodimer [28]. POT1 binds with high affinity to the G-rich strand overhang [29]. RAP1 (repressor-activator protein 1] incorporates to the shelterin complex via TRF2 interaction [28]. In addition, telomeres and subtelomeric regions are enriched in heterochromatin components including the association of HP1 proteins and histone 3 Lysine 9 and histone 4 lysine 20 trimethylation which further contributes to their stability [30].

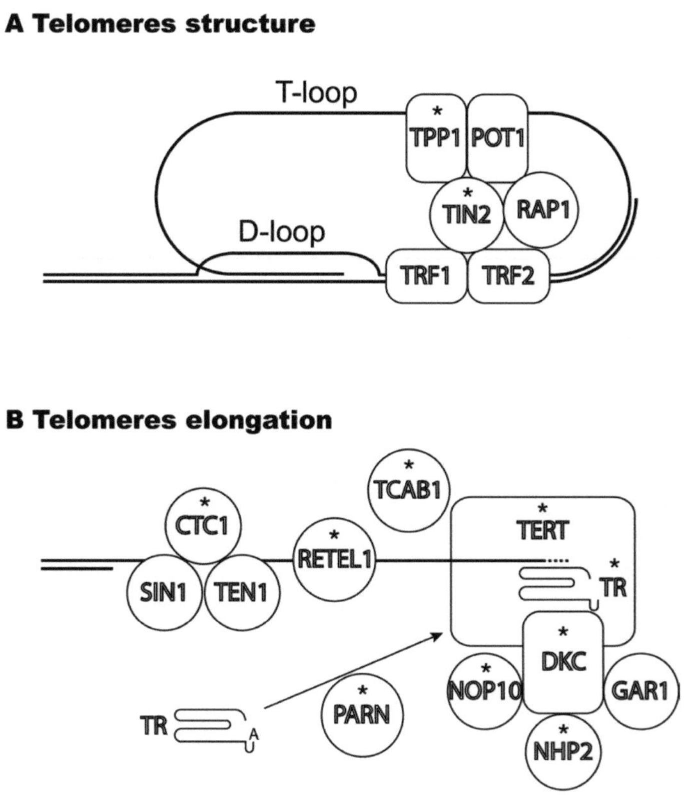


**Figure 1.** Telomere structure and elongation mechanism.

The shelterin complex is required for telomere maintenance and function and prevents the recognition of telomeres as damaged DNA. TRF2 inhibits the ATM kinase that induces the canonical non-homologous-end-joining DNA repair pathway that would result in telomere-telomere fusions [31]. In addition, POT1 inhibits signalling by the ATR kinase in response to DNA damage by double-strand and single-strand breaks and alkylating agents [32]. POT1 also inhibits sister-telomere associations [33].

Telomere structure is schematically shown in upper panel A of the figure. Telomeric DNA is formed by repetitions of the TTAGGG hexanucleotide and is represented as two lines in the figure. The upper line represents the leading, G-rich strand. The 3′ end of this strand is single-stranded and forms a loop (T-loop) to hybridize to a region of the upstream double-stranded DNA forming a smaller loop (D-loop). The lower line represents the lagging DNA strand. Proteins of the shelterin complex, which binds to telomeric DNA, are represented as boxes. Asterisks indicate the proteins whose encoding gene have been found mutated in patients with telomere biology disorders. Panel B represent the components involved in telomere elongation. DNA is represented as two lines and proteins as boxes, as indicated on panel A. The DNA leading strand is the upper one and the DNA being synthesized is represented as a broken line. The components of the telomerase complex that catalyzes telomere elongation are represented on the right of the panel. Telomerase complex is composed by the TERT, DKC, NOP10, NHP2 and GAR1 proteins and the RNA molecule TR. The protein TCAB1 is required for telomerase recruitment to telomeres. PARN is required for TR RNA processing. The RETEL1 helicase and the CTC1/SIN1/TEN1 complex facilitate telomere elongation by disrupting DNA secondary structures. Asterisks indicate the proteins whose encoding genes have been found mutated in patients with telomere biology disorders.

### 2.2. Telomere elongation

In this section a brief summary of the telomere elongation process and its regulation will be presented because many of the proteins involved are related to telomere biology disorders. A schematic representation of the process is shown at the lower panel of Figure 1. Genes mutated in telomere biology disorders, as described in next sections, are indicated by asterisks. Telomere replication has been reviewed recently by several authors [18, 19, 34-36]. Cellular DNA polymerases cannot complete the replication of DNA double-strand ends which is know as the end-replication problem [37], as mentioned in the Introduction section. In mammals, telomere DNA 3′ ends are elongated by the telomerase complex through reverse transcription. The catalytic activity of the complex resides in the TERT (telomerase reverse transcriptase) protein [6] while the 454 nucleotides long TR (telomerase RNA, encoded by the TERC gene) is used as template [38] (Figure 1, lower panel) [36]. This is because TR has an internal region complementary to the TTAGGG repeats that allows hybridization to the 3′ end of the telomere DNA [36]. The TR RNA has similarity to other small nucleolar RNAs and contains a H/ACA motif [39]. It is transcribed by RNA polymerase II and contains a Cap structure and its 5′end and a 3′ oligo-Adenosine tail [40]. It has been recently shown that the 3′ end of TR has to be processed through exonuclease cleavage and that the Poly(A)-specific ribonuclease (PARN) is required for this maturation process [41].

Additional proteins form part of the telomerase complex and are required for its assembly and stability. Among them, dyskerin (encoded by the DKC1 gene) binds to TR through its interaction with the dyskerin PUA RNA binding domain [42]. Dyskerin binding is required for TR stability and for its recruitment to the telomerase complex. The proteins NHP2 and NOP10 associate to dyskerin and are also required for telomerase assembly [43].

Telomerase activity is dependent on TERT gene expression that is tissue-dependent and developmentally regulated, as mentioned in the Introduction section. In addition, it is dependent on protein-protein interactions that regulate telomerase-complex assembly and its recruitment to telomeres. One of the proteins involved is TCAB1 (encoded by the WRAP53 gene) that is an essential component of the subnuclear Cajal body structures. TACB1associates to TR, contributing to telomerase assembly in these structures [44]. Depletion of TCAB1 results in a relocation of the telomerase complex to the nucleolus and reduced recruitment to telomeres [44]. The shelterin-complex component TPP1 is also required for the recruitment of telomerase to telomeres. The TEL patch of TPP1, rich in Glutamate and Leucine residues, interacts with the TEN domain of TERT to mediate telomerase recruitment [45]. This interaction also promotes the telomerase ability to catalyze repeated cycles of DNA synthesis at the telomeres [46].

After elongation of the G-rich overhanging strand by the telomerase complex the C-rich strand is synthesized by the activity of the primase/DNA polymerase complex [35]. Proteins with helicase activity are required to facilitate telomere elongation through disruption of DNA structures that impair telomerase and DNA polymerase activity. The G-rich nature of the overhanging strand favours the formation of secondary structures such as G-quartets [47]. In addition, the D-loop structure of telomeres can also impair DNA synthesis. One of the proteins involved in solving DNA structures at the telomeres is RETEL1 (regulator of telomere length 1], a DNA helicase with D-loop-disrupting activity that has been proposed to facilitate T loop unwinding and to counteract the formation of G-quartets [48, 49]. In addition, RETEL1 has additional functions at other DNA loci [50]. The CST complex, formed by the CTC1, STN1 and TEN1 proteins promotes the initiation of the lagging C-rich strand synthesis [51]. CTC1 binds to the single-stranded G-rich DNA strand and recruits the initiator Pol$\alpha$ primase complex to accomplish C-rich strand synthesis [52].

Once DNA synthesis is completed at telomeres, DNA is further processed to generate the G-strand overhangs [35]. This is a highly regulated process so that G-strands overhangs are between 30 and 400 nucleotides long and the C-rich strand ends at the 3′-CCAATC-5′ sequence in most telomeres [53]. Processing requires the activity of several factors: the Apollo/SNMB1 nuclease, Exonuclease I, the CST complex and two shelterin proteins, POT1 and TRF2 [54].

It is important to enforce that although telomere structure and replication have been presented separately for simplicity they are highly interconnected processes. For example, proteins of the shelterin complex play essential roles in telomere elongation through recruitment of the telomerase complex and proteins involved in the regulation of telomere length.

### 2.3. Telomere biology disorders

Several diseases related to telomere biology will be described in this section. The clinical manifestations of each disease will be described together with their molecular bases. These

http://dx.doi.org/10.5772/65353

diseases are multisystem genetic disorders that share many of the affected genes (see [12, 13, 18, 19, 55-58] for recent reviews). They also have in common the presence of very short telomeres in the affected patients. However, time of onset, phenotype and clinical severity of these diseases are very heterogeneous. Some of the disorders manifest in young children as it is the case of Dyskeratosis congenita, Hoyeraal-Hreidarsson syndrome, Revesz syndrome and Coats plus syndrome that are rare diseases presented with very low frequency in the population. Other diseases that manifest at older ages, generally in adults, are less severe and more frequent in the population. Among these are Aplastic anemia, Lung disease and Non-alcoholic, non-infectious liver disease. A summary of these diseases, their clinical manifestations, time of presentation and the genes that have been found mutated is shown in Table 1.

| Disease | Symptoms | Presentation time | Mutated genes (inheritance)* |
|---|---|---|---|
| Dyskeratosis congenita | Nail dysplasia | Childhood | DKC1 (XL) |
| | Abnormal skin pigmentation | | TERT (AD,AR) |
| | Oral leukoplakia | | TERC (AD) |
| | Bone marrow failure | | TINF2 (AD) |
| | Pulmonary fibrosis | | WRAP53 (AR) |
| | Liver abnormalities | | NOP10 (AR) |
| | Avascular necrosis of the hips | | NHP2 (AR) |
| | Stenosis of the exophagus, lacrimal ducts and/or uretra | | CTC1 (AR) |
| | Increased cancer risk | | RTEL1 (AD,AR) |
| | Osteopenia, risk of bone fractures | | PARN (AR) |
| | Psychiatric disorders | | |
| Hoyeraal-Hreidarsson syndrome | Intrauterine growth retardation | Early childhood | DKC1 (XL) |
| | Microcephaly | | TINF2 (AD) |
| | Cerebellar hypoplasia | | TERT (AR) |
| | Thrombocytopenia | | RTEL1 (AR) |
| | Immunodeficiency | | TPP1 (AR) |
| | Nonspecific enteropathies | | PARN (AR) |
| | Bone marrow failure | | |
| Revesz syndrome | Bilateral exudative retinopathy | Early childhood | TINF2 (AD) |
| | Bone marrow failure | | |
| | Intrauterine growth retardation | | |
| | Intracraneal calcifications | | |

| Disease | Symptoms | Presentation time | Mutated genes (inheritance)* |
|---|---|---|---|
| | Developmental delay | | |
| | Fine, sparse hair | | |
| | Nail dystrophy | | |
| Coats plus syndrome | Bilateral exudative retinopathy | Early childhood | CTC1 (AR) |
| | Retinal telangiectasias | | |
| | Intrauterine growth retardation | | |
| | Bone abnormalities with poor healing | | |
| | Gastrointestinal vascular ectasias | | |
| Aplastic anemia | Bone marrow failure | Middle age | TERC (AD)<br>TERT (AD) |
| Idiopathic pulmonary fibrosis | Pulmonary fibrosis | Middle age | TERC (AD) |
| | Emphysema | | TERT (AD) |
| | Interstitial pneumonitis | | PARN (AD) |
| | Honeycombing in high resolution computarized tomography | | RTEL1 (AD) |
| Nonalcoholic, noninfectious liver disease | Hepatic fibrosis | Middle age | TERC (AD) |
| | Noncirrhotic portal hypertension | | TERT (AD) |
| | Hepatopulmonary syndrome | | |

*XL: X-linked; AD: autosomal dominant; AR: Autosomal recesive

**Table 1.** Clinical characteristics of telomere biology disorders.

### *2.3.1. Dyskeratosis congenita*

Dyskeratosis congenita (DC) was the first telomere biology disease described in early 1900s [59]. It is an inherited disorder that is usually diagnosed in early childhood. The most characteristic clinical feature is a triad of mucocutaneous features: leukoplakia, reticulated skin pigmentation and nail dystrophy, as shown in Table 1. Lacy reticular pigmentation use to be observed at neck and upper chest. However, DC symptoms have variable expressivity and/or incomplete penetrance and this triad is not always present. Some patients worsen with age and the triad might not be evident in the firsts examinations. The median age of appearance of the triad is approximately 8 years [59]. The variability in the nail phenotype can go from ridging to complete nail loss and can involve both the finger and toenails. The skin may be hyper or hypo pigmented. Leukoplakia may affect other mucosa surfaces. However, additional reports expanded the phenotype and it is now recognized as a multisystem disease. One of the most common haematological manifestations is bone marrow failure that is the most significant cause of mortality in DC patients, up to 60-70% [60]. Patients present hypocellular bone marrow and severe cytopenias.

DC patients frequently show other skin manifestations, some of them are atrophy of the dorsal surface of hands and feet,hyperhydrosis and hyperkeratosis of palms and soles. Other mucosal surfaces can also be affected leading to stenosis of the oesophagus, urethra or lacrimal duct. Oesophageal strictures and non-specific enteropathies are common. Dental abnormalities can be also observed including extensive caries in 13-17% of the patients [61]. Early greying and loss of hair also occur. Skeletal abnormalities are also observed in up to 5% of the patients [62] including osteoporosis and avascular necrosis. Osteoporosis resembles that seen in natural aging and can led to fractures [63].

Respiratory abnormalities are also a significant cause of morbidity and mortality and cause the death of 10-15% of DC patients [64]. The main clinical manifestation is pulmonary fibrosis that usually is posterior to the mucocutaneous or bone marrow features. Hepatic disease can be also observed including cirrhosis, fibrosis, portal hypertension and portal vein thrombosis and several cases of non-alcoholic, non-infectious liver diseases have been reported [65].

Neuropsychiatric disorders were recently described in 55% of children and 75% of adult DC patients [66]. These disorders include mood, anxiety, psychotic and adjustment disorders, attention deficit/hyperactivity, intellectual disability, learning disabilities and pervasive developmental disorders.

DC patients also present increased risk of cancer development. Co-occurrence of Myelodysplastic syndrome (MDS), Acute myelogenous leukemia (AML) and head and neck squamous cell cancer has been described. A literature review reported a 11-fold increased risk of cancer in DC patients including AML, MDS, tongue cancer, cervical squamous cell carcinoma and non-Hodgkin's lymphoma, with a risk of 40% of developing any cancer by the age of 50 [67].

This diversity in clinical manifestations makes the diagnosis of DC challenging. When the mucocutaneous triad is observed the diagnosis is relatively clear but this is not always the case. Vulliamy et al proposed in 2006 clinical criteria for the diagnosis of DC [68]. These criteria require the presence of the three components of the mucocutaneous triad or one feature of the triad, bone marrow failure and two other clinical manifestations usually found in DC patients, as described above. However, the diagnosis of some patients can still be difficult because the triad might evolve late in time and other clinical manifestations might not be associated to DC because of their diversity.

#### *2.3.1.1. Dyskeratosis congenita as a telomere biology disease, implications in diagnosis*

Dyskeratosis congenita may have X-linked inheritance which allowed the identification of one X-chromosome gene that presented missense mutations in several unrelated DC patient. The encoded protein was named dyskerin and the gene DKC1 [60, 69]. Dyskerin was characterized as a highly conserved protein with possible nucleolar functions [60]. Soon afterwards, fibroblasts derived from DC patients were shown to have very short telomeres [70]. These cells also presented reduced telomerase activity and decreased levels of TERC expression. The correlation between Dyskeratosis and telomere length was strengthened when a large family was found carrying an autosomal dominant mutation in the TERC gene [71].

The recognition of DC as a telomere biology disease helped to understand the biology of this disease. As mentioned in the Introduction, critically short telomeres are recognized as damaged DNA by DNA-damage response pathways that involve the ATM and ATR protein kinases and the p53 protein. Activation of these pathways induces apoptotic cell death and cellular senescence. Telomere shortening is associated to DNA replication, which is specially relevant in cells that have impaired systems of telomere elongation and protection, as is the case of DC patients cells. Therefore, highly proliferative cells are expected to be the firstly affected by telomere shortening. Some of these highly proliferative cells are the stem cells of tissues with high capacity of renewal such epithelia, bone marrow cells and lymphocytes. These cells types are characterized by the expression of high telomerase activity in healthy individuals. Depletion of these stem cell populations can explain the main clinical manifestations of DC patients. Among them are the deficit observed in epithelial tissues such as different mucosa and skin that could be due to insufficient cell renewal because of exhaustion of stem cell populations. Impaired proliferation of bone marrow stem cells also could explain the existence of hypocellular bone marrow and severe cytopenia. Pulmonary alveolar stem cell failure has also been recently described in patients with telomere dysfunction [72]. The reduction in the number and proliferative capacity of stem cells can also explain the premature aging of DC patients as manifested by hair loss and early greying. These data would recognize DC as a stem cell disease.

A second clinical characteristic associated to progressive telomere shortening is the existence of genetic anticipation. It is defined by the occurrence of increasing disease severity and early onset with successive generations, as observed in multigenerational families with autosomal dominant DC [73-75]. Genetic anticipation is due, in these diseases, to non-complete telomere replication in germinal cells due to impaired telomerase activity. Successive generations inherit progressively short telomeres and, therefore, critically short telomeres appear at an early age in highly proliferative tissues of the affected patients.

The identification of telemere shortening also provides one important diagnostic criteria. DC patients are characterized by the presence of very short telomeres in peripheral blood cells. Usually bellow the 1% of the telomere size of control populations of the same age as the patient. Measuring telomere length provides one differential diagnostic criteria for telomere biology diseases. The length of telomeres can be determined by different methods in patient samples [76] and compared with controls of the same age. Variation of telomere length with ethnicity has also been described [77]. One of the methods estimates telomere length by Southern blot. Purified DNA is digested with a restriction enzyme that has recognition sites close to the telomeres (sub-telomeric region) but not at the telomere. Digestion products are separated in agarose gels and blotted to membranes that are hybridized to telomere-specific probes. The distribution of telomeres size and average length can be determined by comparison to the migration of DNA molecular weight markers. The use of this technique requires relatively high amounts of pure DNA.

Telomere length can also be determined by quantitative PCR methods from clinical samples. Some of these methods use telomere-specific oligonucleotides to determine the amount of telomeric DNA in comparison to non-telomeric DNA in each sample. This method has the advantage that a large number of samples can be easily analyzed but it gives and average length of all the cellular telomeres. However, variation in the length of individual chromosomes can be also important in disease progression [78]. Telomeres rearrangements can also have a large effect on the cell [79] and would not be detected by measuring average telomeric DNA content. A PCR-based method that determines single telomere length (Single telomere length assay, STELA) has also been developed [80]. Telomere length can also be determined by flow fluorescence in situ hybridization (flow-FISH) using peripheral blood lymphocytes [81]. This technique can be used in clinical settings and has been shown to be highly sensitive and specific in identifying patients with DC from their unaffected relatives and healthy controls [81, 82]. Flow-FISH is presently the only clinically certified test for DC.

*2.3.1.2. Molecular genetics of Dyskeratosis congenita*

DC is a rare inherited disease caused by mutations in genes coding for proteins involved in telomere synthesis and protection. Mutations in ten genes have been identified to date in DC patients [55]. Mutations in these genes explain about 60% of the cases of DC so that there are many cases where the causative gene has not been identified. Until few years ago, molecular diagnosis was made through PCR amplification and DNA sequencing of each exon of the candidate genes, pre-analyzed by High Resolution Melting [83]. Discovery of new genes involved in DC and related telomeropathies required positional cloning and were challenging projects. The development of techniques of massive parallel DNA sequencing makes now possible to sequence either all the genes of a patient (genome sequencing) or all the gene exons (exome sequencing) [84]. Analyses of massive sequencing data greatly facilitates molecular diagnosis as well as the discovery of genes whose causative relationship with the disease was previously unknown. One example is the recent identification of mutations in the PARN gene, coding for a Poly(A)-specific ribonuclease in DC patients [85]. The genetic mutations found in DC patients will be reviewed in this section of the chapter and have been described in recent reviews [18, 86]. A summary is also presented in Table 1. Detailed updated information on the nucleotide variants found in DC-related genes can also be found at the Telomerase Database (http://telomerase.asu.edu/diseases.html).

2.3.1.2.1 Dyskerin (DKC1]

Dyskerin is a 524 amino acids long protein that is highly conserved during evolution. It is an essential nucleolar protein that is expressed in all tissues [42]. Dyskerin participates in two very relevant cellular activities, telomere maintenance and RNA pseudouridylation. The first activity has been described in the Telomere elongation section of this chapter (section 2.2]. For the second activity dyskerin binds to small nucleolar RNAs containing the H/ACA box to form small nucleolar RNP (snoRNP) complexes. The proteins NHP2, NOP10 and GAR1, involved in telomerase assembly are also part of these complexes [42]. Small nucleolar RNAs guide snoRNPs to specific uridine residues that are converted to pseudouridines by dyskerin. Pseudouridylation takes place in many cellular RNAs including ribosomal RNAs but also small nuclear and nucleolar RNAs and mRNAs, as recently described [87]. This modification is important for folding and processing of these RNAs [88]. One subset of snoRNPs (Cajal body RNPs, scaRNPs) is directed to Cajal bodies by the TCAB1 protein [89]. The telomerase RNA, TR, assembles as a typical scaRNP, which is important for TR stability and telomerase recruitment [39, 70] as previously indicated (section 2.1]. Because of this pseudouridylation activity of rRNAs, dyskerin is important for ribosome biogenesis and function, and dyskerin mutations could impair protein synthesis. However, human cells obtained from X-linked DC patients showed intact or only slightly affected ribosome biogenesis and function and very reduced TR levels [90, 91]. These data support the hypothesis that impaired TR stability and telomerase activity are the main cause of DC. However, Bellodi et al. have reported that impaired protein synthesis could contribute to the cancer predisposition of DC patients [92].

Sequence analyses in the Pfam databank identified three functional domains in dyskerin: the dyskerin-like domain (amino acids 48-106] with a yet unknown function; the TruB pseudouridine synthase catalytic domain (aa 110-126], and the PUA RNA binding domain (aa 297-370]. To date, over 50 different DKC1 mutations have been found in association with DC. Many of them were inherited but there were some that were generated de novo in the patients. Not all these mutations show the same severe phenotype and 13 of them cause the Hoyeraal-Hreidarsson syndrome, a more severe manifestation that will be described in the section 2.3.2 of this chapter. Two of the DKC1 mutations are only found in this syndrome. Most DKC1 mutations cluster in two regions of the gene: the region coding amino acids 2-72, at the N-terminus of the protein, and the region coding amino acids 314-420, at the PUA domain [68, 86]. These two domains are contiguous in the three-dimensional structure of the protein and might form a binding site for other proteins [93]. Some disease-causing mutations have been show to alter dyskerin-TR binding because they affect binding of the RNP assembly factor SHQ1 [94]. N-terminal DKC1 mutations overlap a SUMOylation motif and Brault et al have shown that impaired SUMOylation leads to reduced dyskerin, and TR, levels [95]. A mutation in the promoter region of DKC1 that affected dyskerin expression was also identified in a DC patient [96] suggesting that protein levels could have an important role in DC pathogenesis. DKC1 is encoded in the X-chromosome and dyskerin mutations have X-linked transmission with affected males and carrier mothers. In most of the cases carriers do not show any clinical manifestation but carriers of some mutations can manifest late onset diseases such as pulmonary fibrosis that will be described in section 2.3.6.

2.3.1.2.2 Telomerase Reverse Transcriptase (TERT)

The catalytic protein component of the telomerase complex is one 1132 amino acid long protein that contains three major functional domains conserved trough evolution [97]. The telomerase essential N-terminal (TEN) domain is highly conserved among vertebrate proteins and has been implicated in telomere DNA binding upstream of the primer-template interaction [98]. The TEN domain contains a DAT motif involved in telomerase recruitment to the telomeres through interaction with the TEL patch of TPP1 shelterin component. The TERT RNA-binding domain (TRBD) is located next to the TEN domain and precedes the reverse transcriptase domain, which contains the active site for reverse transcription. In addition, the reverse transcriptase motif also participates in TR RNA binding ensuring the maintenance of a stable telomerase complex [99]. Finally, TERT contains a less-conserved C-terminal extension region.

Comparative analysis of the TERT gene in healthy individuals and telomere biology disorder patients has shown a high degree of nucleotide variation. More than 200 distinct missense nucleotide variants are described in the TERT gene at the Exome Aggregation Consortium (ExAC) database (http://exac.broadinstitute.org/). This database compiles all the nucleotides variants found in the different Exome sequencing projects and presently accumulates information from about 60.700 individuals [121.400 alleles for each gene). Data from both healthy individuals and patients from different diseases are incorporated to this database. Over 75 TERT mutations, most of them novel, have been reported in telomere biology disorders diseases [100], including missense, stop gain, frameshift and splice site mutations. However, the existence of a given mutation in a patient does not imply that it is causative of the disease. It might be a mutation that does not affect protein functionality. The existence of a familiar history showing a strong correlation between the presence of the mutation and disease manifestation would support the causative role of this mutation. However, if it is a novel mutation, or the family history is short, experimental assay of the activity of the mutated protein is required to ascertain the possible causal role. For this purpose, mutated TERT proteins are expressed in cells that have very low telomerase activity, if any. The activity of the mutated protein can be consequently tested on this background using the telomere repeat amplification protocol (TRAP) or primer extension assays (see Collopy et al [101] for a recent example).

TERT mutations associated with DC and other telomere biology disorders are found all over the protein although their frequency is higher at the reverse transcriptase domain. Most reported patients with TERT mutations are monoallelic heterozygous. The telomerase activity found in cells from these patients is an average of homozygous wild type and mutant cells and might indicate that haploinsufficiency is the cause of the clinical phenotype [74, 102, 103].

2.3.1.2.3 Telomerase RNA, TR (TERC)

The RNA component of the telomerase complex is 454 nucleotides in length and is encoded by the TERC gene. This RNA provides the template sequence for reverse transcription and is involved in assemblage of the RNP complex [104]. The interaction between TR and TERT regulates the catalytic activity, processivity and telomere-binding activity of the telomerase complex [105]. TR presents domains conserved through evolution that are involved in RNA stabilization, accumulation, subcellular localization and telomerase assembly. They are the template/pseudoknot domain and the CR4/5 motif [106]. These two domains are sufficient to restore telomerase activity when combined with TERT [107, 108]. An additional H/ACA domain at the 3′ end of TR allows binding of the proteins required for telomerase biogenesis dyskerin, NOP10, NHP2 and GAR1 [43].

Mutations in TERC are less frequent than in TERT in DC patients and approximately 60 different mutations have been reported [100]. Nucleotide variants are also less frequent in the general population and only 62 are reported in ExAC exomes database. Among the mutations found in DC patients some deleted large segments that affect functional domains while others are nucleotide substitutions. Mutations are particularly frequent at the pseudoknot domains and present an autosomal dominant inheritance (http://telomerase.asu.edu/diseases.html). As indicated for TERT, the functional significance of TERC mutations, specially nucleotide substitutions, has to be determined experimentally. A relevant example determined functional properties such as TR stability, TERT interaction, telomerase activity and processivity of 13 TR mutations [109].

2.3.1.2.4 TERF1- interacting nuclear factor 2 (TINF2]

The gene TINF2 codes for the protein TIN2, component of the shelterin complex that protect the telomere and regulates telomerase recruitment and activity. TIN2 links the double-stranded DNA binding proteins TRF1and TRF2 to the single-stranded DNA binding proteins TPP-1 and POT1 within the shelterin complex. TIN2 also interacts with heterochromatin protein 1 gamma (HP1$\gamma$) [110] through the canonical PTVML binding site [111] which is crucial for sister telomere cohesion.

Over 20 mutations in TINF2 have been described in DC patients. Many of them are novel mutations and results in early-onset disease. Familiar mutations are usually inherited in autosomal-dominant manner [111, 112]. All TINF2 mutations reported to date cluster in a segment coding for 34 amino acids centrally located in the gene. The function of this short protein fragment is not clear at the present time. One of the functions affected in some TINF2 mutants is HP1$\gamma$ binding [110] which could be explained because the PTVML binding site is located within the mutation cluster [111]. Impaired HP1$\gamma$ binding resulted in reduced sister telomere cohesion. On the contrary, the interaction of TIN2 with TERF1 is not affected in most of the mutated proteins [112, 113]. Impairment of telomerase recruitment to telomeres in a TIN2 mutant has been reported [114]. However, the telomere shortening observed in a mouse model of TINF2 mutation was recently reported to be telomerase independent [115].

2.3.1.2.5 TCAB1: Driving telomerase to Cajal bodies (WRAP53]

The protein TCAB1 (encoded by the WRAP53 gene) [116] binds to the telomerase RNA, TR, through the 4 nucleotides CAB box, present on small Cajal body-associated RNAs. Telomerase recruitment to Cajal Bodies is required for consequent assembly on the telomeres [44, 117].

Compound heterozygous mutations in WRAP53 have been identified in DC patients [118]. Telomerase localization to Cajal Bodies was disrupted in this patients leading to TR accumulation in the nucleoli. Mutations map to a region that mediates interaction between TCAB1 and the TCP-1 Ring Complex (TRiC) that is required for TCAB1 folding.

2.3.1.2.6 Nucleolar protein 10 (NOP10, Nola3]

Nucleolar protein 10 (NOP10] is encoded by the Nola3 gene (nucleolar protein family A, member 3]. This protein is a H/ACA snoRNA-binding protein that binds the TR RNA in association with dyskerin and NHP2 [43]. One homozygous mutation has been found in a DC patient that impaired TR binding and RNP assembly [119].

2.3.1.2.7 NHP2 ribonucleoprotein (Nola 2]

Similarly to NOP10, the NHP2 protein, encoded by the NHP2 gene, also named Nola2, is a H/ ACA snoRNA-binding protein that associates to TR together with dyskerin [43]. One homozygous missense mutation in the NHP2 gene was described in a patient with severe DC while compound heterozygous mutations were described in a second DC patient [120]. These patients had decreased TR levels and short telomeres because of impaired telomerase assembly and stability [119].

2.3.1.2.8 Conserved telomere maintenance component 1 (CTC1]

The protein CTC1 is one of the components of the CST complex (CTC1, STN1, TEN1] that promotes re-start of the telomere lagging strand synthesis and fill-in C-rich strand synthesis at the telomeres [51, 52]. CTC1 binds to single-stranded DNA at telomeres and associates with the replication initiator pol$\alpha$ primase complex.

Biallelic, compound heterozygous, CTC1 mutations were identified in a group of DC patients [121, 122]. These mutations impaired the association of CSC1 with STN1, TEN1 and pol$\alpha$ primase, telomeric DNA binding and cellular localization [123]. To date, 10 CTC1 mutations have been associated with DC patients [122].

2.3.1.2.9 Regulator of telomere elongation helicase 1 (RTEL1]

Regulator of telomere elongation helicase 1 is an essential DNA helicase that belongs to a small family of these proteins involved in different genomic instability diseases [124]. At telomeres, RTEL1 disrupts the D-loops resolving the T-loop structure [48]. RTEL1 is recruited to telomeres by TRF2 in late S phase and is essential to prevent nuclease-dependent excision of telomere T-circles [49]. RTEL1 also show G-quartet unwinding activity required for telomeric DNA replication although this activity is independent of TRF2 [50]. In addition, RTEL1 has important non-telomeric functions in processes such as DNA-replication, DNA repair and homologous recombination [125].

Whole-exome sequencing in DC patients and their families identified RTEL1 mutations that could cause DC and related telomere biology disease such as the Hoyeraal–Hreidarsson syndrome and Pulmonary Fibrosis, that will be described later (sections 2.3.2 and 2.3.6] [126-128]. To date almost 30 RTEL1 variants have been reported in telomere biology diseases patients. Most RTEL1 mutations are transmitted in autosomal recessive manner but autosomal dominance has been also reported [126]. Some mutations map to functional protein domains such as the helicase, harmonin homology or the C4C4 metal-binding motifs [129]. The RTEL1 R1264H mutation, that impairs RTEL1 interaction with TRF2, has been found in 1% of the Ashkenazi Jewish population [130].

2.3.1.2.10 Poly(A)-specific 3′ exoribonuclease (PARN)

Poly(A)-specific 3′ exoribonuclease is a widely expressed protein with Poly(A) deadenylase activity that participates in the regulation of global mRNA levels during development [131]. In addition, PARN also deadenylates small nucleolar RNAs [40]. A recent exome sequencing study linked PARN mutations with pulmonary fibrosis and telomere shortening [128].

A subsequent study, also based on exome sequencing, identified bialelic mutations in the PARN gene in three families with individuals exhibiting severe DC [85]. Two of the families were homozygous for one missense variant and one Splicing-altering variant, respectively. The third affected patient was a compound heterozygous. These patients exhibited reduced TERC, DKC1, RTEL1 and TERF1 mRNA levels. Cells from these patients showed activated DNA-damage response associated to nuclear p53 regulation, cell-cycle arrest and reduced cell viability upon UV treatment [85]. These results supported a potential link between PARN, the p53-dependent pathway and telomere shortening [132]. A subsequent study using cells derived from these patients has shown that PARN is required for the 3'-maturation of the telomerase RNA component [41]. Specifically, PARN is required for removal of the oligo(A) tails post-transcriptionally added to the TR 3' end and that target nuclear RNAs for degradation.

*2.3.2. Hoyeraal-Hreidarsson syndrome*

The Hoyeraal-Hreidarsson syndrome (HH) is frequently considered a severe variant of DC, typically presented in infancy [133]. The first patients with this syndrome were described by Hoyeraal et al [134] and Hreidarsson et al [135]. However, the eponym was first proposed in 1995 in a case report of a child with clinical features very similar to those described by Hoyeraal and Hreidarsson [136]. About 50 cases of HH have been reported since the first description [86]. HH is a multisystem genetic disorder and represents the extreme phenotype of the telomere biology disorders. Peripheral blood cells from these patients present very short telomeres, below the first percentile for their age. Clinical manifestations typically present early in childhood. These patients present developmental problems such as cerebellar hypoplasia, microcephaly, developmental delay and intrauterine growth retardation (IUGR). In addition, typically present immunodeficiency and progressive bone marrow failure. In addition to these specific symptoms, HH patients can also present clinical manifestations found in DC patients. For example, the typical triad of mucocutaneous alterations shown in DC patients can also be present at diagnosis or develop with time in HH patients. Other DC-associated symptoms that are also present in some HH patients include immunodeficiency, prematurity, dysmorphology, gastrointestinal features and neurological symptoms. Among these symptoms, cerebellar hypoplasia is considered a requirement for the diagnosis of HH [75, 137]. Other neurological complications include impaired myelination, seizures, hypoplastic corpus callosum and intracranial calcifications (reviewed in Glousker et al. [86]). Immunodeficiency is observed in a large proportion of HH patients with increased susceptibility to life-threatening infections. Over half of the patients present with lymphopenia [86]. The T cell compartment is less frequently affected although abnormalities of T cell proliferation have been observed [138]. There are also some reports of severe combined immunodeficiency [139]. Therefore, any child presenting with humoral deficiency or combined immunodeficiency and neurological features (microcephaly, cerebellar hypoplasia) should be considered a possible HH patient. Digestive tract anomalies are frequent in HH patients and include oesophageal strictures, severe enteropathy and colitis [140]. Other clinical complications include skeletal malformations [141], urinary tract abnormalities [136, 142], and ophthalmological signs [136, 142].

http://dx.doi.org/10.5772/65353

#### 2.3.2.1. *Molecular genetics of Hoyeraal-Hreidarsson syndrome*

As mentioned above, HH can be considered as severe form of DC and, in agreement with this consideration, some of the genes mutated in DC are also found mutated in HH patients [86]. The specific mutations present in HH patients can be different to those found in DC so that mutations that affect more importantly protein function are associated to HH. In other cases the difference is found in allele composition so that some mutations are found in homozygosis or compound heterozygosis in HH and in heterozygosis in DC. The mutations presently associated to HH will be briefly described in the following paragraphs and the genes affected are indicated in Table 1.

2.3.2.1.1 Dyskerin (DKC1]

DKC1 mutations cause DC and also HH so that 13 out of the over 50 different mutations presently known cause DC and HH and two of them are only found in HH (T49M and S304N) [68, 143]. No clear correlation has been found between the location of the mutation on dyskerin functional domains and the severity of the disease. Indeed, some mutations are associated with variable severity from mild DC to HH, like the A353V mutation [144]. The two HH-associated mutations are located to the catalytic TruB domain suggesting that pseudouridylation activity is important for telomerase function [143].

2.3.2.1.2 Telomerase Reverse Transcriptase (TERT)

Mutations in the TERT gene have been found in HH patients but not as frequently as in DC patients. From the more than 50 TERT mutations related to telomere biology disorders only five are implicated in HH. Four of them cause HH in homozygosis (T567M, R901W) [145, 146] or compound heterozygosis (P530L, A880T) [147]. Carriers of these mutations have short telomeres without reported clinical manifestations. The A880T and R901W mutations fall into the TERT catalytic reverse transcriptase domain and the T576M mutation in the RNA-binding domain. These mutations greatly impair telomerase activity and processivity, respectively [146]. Only one autosomal dominant TERT mutation has been associated with HH (F1127L) but it was also found in the healthy mother with could indicate the presence of a second, paternal, mutation or disease anticipation [148].

2.3.2.1.3 TERF1- interacting nuclear factor 2 (TINF2]

The shelterin component TIN2 is encoded by the gene TINF2 and has an important role by interacting with the double-stranded DNA binding proteins TRF1/TRF2 and the single-stranded DNA binding heterodimer TPP1/POT1, as mentioned above. Three of the over 20 DC-associated TINF2 mutations have been found in HH patients. These mutations were de novo or inherited in an autosomal-dominant manner [100, 111].

2.3.2.1.4 Regulator of telomere elongation helicase 1 (RTEL1]

The RTEL1 protein is a DNA helicase required for telomere replication, as mentioned above. Presently, 18 RTEL1 mutations have been described in 17 HH patients. Most RTEL1 mutations were biallelic, with either homozygous or compound heterozygous recessive inheritance. The mutations were located in domains involved in protein-protein interaction or ubiquitin transfer [127, 142].

2.3.2.1.5 TPP1 (ACD)

The protein TPP1 (TINT1, PTOP, PIP1] is encoded by the Adrenocortical Dysplasia Homolog (ACD) gene and is a component of the shelterin complex, as previously described (Section 2.1]. Three functional domains have been identified in this protein. The N-terminal OB domain is involved in the interaction of TPP1 with TERT that participates in the recruitment of the telomerase complex to telomeres through the TEL patch and increases telomerase processivity [45, 46]. The central domain is required for heterodimer formation with POT1 [28, 149]. The C-terminal domain binds TIN2 to form the shelterin complex, as mentioned above [150]. Whole exome sequencing discovered a mutation at the TEL patch of TPP1 together with a missense mutation in this same gene in a compound heterozygous HH patient [151]. The TEL patch mutation was a single amino acid deletion and resulted in a reduction of telomerase processivity and recruitment to telomeres. This same mutation has been identified in a family with aplastic anemia and other DC symptoms and was transmitted in a dominant inheritance manner [152].

2.3.2.1.6 Poly(A)-specific 3′ exoribonuclease PARN

The Poly(A)-specific 3′ exoribonuclease is involved in processing of the telomerase RNA, TR, as mentioned above. A recent work identified PARN mutations in three families with individuals exhibiting severe DC [85]. Actually, some of these patients had a disease classified as HH syndrome associating PARN mutations to this disease [132]. These patients presented biallelic mutations in the PARN gene indicating a recessive manner of inheritance.

### *2.3.3. Revesz syndrome*

The syndrome of Revesz (RS) is a telomere biology disorder that affects young children. This disease was first reported by Revesz et al as a case of a 6-month-old children with bilateral exudative retinopathy that developed a severe bone marrow failure [153]. This and subsequent reports indicated the following symptoms, summarized in Table 1: intrauterine growth retardation, intracranial calcifications, developmental delay, fine spare hair and nail dystrophy. The clinical presentations have several symptoms in common with DC and the specific diagnosis of RS requires identification of bilateral exudative retinopathy [154]. Besides common manifestations, the relation of RS with DC and other telomere biology disorders was confirmed because RS patients have very short telomeres and present mutations in the TINF2 gene, that encodes the TIN2 shelterin component [111].

### *2.3.4. Coats plus syndrome/CRMCC*

The Coats plus syndrome (CPS) is also known as cerebroretinal microangiopathy with calcifications and cysts (CRMCC). Coats plus patients have bilateral exudative retinopathy, retinal telangiectasias, intrauterine growth retardation, intracranial calcifications, bone abnormalities with poor healing, and gastrointestinal vascular ectasias (Table 1). Some patients also present DC-related features such as dystrophic nails, sparse or greying hair and anemia. Intracranial calcifications and bilateral exudative retinopathy are also present in RS patients but Coats plus patients also present cerebellar and hematologic manifestations [12, 56].

Autosomal recessive compound heterozygous mutations in CTC1 have been described in CPS identifying this syndrome as a telomere biology disorder [155-157]. As mentioned above, the protein Conserved telomere maintenance component 1 (CTC1] is required for telomere elongation. Actually, mutations in CTC1 probably account for most of the CTS cases. In addition, telomeres that are bellow the first percentile for age have been found in CTS patients and telomeres from heterozygous carriers have a length bellow average [155].

### 2.3.5. *Aplastic anemia*

Aplastic anemia is one of the clinical manifestations of telomere biology disorders in adults usually associated to mutations in TERT and TERC. Symptoms in these patients are milder than in children and mucocutaneous features are infrequent [12, 56]. Aplastic anemia can have very different causes and there are inherited and acquired forms of the disease. Acquired forms can be related to environmental exposures and infectious, among other factors, and is immune-mediated. Inherited aplastic anemia has been reported to occur in patients with Fanconi anemia, Shwachman-Diamond syndrome and other inherited bone marrow failures, including DC. It has been described that approximately 10% of patients with isolated aplastic anemia have mutations in TERC and TERT genes [158]. These mutations usually present an autosomal dominant manner of inheritance. Telomere length in these patients is usually bellow the 10% percentile for age [159]. The existence of symptoms related to telomere biology disorders in relatives of these patients, such as pulmonary fibrosis, mild cytopenias, leukemia and squamous cell cancer, can be of great help for their diagnosis [12].

### 2.3.6. *Pulmonary fibrosis*

Idiopathic pulmonary fibrosis (IPF) is a lung disease characterized by progressive interstitial fibrosis that has a poor prognosis (median survival time of 2-3 years) [160]. Diagnosis of pulmonary fibrosis, also known as interstitial pneumonia, is made by the presence of honeycombing on high-resolution computarized tomography (HRCT). In addition to pulmonary fibrosis, these patients can present a range of pulmonary pathologies, including bronchiolitis, obliterans organizing pneumonia, chronic hypersensitive pneumonia and emphysema alone or combined with pulmonary fibrosis (Table 1) [56]. Familial forms of pulmonary fibrosis have been also described and might represent up to 20% of the cases [161]. The study of these familial forms identified mutations in TERT and TERC in 8-15 % of the cases [162, 163], establishing IPF as a telomere biology disorder. IPF is inherited in these families as an autosomal dominant trail. This observation is supported by animal models since TERT null mice have decreased number or alveolar epithelial cells [164]. TRF1 deletion in type II alveolar cells also causes pulmonary fibrosis in mice [165].

Heterozygous mutations in genes coding for telomere-related proteins have been found in 15-20% of IPF families without a history of DC [162, 163, 166] and 1-3% of sporadic cases of IPF [167]. In addition, 20% of patients with DC develop pulmonary fibrosis [57, 58]. In agreement with these observations, IPF patients have significantly shorter telomeres than age-matched controls. Actually, IPF is the most common manifestation of telomere biology disorders since DC and AA have much lower prevalence [168]. IPF due to telomere disfunction presents in adulthood, into middle age [164]. The gene most frequently mutated in IPF patients is TERT [8-15% of familial cases) but mutations have been also found in TERC (<1%), DKC1 (<1%)[169], TINF2 (<1%)[170], RTEL1 [5%)[128, 166] and PARN [4%) [128]. TERT mutations have been also found in smokers with severe emphysema at a frequency of 1% [171]. Telomere dysfunction due to these genetic mutations can originate irreversible alveolar stem cell failure that would be at the origin of pulmonary fibrosis and emphysema [72, 162]. IPF patients that carry mutations in telomere-related genes can also present extra-pulmonary manifestations related to telomere biology disorders such as bone marrow failure including red blood cells, single lineage cytopenias or aplastic anemia [164]. Actually, the complex syndrome of IPF and bone marrow failure predicted the presence of TERT or TERC mutations in 10 families that presented these diseases in consecutive generations [172].

Short telomere length is a common finding in IPF patients, even in those without mutations in telomere-related genes [167]. These results could indicate that IPF may be more likely to develop in those individuals that naturally present shorter telomeres in the general population. These individuals might also have increased incidence of other telomere-related disorders such as cryptogenic liver cirrhosis and diabetes [58].

*2.3.7. Liver disease*

The study of five families with liver disease in combination with hematologic and autoimmune disorders identified mutations in TERT and TERC [65]. A subsequent study of patients with idiopathic live cirrhosis also found an increased frequency of TERT and TERC mutations [3.7% vs 0,85% in the control population) [173]. Affected patients presented reduced telomerase activity and short telomere length in peripheral blood cells. They also have increased probability to progress to end-stage liver disease. In addition, liver disease, including hepatic fibrosis, noncirrhotic portal hypertension, and hepatopulmonary syndrome has been reported in DC patients (Table 1) [62, 64].

## 2.4. Treatment of telomere biology disorders

Treatment of diseases with several organs potentially compromised has many practical complications. Presently, there are no curative therapies for many of the clinical manifestations of telomere biology disorders. The major causes of decease in these patients are bone marrow failure and pulmonary fibrosis and in this section we will summarize the present treatment of these pathologies. In the second part we will describe some of the experimental strategies that are being used to generate new therapies for telomere biology disorders.

*2.4.1. Present treatment of telomere biology diseases*

Hematopoietic stem cells transplantation (HSCT) is the only treatment than can cure bone marrow failure in these patients. Donor's selection requires special attention in telomere biology disorders since relatives might be silent carriers of the mutations, given the clinical heterogeneity of these diseases. This circumstance has been reported in two cases and there was a failure either to engraft or to mobilize stem cells from the graft [174]. Analysis of the outcome of 34 DC patients transplanted with bone marrow indicated higher rates of mortality and morbidity due to respiratory complications and graft failure [175]. Best results were obtained transplanting grafts from HLA-matched siblings but the 10-year probability of survival was 30% in this study. Conditioning of transplanted DC patients may also contribute to long-term development of pulmonary fibrosis and liver disease. Therefore, the use of reduced intensity conditioning, avoiding radiotherapy, busulfan and high dose of cyclophosphamide might benefit to these patients [176].

Androgen therapy has been also used for telomere biology disorder patients with bone marrow failure. These patients seem to be responsive to male hormones [177]. The mechanism involved seems to be that male hormones modulate TERT gene expression and increase telomerase activity [178]. In a retrospective analysis of 16 DC patients treated with androgens, 11 achieved clinically significant hematologic response [179]. Telomere elongation after androgen treatment has been reported in one case [180]. However, androgens can have side effects such as masculinisation, liver function abnormalities, hyperlipidemia and splenic peliosis (when androgens are used in conjunction with GCSF) and telomere biology disorders patients can be specially sensitive to these effects [181]. The androgen-stimulating hormone Danazol has less masculinising side effects and has been also used for treatment of DC patients [182].

Treatment of idiopathic pulmonary fibrosis is presently mainly supportive with pulmonary rehabilitation therapy and the administration of supplemental oxygen. Recently, two pharmacological agents, pirfenidone [183] and nintedanib [184] were shown to reduce lung function decline in IPF patients. Danazol administration has also been described to slow down the progression of pulmonary fibrosis in DC patients [182]. However, lung transplantation is the only curative strategy available. Lung transplantation was successfully used in a patient after HSCT [185]. The study of a small series of IPF patients with TERC or TERT mutations showed a favourable short term output with 7 of 8 patients alive after a median follow-up of 1,9 years. However, frequent haematological, renal and infectious complications were observed [186].

Because of the lack of curative therapies, telomere biology disorder's management are presently based on supportive measures and close follow-up for medium and long term complications [55]. Regular clinical review to monitor organ-specific disease progression, such as haematological analysis and pulmonary function testing must be performed. Surveillance for the appearance of dermatological and digestive tumours is important for early detection and complete surgical resection. Preventive measures such as avoidance of potential carcinogens (tobacco smoke, sun exposure) and adequate dental hygiene are also very important.

### 2.4.2. *Experimental strategies for treatment of telomere biology disorders*

Important efforts for the development of mice models of telomere biology disorders aimed to the development of novel therapies have been made in the last years [187]. However, the existence of very long telomeres in the mice strains used for experimentation [50-100 kb) has made of this a difficult task. Mice strains with defective telomerase activity have been generated [187, 188] but they have to be crossed for 4-5 generations before their telomeres are sufficiently short to manifest telomere-associated defects [189]. The use of mice with short telomeres to generate telomerase-deficient strains provided a better experimental model [190]. Mouse models carrying mutations in DKC1 have been also generated [191]. More recently, tissue-specific inactivation of genes related to telomere biology has been used to generate mice models of these diseases. For example, mice models of bone marrow failure and pulmonary fibrosis were generated by deleting the TRF1 gene in the hematopoietic compartment and type II alveolar cells, respectively [165, 192]. However, these mouse models did not completely reproduce the human disease and telomere size was not reduced [190, 191]. Mice lacking the p53 C-terminal domain had short telomeres and suffer from aplastic anemia and pulmonary fibrosis and could be a useful model for the study of telomere biology disorders [193].

Telomere biology disorders are caused by mutations in a single gene in most patients and could be, therefore, amenable for gene therapy strategies. An important caveat is that telomere length is narrowly controlled and excessively long telomeres increase the probability of developing some cancers such as melanoma [13]. Mice over-expressing TERT also develop a large number of tumors unless the tumor-suppressor protein p53 is also overexpressed [194]. Raval et al recently showed that inducible reactivation of telomerase activity could reverse defective hematopoiesis caused by telomere shortening in TERT-deleted mice [189] opening new perspectives to gene therapy approaches. Transient expression of TERT also extends telomeres in human cells [195]. Recent reports indicate that TERT plays roles beyond telomeres and contributes to stem cells maintenance and cell reprogramming which might offer new therapeutics targets for telomere biology disorders [196].

Telomere shortening results in the accumulation of DNA damage at telomeres and the activation of the p53 pathway, as mention above. A DC mouse model in which mice carries a DKC1 exon 15 deletion demonstrated that mutant cells had a growth retardation compared to wild-type cells [191]. Mutant cells accumulated increased levels of DNA damage. In addition, these cells are hypersensitive to oxygen and accumulate reactive oxygen species. Treatment of these cells with the antioxidant N-acetyl cysteine increased cell growth, both in vitro and in vivo. Competitive bone marrow repopulation studies showed that the DCK1 mutation is associated with a functional stem cell defect consistent with accelerated senescence. This stem cell defect was partially reverted by N-acetyl cystein treatment of the animals [197]. These results suggest that antioxidant treatment may prevent or delay some DC manifestations.

A new therapeutic opportunity came from the observation that a dyskerin motif, corresponding to the TruB domain of the protein (GSE24.2], reactivated telomerase activity in DC-patients and human telomerase-deficient cells [198]. This peptide activated human TERT promoter in a c-myc expression-dependent manner. GSE24.2 rescued DC-fibroblasts from premature senescence. The peptide also increased the telomerase RNA, TR, expression trough stabilization of the molecule [199]. DC-cells presented increased DNA damage at the telomeres and increased levels of oxidative stress. Expression of GSE24.2 decreased both DNA damage and oxidative stress of the cells that expressed a DKC1 mutant protein [200]. Subsequent studies demonstrated that a shorter fragment of GSE24.2, named GSE4, maintained the same biological activity and induced telomerase activity and cell proliferation of DKC-mutant cells. In addition, DNA damage, oxidative stress and cell senescence were reduced upon expression of GSE4 [201]. GSE24.2 could be delivered to cells using surface modified biodegradable polymeric nanoparticles, which might facilitate their administration to patients [202]. These results open a new therapeutic opportunity for the treatment of telomere biology disorders and GSE24.2 was recently approved by the EMA as an orphan drug for DC treatment (EU/3/12/1070-EMA/OD/136/11].

## 2.5. Conclusion

Telomere biology disorders, also named telomeropathies, compose a group of diseases with diverse clinical presentations, affecting several systems, but a common genetic etiology. Telomere maintenance or protection is defective in the patients affected by these diseases and, as a consequence, they present short telomeres. Critically short telomeres induce cell death or senescence impairing cell proliferation. Cell renewal in adult tissues depends on the proliferation of stem cells. In patients with defects in telomere biology, telomeres of stem cells are shortened after each cell cycle and get exhausted much earlier than in healthy individuals which impairs tissue renewal. This effect is specially important in highly proliferative tissues such as bone marrow, lymphocytes and epithelial tissues, including lung alveolar epithelia, that are the tissues mainly affected in patients with telomere biology disorders.

The severity of the disease seems to be dependent on the functional alterations that each mutation causes in the biological activity of the corresponding protein. The genetic doses is also very important since patients that are homozygous for the mutation or compound heterozygous for more than one mutation usually present more severe symptoms of the disease that manifest at an early age. These forms of the disease are inherited in a recessive or X-linked manner. Heterozygous patients might be healthy carriers but they can also present milder forms of the disease that present at an older age, generally in adults. These disease manifestations are inherited in an autosomal dominant manner. There is also an association between the severity of the disease and the tissues affected. High-turnover tissues are affected in younger patients and as a more severe disease. For example, the main manifestation in infancy is severe immunodeficiency affecting B cells, T cells and NK cells that have high replication rates. Bone marrow defects manifests later in children and young adults as isolated cytopenias and aplastic anemia. The gastrointestinal epithelium is also affected in children and young adults. In contrast, telomere phenotypes predominantly manifest in slow-turnover tissues such as lung and liver in adults [9]. There is also a strong correlation between the size of the telomeres, as determined in peripheral blood cells, the severity of the disease and the time of presentation so that patients younger and with more severe presentation have shorter telomeres [12].

Genetic anticipation can also have a relevant influence in the presentation and evolution of these diseases. As previously described, patients and healthy carriers of telomere biology disease can transmit shortened telomeres to their descendants. If descendants are affected by the disease, their stem cells will present critically short telomeres at an early age that the previous generation, anticipating the time of onset and increasing the severity of the disease [74]. For example, a large family has been described with several patients manifesting IPF, bone marrow failure or a combined phenotype. There seemed to be a difference of several decades in the onset of the disease between generations with IPF manifesting in older individuals (mean 51 years) and bone marrow failure in younger ones [14 years) [172].

The heterogeneous presentation of telomere biology diseases make difficult their diagnosis as already mentioned in the description of DC (section 2.3.1]. In addition, some of the symptoms also occur in patients with other diseases. For example, inherited bone marrow failure is also observed in patients with Fanconi anemia, Shwachmann-Diammond syndrome and other inherited BMFs. However, differentiating DC-associated BMF is important for patient management since, for example, these patients often do not respond to immunosuppressive therapy. One important criterion for diagnosis of telomere biology disorders is the presence of short telomeres in comparison to the aged healthy population, usually lower than the 1% percentile. However, some IPF patients present short telomeres even in the absence of mutations in telomere biology related genes [167]. Therefore, an accurate diagnosis requires establishing the molecular basis of the disease, identifying the causative mutation. Molecular diagnosis can be done sequencing the exons contained in the genes presently known to be mutated in telomere biology disorders. However, the high number of candidate genes and the large number of exons present in some of them makes this approach time-consuming and expensive. Alternatively, sequencing by exome sequencing techniques all exons of patients and close relatives is becoming a more attractive, faster and cheaper method [84]. In addition, exome sequencing allows the identification of mutations in genes that have not been previously related to telomere biology (see [128] for a recent example).

These diseases can be considered and example of the importance of precision medicine for diagnosis but also for patient managing and genetic counselling. The importance in diagnosis is enforced by the elevated heterogeneity of the clinical presentations in several systems that can create some uncertainty until a genetic analysis is performed. The importance for patient management derives from the possible progressive alteration of different organs, as mentioned above. This progression with time is very characteristic of telomerase biology disorders and can only be predicted by a precise molecular diagnosis. Disease progression also determines the therapeutic treatment. As mentioned above, the only curative alternatives are organ transplantation, either hematopoietic stem cell transplantation (HSCT) or lung transplantation. However, in telomere biology disorders both transplants have specific complications. Reduced intensity conditioning is advised and patients frequently present graft failure. In the case of HSCT respiratory complications have been described. In contrast, haematological, renal and infectious complications were observed after lung transplantation. Both complications could be expected for the multi-systemic nature of these diseases.

Precision medicine is also important for genetic counselling in telomere biology disorders [12]. Depending on the mutation, these diseases can have different manners of inheritance. The phenotypic penetrance of each mutation can be different. Heterozygous clinically silent carriers can be found whose long-term evolution is not yet understood. Patients treated for a symptom can develop a different one later on. As mentioned above, supportive measures and close follow-up of patients and carrier relatives is also very important. All these characteristics, specific to these diseases, might be difficult to transmit to the patients and their relatives what makes even more important to provide appropriate genetic education and counselling to the families.

As mentioned above, presently there are no really curative alternatives for these diseases. Lung transplantation and HSCT are important therapeutic interventions but, unfortunately, with a short time of survival. Some experimental therapies are promising but new curative therapies are urgently needed and should be the focus of intensive research in the near future.

## Acknowledgements

This work was supported by grant PI1401495 from Fondo de Investigaciones Sanitarias, Instituto de Salud Carlos III, Spain, supported by FEDER funds. CM-G is supported by the CIBER de Enfermedades Raras (CIBERER).

## Author details

Rosario Perona[1,2,3*], Laura Iarriccio[1,4], Laura Pintado-Berninches[1,4], Javier Rodriguez-Centeno[1,4], Cristina Manguan-Garcia[1,2], Elena Garcia[4], Blanca Lopez-Ayllón[1,3] and Leandro Sastre[1,2,3]

*Address all correspondence to: lsastre@iib.uam.es

1 Instituto de Investigaciones Biomedicas, CSIC/UAM, Madrid, Spain

2 CIBER de Enfermedades Raras (CIBERER), Valencia, Spain

3 Biomarkers and Experimental Therapeutics in Cancer, IdiPaz, Madrid, Spain

4 Advanced Medical Projects, Madrid, Spain

## References

[1] McElligott R, Wellinger RJ. The terminal DNA structure of mammalian chromosomes. EMBO J. 1997 Jun 16;16(12):3705-14.

[2] de Lange T. Shelterin: the protein complex that shapes and safeguards human telomeres. Genes Dev. 2005 Sep 15;19(18):2100-10.

[3] Karlseder J, Broccoli D, Dai Y, Hardy S, de Lange T. p53- and ATM-dependent apoptosis induced by telomeres lacking TRF2. Science. 1999 Feb 26;283(5406):1321-5.

[4] Harley CB, Futcher AB, Greider CW. Telomeres shorten during ageing of human fibroblasts. Nature. 1990 May 31;345(6274):458-60.

[5] Blackburn EH, Greider CW, Szostak JW. Telomeres and telomerase: the path from maize, Tetrahymena and yeast to human cancer and aging. Nat Med. 2006 Oct;12(10): 1133-8.

[6] Greider CW, Blackburn EH. Identification of a specific telomere terminal transferase activity in Tetrahymena extracts. Cell. 1985 Dec;43(2 Pt 1):405-13.

[7] Kim NW, Piatyszek MA, Prowse KR, Harley CB, West MD, Ho PL, et al. Specific association of human telomerase activity with immortal cells and cancer. Science. 1994 Dec 23;266(5193):2011-5.

[8] Wright WE, Piatyszek MA, Rainey WE, Byrd W, Shay JW. Telomerase activity in human germline and embryonic tissues and cells. Dev Genet. 1996;18(2):173-9.

[9] Armanios M. Telomeres and age-related disease: how telomere biology informs clinical paradigms. J Clin Invest. 2013 Mar;123(3):996-1002.

[10] Lopez-Otin C, Blasco MA, Partridge L, Serrano M, Kroemer G. The hallmarks of aging. Cell. 2013 Jun 6;153(6):1194-217.

[11] Nabetani A, Ishikawa F. Alternative lengthening of telomeres pathway: recombination-mediated telomere maintenance mechanism in human cells. J Biochem. 2010 Jan; 149(1):5-14.

[12] Savage SA. Human telomeres and telomere biology disorders. Prog Mol Biol Transl Sci. 2014;125:41-66.

[13] Stanley SE, Armanios M. The short and long telomere syndromes: paired paradigms for molecular medicine. Curr Opin Genet Dev. 2015 Aug;33:1-9.

[14] Horn S, Figl A, Rachakonda PS, Fischer C, Sucker A, Gast A, et al. TERT promoter mutations in familial and sporadic melanoma. Science. 2013 Feb 22;339(6122):959-61.

[15] Huang FW, Hodis E, Xu MJ, Kryukov GV, Chin L, Garraway LA. Highly recurrent TERT promoter mutations in human melanoma. Science. 2013 Feb 22;339(6122):957-9.

[16] Aoude LG, Pritchard AL, Robles-Espinoza CD, Wadt K, Harland M, Choi J, et al. Nonsense mutations in the shelterin complex genes ACD and TERF2IP in familial melanoma. J Natl Cancer Inst. 2015 Feb;107(2):pli:dju408.

[17] Bainbridge MN, Armstrong GN, Gramatges MM, Bertuch AA, Jhangiani SN, Doddapaneni H, et al. Germline mutations in shelterin complex genes are associated with familial glioma. J Natl Cancer Inst. 2015 Jan;107(1):384.

[18] Bertuch AA. The Molecular Genetics of the Telomere Biology Disorders. RNA Biol. 2016; 13(8):696-706.

[19] Giardini MA, Segatto M, da Silva MS, Nunes VS, Cano MI. Telomere and telomerase biology. Prog Mol Biol Transl Sci. 2014;125:1-40.

[20] Aubert G, Baerlocher GM, Vulto I, Poon SS, Lansdorp PM. Collapse of telomere homeostasis in hematopoietic cells caused by heterozygous mutations in telomerase genes. PLoS Genet. 2012;8(5):e1002696.

[21] Kipling D, Cooke HJ. Hypervariable ultra-long telomeres in mice. Nature. 1990 Sep 27;347(6291):400-2.

[22] Blasco MA. Telomeres and human disease: ageing, cancer and beyond. Nat Rev Genet. 2005 Aug;6(8):611-22.

[23] de Lange T, Shiue L, Myers RM, Cox DR, Naylor SL, Killery AM, et al. Structure and variability of human chromosome ends. Mol Cell Biol. 1990 Feb;10(2):518-27.

[24] de Lange T. T-loops and the origin of telomeres. Nat Rev Mol Cell Biol. 2004 Apr; 5(4):323-9.

[25] Cooper JP, Nimmo ER, Allshire RC, Cech TR. Regulation of telomere length and function by a Myb-domain protein in fission yeast. Nature. 1997 Feb 20;385(6618): 744-7.

[26] Broccoli D, Smogorzewska A, Chong L, de Lange T. Human telomeres contain two distinct Myb-related proteins, TRF1 and TRF2. Nat Genet. 1997 Oct;17(2):231-5.

[27] Ye JZ, Donigian JR, van Overbeek M, Loayza D, Luo Y, Krutchinsky AN, et al. TIN2 binds TRF1 and TRF2 simultaneously and stabilizes the TRF2 complex on telomeres. J Biol Chem. 2004 Nov 5;279(45):47264-71.

[28] Liu D, O'Connor MS, Qin J, Songyang Z. Telosome, a mammalian telomere-associated complex formed by multiple telomeric proteins. J Biol Chem. 2004 Dec 3;279(49): 51338-42.

[29] Chen LY, Redon S, Lingner J. The human CST complex is a terminator of telomerase activity. Nature. 2012 Aug 23;488(7412):540-4.

[30] Garcia-Cao M, O'Sullivan R, Peters AH, Jenuwein T, Blasco MA. Epigenetic regulation of telomere length in mammalian cells by the Suv39h1 and Suv39h2 histone methyltransferases. Nat Genet. 2004 Jan;36(1):94-9.

[31] Karlseder J, Hoke K, Mirzoeva OK, Bakkenist C, Kastan MB, Petrini JH, et al. The telomeric protein TRF2 binds the ATM kinase and can inhibit the ATM-dependent DNA damage response. PLoS Biol. 2004 Aug;2(8):E240.

[32] Wu L, Multani AS, He H, Cosme-Blanco W, Deng Y, Deng JM, et al. Pot1 deficiency initiates DNA damage checkpoint activation and aberrant homologous recombination at telomeres. Cell. 2006 Jul 14;126(1):49-62.

[33] Diotti R, Loayza D. Shelterin complex and associated factors at human telomeres. Nucleus. 2011 Mar-Apr;2(2):119-35.

[34] Nandakumar J, Cech TR. Finding the end: recruitment of telomerase to telomeres. Nat Rev Mol Cell Biol. 2013 Feb;14(2):69-82.

[35] Martinez P, Blasco MA. Replicating through telomeres: a means to an end. Trends Biochem Sci. 2015 Sep;40(9):504-15.

[36] Schmidt JC, Cech TR. Human telomerase: biogenesis, trafficking, recruitment, and activation. Genes Dev. 2015 Jun 1;29(11):1095-105.

[37] Watson JD. Origin of concatemeric T7 DNA. Nat New Biol. 1972 Oct 18;239(94): 197-201.

[38] Greider CW, Blackburn EH. A telomeric sequence in the RNA of Tetrahymena telomerase required for telomere repeat synthesis. Nature. 1989 Jan 26;337(6205):331-7.

[39] Mitchell JR, Cheng J, Collins K. A box H/ACA small nucleolar RNA-like domain at the human telomerase RNA 3' end. Mol Cell Biol. 1999 Jan;19(1):567-76.

[40] Berndt H, Harnisch C, Rammelt C, Stohr N, Zirkel A, Dohm JC, et al. Maturation of mammalian H/ACA box snoRNAs: PAPD5-dependent adenylation and PARN-dependent trimming. RNA. 2012 May;18(5):958-72.

[41] Moon DH, Segal M, Boyraz B, Guinan E, Hofmann I, Cahan P, et al. Poly(A)-specific ribonuclease (PARN) mediates 3'-end maturation of the telomerase RNA component. Nat Genet. 2015 Dec;47(12):1482-8.

[42] Angrisani A, Vicidomini R, Turano M, Furia M. Human dyskerin: beyond telomeres. Biol Chem. 2014 Jun;395(6):593-610.

[43] Egan ED, Collins K. Specificity and stoichiometry of subunit interactions in the human telomerase holoenzyme assembled in vivo. Mol Cell Biol. 2010 Jun;30(11): 2775-86.

[44] Venteicher AS, Abreu EB, Meng Z, McCann KE, Terns RM, Veenstra TD, et al. A human telomerase holoenzyme protein required for Cajal body localization and telomere synthesis. Science. 2009 Jan 30;323(5914):644-8.

[45] Zhong FL, Batista LF, Freund A, Pech MF, Venteicher AS, Artandi SE. TPP1 OB-fold domain controls telomere maintenance by recruiting telomerase to chromosome ends. Cell. 2012 Aug 3;150(3):481-94.

[46] Nandakumar J, Bell CF, Weidenfeld I, Zaug AJ, Leinwand LA, Cech TR. The TEL patch of telomere protein TPP1 mediates telomerase recruitment and processivity. Nature. 2012 Dec 13;492(7428):285-9.

[47] Williamson JR, Raghuraman MK, Cech TR. Monovalent cation-induced structure of telomeric DNA: the G-quartet model. Cell. 1989 Dec 1;59(5):871-80.

[48] Vannier JB, Pavicic-Kaltenbrunner V, Petalcorin MI, Ding H, Boulton SJ. RTEL1 dismantles T loops and counteracts telomeric G4-DNA to maintain telomere integrity. Cell. 2012 May 11;149(4):795-806.

[49] Sarek G, Vannier JB, Panier S, Petrini JH, Boulton SJ. TRF2 recruits RTEL1 to telomeres in S phase to promote t-loop unwinding. Mol Cell. 2015 Feb 19;57(4):622-35.

[50] Vannier JB, Sandhu S, Petalcorin MI, Wu X, Nabi Z, Ding H, et al. RTEL1 is a replisome-associated helicase that promotes telomere and genome-wide replication. Science. 2013 Oct 11;342(6155):239-42.

[51] Stewart JA, Wang F, Chaiken MF, Kasbek C, Chastain PD, 2nd, Wright WE, et al. Human CST promotes telomere duplex replication and general replication restart after fork stalling. EMBO J. 2012 Aug 29;31(17):3537-49.

[52] Wang F, Stewart JA, Kasbek C, Zhao Y, Wright WE, Price CM. Human CST has independent functions during telomere duplex replication and C-strand fill-in. Cell Rep. 2012 Nov 29;2(5):1096-103.

[53] Sfeir AJ, Chai W, Shay JW, Wright WE. Telomere-end processing the terminal nucleotides of human chromosomes. Mol Cell. 2005 Apr 1;18(1):131-8.

[54] Wu P, Takai H, de Lange T. Telomeric 3' overhangs derive from resection by Exo1 and Apollo and fill-in by POT1b-associated CST. Cell. 2012 Jul 6;150(1):39-52.

[55] Barbaro P, Ziegler DS, Reddel RR. The wide-ranging clinical implications of the Short Telomere Syndromes. Intern Med J. 2016; 46(4):393-403.

[56] Townsley DM, Dumitriu B, Young NS. Bone marrow failure and the telomeropathies. Blood. 2014 Oct 30;124(18):2775-83.

[57] Kropski JA, Blackwell TS, Loyd JE. The genetic basis of idiopathic pulmonary fibrosis. Eur Respir J. 2015 Jun;45(6):1717-27.

[58] Armanios M. Telomerase and idiopathic pulmonary fibrosis. Mutat Res. 2012 Feb 1;730(1-2):52-8.

[59] Dokal I. Dyskeratosis congenita in all its forms. Br J Haematol. 2000 Sep;110(4): 768-79.

[60] Heiss NS, Knight SW, Vulliamy TJ, Klauck SM, Wiemann S, Mason PJ, et al. X-linked dyskeratosis congenita is caused by mutations in a highly conserved gene with putative nucleolar functions. Nat Genet. 1998 May;19(1):32-8.

[61] Atkinson JC, Harvey KE, Domingo DL, Trujillo MI, Guadagnini JP, Gollins S, et al. Oral and dental phenotype of dyskeratosis congenita. Oral Dis. 2008 Jul;14(5):419-27.

[62] Ballew BJ, Savage SA. Updates on the biology and management of dyskeratosis congenita and related telomere biology disorders. Expert Rev Hematol. 2013 Jun;6(3): 327-37.

[63] Pignolo RJ, Suda RK, McMillan EA, Shen J, Lee SH, Choi Y, et al. Defects in telomere maintenance molecules impair osteoblast differentiation and promote osteoporosis. Aging Cell. 2008 Jan;7(1):23-31.

[64] Dokal I. Dyskeratosis congenita. Hematology Am Soc Hematol Educ Program. 2011;2011:480-6.

[65] Calado RT, Regal JA, Kleiner DE, Schrump DS, Peterson NR, Pons V, et al. A spectrum of severe familial liver disorders associate with telomerase mutations. PLoS One. 2009;4(11):e7926.

[66] Rackley S, Pao M, Seratti GF, Giri N, Rasimas JJ, Alter BP, et al. Neuropsychiatric conditions among patients with dyskeratosis congenita: a link with telomere biology? Psychosomatics. 2012 May-Jun;53(3):230-5.

[67] Alter BP, Giri N, Savage SA, Rosenberg PS. Cancer in dyskeratosis congenita. Blood. 2009 Jun 25;113(26):6549-57.

[68] Vulliamy TJ, Marrone A, Knight SW, Walne A, Mason PJ, Dokal I. Mutations in dyskeratosis congenita: their impact on telomere length and the diversity of clinical presentation. Blood. 2006 Apr 1;107(7):2680-5.

[69] Knight SW, Heiss NS, Vulliamy TJ, Greschner S, Stavrides G, Pai GS, et al. X-linked dyskeratosis congenita is predominantly caused by missense mutations in the DKC1 gene. Am J Hum Genet. 1999 Jul;65(1):50-8.

[70] Mitchell JR, Wood E, Collins K. A telomerase component is defective in the human disease dyskeratosis congenita. Nature. 1999 Dec 2;402(6761):551-5.

[71] Vulliamy T, Marrone A, Goldman F, Dearlove A, Bessler M, Mason PJ, et al. The RNA component of telomerase is mutated in autosomal dominant dyskeratosis congenita. Nature. 2001 Sep 27;413(6854):432-5.

[72] Alder JK, Barkauskas CE, Limjunyawong N, Stanley SE, Kembou F, Tuder RM, et al. Telomere dysfunction causes alveolar stem cell failure. Proc Natl Acad Sci U S A. 2015 Apr 21;112(16):5099-104.

[73] Vulliamy T, Marrone A, Szydlo R, Walne A, Mason PJ, Dokal I. Disease anticipation is associated with progressive telomere shortening in families with dyskeratosis congenita due to mutations in TERC. Nat Genet. 2004 May;36(5):447-9.

[74] Armanios M, Chen JL, Chang YP, Brodsky RA, Hawkins A, Griffin CA, et al. Haploinsufficiency of telomerase reverse transcriptase leads to anticipation in autosomal dominant dyskeratosis congenita. Proc Natl Acad Sci U S A. 2005 Nov 1;102(44): 15960-4.

[75] Savage SA, Bertuch AA. The genetics and clinical manifestations of telomere biology disorders. Genet Med. 2010 Dec;12(12):753-64.

[76] Aubert G, Hills M, Lansdorp PM. Telomere length measurement-caveats and a critical assessment of the available technologies and tools. Mutat Res. 2012 Feb 1;730(1-2): 59-67.

[77] Diez Roux AV, Ranjit N, Jenny NS, Shea S, Cushman M, Fitzpatrick A, et al. Race/ethnicity and telomere length in the Multi-Ethnic Study of Atherosclerosis. Aging Cell. 2009 Jun;8(3):251-7.

[78] Hemann MT, Strong MA, Hao LY, Greider CW. The shortest telomere, not average telomere length, is critical for cell viability and chromosome stability. Cell. 2001 Oct 5;107(1):67-77.

[79] Letsolo BT, Rowson J, Baird DM. Fusion of short telomeres in human cells is characterized by extensive deletion and microhomology, and can result in complex rearrangements. Nucleic Acids Res. 2010 Apr;38(6):1841-52.

[80] Baird DM, Rowson J, Wynford-Thomas D, Kipling D. Extensive allelic variation and ultrashort telomeres in senescent human cells. Nat Genet. 2003 Feb;33(2):203-7.

[81] Alter BP, Baerlocher GM, Savage SA, Chanock SJ, Weksler BB, Willner JP, et al. Very short telomere length by flow fluorescence in situ hybridization identifies patients with dyskeratosis congenita. Blood. 2007 Sep 1;110(5):1439-47.

[82] Alter BP, Rosenberg PS, Giri N, Baerlocher GM, Lansdorp PM, Savage SA. Telomere length is associated with disease severity and declines with age in dyskeratosis congenita. Haematologica. 2012 Mar;97(3):353-9.

[83] Carrillo J, Martinez P, Solera J, Moratilla C, Gonzalez A, Manguan-Garcia C, et al. High resolution melting analysis for the identification of novel mutations in DKC1 and TERT genes in patients with dyskeratosis congenita. Blood Cells Mol Dis. 2012 Oct 15-Dec 15;49(3-4):140-6.

[84] Sastre L. Exome sequencing:what clinicians need to know. Advances in Genomics and Genetics. 2014;4:15-27.

[85] Tummala H, Walne A, Collopy L, Cardoso S, de la Fuente J, Lawson S, et al. Poly(A)-specific ribonuclease deficiency impacts telomere biology and causes dyskeratosis congenita. J Clin Invest. 2015 May;125(5):2151-60.

[86] Glousker G, Touzot F, Revy P, Tzfati Y, Savage SA. Unraveling the pathogenesis of Hoyeraal-Hreidarsson syndrome, a complex telomere biology disorder. Br J Haematol. 2015 Aug;170(4):457-71.

[87] Schwartz S, Bernstein DA, Mumbach MR, Jovanovic M, Herbst RH, Leon-Ricardo BX, et al. Transcriptome-wide mapping reveals widespread dynamic-regulated pseudouridylation of ncRNA and mRNA. Cell. 2014 Sep 25;159(1):148-62.

[88] Kiss T, Fayet-Lebaron E, Jady BE. Box H/ACA small ribonucleoproteins. Mol Cell. 2010 Mar 12;37(5):597-606.

[89] Tycowski KT, Shu MD, Kukoyi A, Steitz JA. A conserved WD40 protein binds the Cajal body localization signal of scaRNP particles. Mol Cell. 2009 Apr 10;34(1):47-57.

[90] Wong JM, Collins K. Telomerase RNA level limits telomere maintenance in X-linked dyskeratosis congenita. Genes Dev. 2006 Oct 15;20(20):2848-58.

[91] Carrillo J, Gonzalez A, Manguan-Garcia C, Pintado-Berninches L, Perona R. p53 pathway activation by telomere attrition in X-DC primary fibroblasts occurs in the absence of ribosome biogenesis failure and as a consequence of DNA damage. Clin Transl Oncol. 2013 Jun;16(6):529-38.

[92] Bellodi C, Kopmar N, Ruggero D. Deregulation of oncogene-induced senescence and p53 translational control in X-linked dyskeratosis congenita. EMBO J. 2010 Jun 2;29(11):1865-76.

[93] Walbott H, Machado-Pinilla R, Liger D, Blaud M, Rety S, Grozdanov PN, et al. The H/ACA RNP assembly factor SHQ1 functions as an RNA mimic. Genes Dev. 2011 Nov 15;25(22):2398-408.

[94] Grozdanov PN, Fernandez-Fuentes N, Fiser A, Meier UT. Pathogenic NAP57 mutations decrease ribonucleoprotein assembly in dyskeratosis congenita. Hum Mol Genet. 2009 Dec 1;18(23):4546-51.

[95] Brault ME, Lauzon C, Autexier C. Dyskeratosis congenita mutations in dyskerin SUMOylation consensus sites lead to impaired telomerase RNA accumulation and telomere defects. Hum Mol Genet. 2013 Sep 1;22(17):3498-507.

[96] Salowsky R, Heiss NS, Benner A, Wittig R, Poustka A. Basal transcription activity of the dyskeratosis congenita gene is mediated by Sp1 and Sp3 and a patient mutation in a Sp1 binding site is associated with decreased promoter activity. Gene. 2002 Jun 26;293(1-2):9-19.

[97] Lingner J, Hughes TR, Shevchenko A, Mann M, Lundblad V, Cech TR. Reverse transcriptase motifs in the catalytic subunit of telomerase. Science. 1997 Apr 25;276(5312): 561-7.

[98] Moriarty TJ, Ward RJ, Taboski MA, Autexier C. An anchor site-type defect in human telomerase that disrupts telomere length maintenance and cellular immortalization. Mol Biol Cell. 2005 Jul;16(7):3152-61.

[99] Bryan TM, Goodrich KJ, Cech TR. Telomerase RNA bound by protein motifs specific to telomerase reverse transcriptase. Mol Cell. 2000 Aug;6(2):493-9.

[100] Podlevsky JD, Bley CJ, Omana RV, Qi X, Chen JJ. The telomerase database. Nucleic Acids Res. 2008 Jan;36(Database issue):D339-43.

[101] Collopy LC, Walne AJ, Cardoso S, de la Fuente J, Mohamed M, Toriello H, et al. Triallelic and epigenetic-like inheritance in human disorders of telomerase. Blood. 2015 Jul 9;126(2):176-84.

[102] Xin ZT, Beauchamp AD, Calado RT, Bradford JW, Regal JA, Shenoy A, et al. Functional characterization of natural telomerase mutations found in patients with hematologic disorders. Blood. 2007 Jan 15;109(2):524-32.

[103] Zaug AJ, Crary SM, Jesse Fioravanti M, Campbell K, Cech TR. Many disease-associated variants of hTERT retain high telomerase enzymatic activity. Nucleic Acids Res. 2013 Oct;41(19):8969-78.

[104] Stone MD, Mihalusova M, O'Connor C M, Prathapam R, Collins K, Zhuang X. Stepwise protein-mediated RNA folding directs assembly of telomerase ribonucleoprotein. Nature. 2007 Mar 22;446(7134):458-61.

[105] Lai CK, Miller MC, Collins K. Roles for RNA in telomerase nucleotide and repeat addition processivity. Mol Cell. 2003 Jun;11(6):1673-83.

[106] Chen JL, Opperman KK, Greider CW. A critical stem-loop structure in the CR4-CR5 domain of mammalian telomerase RNA. Nucleic Acids Res. 2002 Jan 15;30(2):592-7.

[107] Tesmer VM, Ford LP, Holt SE, Frank BC, Yi X, Aisner DL, et al. Two inactive fragments of the integral RNA cooperate to assemble active telomerase with the human protein catalytic subunit (hTERT) in vitro. Mol Cell Biol. 1999 Sep;19(9):6207-16.

[108] Mitchell JR, Collins K. Human telomerase activation requires two independent interactions between telomerase RNA and telomerase reverse transcriptase. Mol Cell. 2000 Aug;6(2):361-71.

[109] Robart AR, Collins K. Investigation of human telomerase holoenzyme assembly, activity, and processivity using disease-linked subunit variants. J Biol Chem. 2009 Feb 12;285(7):4375-86.

[110] Canudas S, Houghtaling BR, Bhanot M, Sasa G, Savage SA, Bertuch AA, et al. A role for heterochromatin protein 1gamma at human telomeres. Genes Dev. 2011 Sep 1;25(17):1807-19.

[111] Walne AJ, Vulliamy T, Beswick R, Kirwan M, Dokal I. TINF2 mutations result in very short telomeres: analysis of a large cohort of patients with dyskeratosis congenita and related bone marrow failure syndromes. Blood. 2008 Nov 1;112(9):3594-600.

[112] Sasa GS, Ribes-Zamora A, Nelson ND, Bertuch AA. Three novel truncating TINF2 mutations causing severe dyskeratosis congenita in early childhood. Clin Genet. 2012 May;81(5):470-8.

[113] Xin ZT, Ly H. Characterization of interactions between naturally mutated forms of the TIN2 protein and its known protein partners of the shelterin complex. Clin Genet. 2012 Mar;81(3):301-2.

[114] Yang D, He Q, Kim H, Ma W, Songyang Z. TIN2 protein dyskeratosis congenita missense mutants are defective in association with telomerase. J Biol Chem. 2011 Jul 1;286(26):23022-30.

[115] Frescas D, de Lange T. A TIN2 dyskeratosis congenita mutation causes telomerase-independent telomere shortening in mice. Genes Dev. 2014 Jan 15;28(2):153-66.

[116] Henriksson S, Farnebo M. On the road with WRAP53beta: guardian of Cajal bodies and genome integrity. Front Genet. 2015;6:91.

[117] Stern JL, Zyner KG, Pickett HA, Cohen SB, Bryan TM. Telomerase recruitment requires both TCAB1 and Cajal bodies independently. Mol Cell Biol. 2012 Jul;32(13): 2384-95.

[118] Zhong F, Savage SA, Shkreli M, Giri N, Jessop L, Myers T, et al. Disruption of telomerase trafficking by TCAB1 mutation causes dyskeratosis congenita. Genes Dev. 2011 Jan 1;25(1):11-6.

[119] Trahan C, Martel C, Dragon F. Effects of dyskeratosis congenita mutations in dyskerin, NHP2 and NOP10 on assembly of H/ACA pre-RNPs. Hum Mol Genet. 2009 Mar 1;19(5):825-36.

[120] Vulliamy T, Beswick R, Kirwan M, Marrone A, Digweed M, Walne A, et al. Mutations in the telomerase component NHP2 cause the premature ageing syndrome dyskeratosis congenita. Proc Natl Acad Sci U S A. 2008 Jun 10;105(23):8073-8.

[121] Keller RB, Gagne KE, Usmani GN, Asdourian GK, Williams DA, Hofmann I, et al. CTC1 Mutations in a patient with dyskeratosis congenita. Pediatr Blood Cancer. 2012 Aug;59(2):311-4.

[122] Walne AJ, Bhagat T, Kirwan M, Gitiaux C, Desguerre I, Leonard N, et al. Mutations in the telomere capping complex in bone marrow failure and related syndromes. Haematologica. 2013 Mar;98(3):334-8.

[123] Chen LY, Majerska J, Lingner J. Molecular basis of telomere syndrome caused by CTC1 mutations. Genes Dev. 2013 Oct 1;27(19):2099-108.

[124] White MF. Structure, function and evolution of the XPD family of iron-sulfur-containing 5'-->3' DNA helicases. Biochem Soc Trans. 2009 Jun;37(Pt 3):547-51.

[125] Uringa EJ, Lisaingo K, Pickett HA, Brind'Amour J, Rohde JH, Zelensky A, et al. RTEL1 contributes to DNA replication and repair and telomere maintenance. Mol Biol Cell. 2012 Jul;23(14):2782-92.

[126] Ballew BJ, Yeager M, Jacobs K, Giri N, Boland J, Burdett L, et al. Germline mutations of regulator of telomere elongation helicase 1, RTEL1, in Dyskeratosis congenita. Hum Genet. 2013 Apr;132(4):473-80.

[127] Le Guen T, Jullien L, Touzot F, Schertzer M, Gaillard L, Perderiset M, et al. Human RTEL1 deficiency causes Hoyeraal-Hreidarsson syndrome with short telomeres and genome instability. Hum Mol Genet. 2013 Aug 15;22(16):3239-49.

[128] Stuart BD, Choi J, Zaidi S, Xing C, Holohan B, Chen R, et al. Exome sequencing links mutations in PARN and RTEL1 with familial pulmonary fibrosis and telomere shortening. Nat Genet. 2015 May;47(5):512-7.

[129] Stanley SE, Noth I, Armanios M. What the genetics "RTEL"ing us about telomeres and pulmonary fibrosis. Am J Respir Crit Care Med. 2015 Mar 15;191(6):608-10.

[130] Fedick AM, Shi L, Jalas C, Treff NR, Ekstein J, Kornreich R, et al. Carrier screening of RTEL1 mutations in the Ashkenazi Jewish population. Clin Genet. 2014 Aug;88(2): 177-81.

[131] Korner CG, Wahle E. Poly(A) tail shortening by a mammalian poly(A)-specific 3'-exoribonuclease. J Biol Chem. 1997 Apr 18;272(16):10448-56.

[132] Mason PJ, Bessler M. mRNA deadenylation and telomere disease. J Clin Invest. 2015 May;125(5):1796-8.

[133] Ohga S, Kai T, Honda K, Nakayama H, Inamitsu T, Ueda K. What are the essential symptoms in the Hoyeraal-Hreidarsson syndrome? Eur J Pediatr. 1997 Jan;156(1): 80-1.

[134] Hoyeraal HM, Lamvik J, Moe PJ. Congenital hypoplastic thrombocytopenia and cerebral malformations in two brothers. Acta Paediatr Scand. 1970 Mar;59(2):185-91.

[135] Hreidarsson S, Kristjansson K, Johannesson G, Johannsson JH. A syndrome of progressive pancytopenia with microcephaly, cerebellar hypoplasia and growth failure. Acta Paediatr Scand. 1988 Sep;77(5):773-5.

[136] Aalfs CM, van den Berg H, Barth PG, Hennekam RC. The Hoyeraal-Hreidarsson syndrome: the fourth case of a separate entity with prenatal growth retardation, progressive pancytopenia and cerebellar hypoplasia. Eur J Pediatr. 1995 Apr;154(4):304-8.

[137] Savage SA, Alter BP. Dyskeratosis congenita. Hematol Oncol Clin North Am. 2009 Apr;23(2):215-31.

[138] Sznajer Y, Baumann C, David A, Journel H, Lacombe D, Perel Y, et al. Further delineation of the congenital form of X-linked dyskeratosis congenita (Hoyeraal-Hreidarsson syndrome). Eur J Pediatr. 2003 Dec;162(12):863-7.

[139] Cossu F, Vulliamy TJ, Marrone A, Badiali M, Cao A, Dokal I. A novel DKC1 mutation, severe combined immunodeficiency (T+B-NK- SCID) and bone marrow transplantation in an infant with Hoyeraal-Hreidarsson syndrome. Br J Haematol. 2002 Dec;119(3):765-8.

[140] Borggraefe I, Koletzko S, Arenz T, Fuehrer M, Hoffmann F, Dokal I, et al. Severe variant of x-linked dyskeratosis congenita (Hoyeraal-Hreidarsson Syndrome) causes significant enterocolitis in early infancy. J Pediatr Gastroenterol Nutr. 2009 Sep;49(3): 359-63.

[141] Malbora B, Avci Z, Ozbek N. Aplastic anemia and Hoyeraal-Hreidarsson syndrome. Skinmed. 2014 Mar-Apr;12(2):117-8.

[142] Ballew BJ, Joseph V, De S, Sarek G, Vannier JB, Stracker T, et al. A recessive founder mutation in regulator of telomere elongation helicase 1, RTEL1, underlies severe immunodeficiency and features of Hoyeraal Hreidarsson syndrome. PLoS Genet. 2013 Aug;9(8):e1003695.

[143] Knight SW, Heiss NS, Vulliamy TJ, Aalfs CM, McMahon C, Richmond P, et al. Unexplained aplastic anaemia, immunodeficiency, and cerebellar hypoplasia (Hoyeraal-Hreidarsson syndrome) due to mutations in the dyskeratosis congenita gene, DKC1. Br J Haematol. 1999 Nov;107(2):335-9.

[144] Lai W, Deng WP, Liu X, Chen HM, Dai Sh X. A recurrent p. A353V mutation in DKC1 responsible for different phenotypes of dyskeratosis congenita in a Chinese family. J Dermatol Sci. 2011 Aug;63(2):122-4.

[145] Marrone A, Sokhal P, Walne A, Beswick R, Kirwan M, Killick S, et al. Functional characterization of novel telomerase RNA (TERC) mutations in patients with diverse clinical and pathological presentations. Haematologica. 2007 Aug;92(8):1013-20.

[146] Gramatges MM, Qi X, Sasa GS, Chen JJ, Bertuch AA. A homozygous telomerase T-motif variant resulting in markedly reduced repeat addition processivity in siblings with Hoyeraal Hreidarsson syndrome. Blood. 2013 May 2;121(18):3586-93.

[147] Vogiatzi P, Perdigones N, Mason PJ, Wilson DB, Bessler M. A family with Hoyeraal-Hreidarsson syndrome and four variants in two genes of the telomerase core complex. Pediatr Blood Cancer. 2013 Jun;60(6):E4-6.

[148] Vulliamy TJ, Walne A, Baskaradas A, Mason PJ, Marrone A, Dokal I. Mutations in the reverse transcriptase component of telomerase (TERT) in patients with bone marrow failure. Blood Cells Mol Dis. 2005 May-Jun;34(3):257-63.

[149] Ye JZ, Hockemeyer D, Krutchinsky AN, Loayza D, Hooper SM, Chait BT, et al. POT1-interacting protein PIP1: a telomere length regulator that recruits POT1 to the TIN2/TRF1 complex. Genes Dev. 2004 Jul 15;18(14):1649-54.

[150] Takai KK, Kibe T, Donigian JR, Frescas D, de Lange T. Telomere protection by TPP1/POT1 requires tethering to TIN2. Mol Cell. 2011 Nov 18;44(4):647-59.

[151] Kocak H, Ballew BJ, Bisht K, Eggebeen R, Hicks BD, Suman S, et al. Hoyeraal-Hreidarsson syndrome caused by a germline mutation in the TEL patch of the telomere protein TPP1. Genes Dev. 2014 Oct 1;28(19):2090-102.

[152] Guo Y, Kartawinata M, Li J, Pickett HA, Teo J, Kilo T, et al. Inherited bone marrow failure associated with germline mutation of ACD, the gene encoding telomere protein TPP1. Blood. 2014 Oct 30;124(18):2767-74.

[153] Revesz T, Fletcher S, al-Gazali LI, DeBuse P. Bilateral retinopathy, aplastic anaemia, and central nervous system abnormalities: a new syndrome? J Med Genet. 1992 Sep; 29(9):673-5.

[154] Tsilou ET, Giri N, Weinstein S, Mueller C, Savage SA, Alter BP. Ocular and orbital manifestations of the inherited bone marrow failure syndromes: Fanconi anemia and dyskeratosis congenita. Ophthalmology. 2010 Mar;117(3):615-22.

[155] Anderson BH, Kasher PR, Mayer J, Szynkiewicz M, Jenkinson EM, Bhaskar SS, et al. Mutations in CTC1, encoding conserved telomere maintenance component 1, cause Coats plus. Nat Genet. 2012 Mar;44(3):338-42.

[156] Polvi A, Linnankivi T, Kivela T, Herva R, Keating JP, Makitie O, et al. Mutations in CTC1, encoding the CTS telomere maintenance complex component 1, cause cerebroretinal microangiopathy with calcifications and cysts. Am J Hum Genet. 2012 Mar 9;90(3):540-9.

[157] Savage SA. Connecting complex disorders through biology. Nat Genet. 2012 Mar; 44(3):238-40.

[158] Yamaguchi H, Baerlocher GM, Lansdorp PM, Chanock SJ, Nunez O, Sloand E, et al. Mutations of the human telomerase RNA gene (TERC) in aplastic anemia and myelodysplastic syndrome. Blood. 2003 Aug 1;102(3):916-8.

[159] Scheinberg P, Cooper JN, Sloand EM, Wu CO, Calado RT, Young NS. Association of telomere length of peripheral blood leukocytes with hematopoietic relapse, malignant transformation, and survival in severe aplastic anemia. JAMA. 2010 Sep 22;304(12):1358-64.

[160] Kim HJ, Perlman D, Tomic R. Natural history of idiopathic pulmonary fibrosis. Respir Med. 2015 Jun;109(6):661-70.

[161] Loyd JE. Pulmonary fibrosis in families. Am J Respir Cell Mol Biol. 2003 Sep;29(3 Suppl):S47-50.

[162] Armanios MY, Chen JJ, Cogan JD, Alder JK, Ingersoll RG, Markin C, et al. Telomerase mutations in families with idiopathic pulmonary fibrosis. N Engl J Med. 2007 Mar 29;356(13):1317-26.

[163] Tsakiri KD, Cronkhite JT, Kuan PJ, Xing C, Raghu G, Weissler JC, et al. Adult-onset pulmonary fibrosis caused by mutations in telomerase. Proc Natl Acad Sci U S A. 2007 May 1;104(18):7552-7.

[164] Diaz de Leon A, Cronkhite JT, Katzenstein AL, Godwin JD, Raghu G, Glazer CS, et al. Telomere lengths, pulmonary fibrosis and telomerase (TERT) mutations. PLoS One. 2010;5(5):e10680.

[165] Povedano JM, Martinez P, Flores JM, Mulero F, Blasco MA. Mice with Pulmonary Fibrosis Driven by Telomere Dysfunction. Cell Rep. 2015 Jul 14;12(2):286-99.

[166] Cogan JD, Kropski JA, Zhao M, Mitchell DB, Rives L, Markin C, et al. Rare variants in RTEL1 are associated with familial interstitial pneumonia. Am J Respir Crit Care Med. 2015 Mar 15;191(6):646-55.

[167] Alder JK, Chen JJ, Lancaster L, Danoff S, Su SC, Cogan JD, et al. Short telomeres are a risk factor for idiopathic pulmonary fibrosis. Proc Natl Acad Sci U S A. 2008 Sep 2;105(35):13051-6.

[168] Armanios M. Syndromes of telomere shortening. Annu Rev Genomics Hum Genet. 2009;10:45-61.

[169] Kropski JA, Mitchell DB, Markin C, Polosukhin VV, Choi L, Johnson JE, et al. A novel dyskerin (DKC1) mutation is associated with familial interstitial pneumonia. Chest. 2014 Jul;146(1):e1-7.

[170] Fukuhara A, Tanino Y, Ishii T, Inokoshi Y, Saito K, Fukuhara N, et al. Pulmonary fibrosis in dyskeratosis congenita with TINF2 gene mutation. Eur Respir J. 2013 Dec; 42(6):1757-9.

[171] Stanley SE, Chen JJ, Podlevsky JD, Alder JK, Hansel NN, Mathias RA, et al. Telomerase mutations in smokers with severe emphysema. J Clin Invest. 2015 Feb;125(2): 563-70.

[172] Parry EM, Alder JK, Qi X, Chen JJ, Armanios M. Syndrome complex of bone marrow failure and pulmonary fibrosis predicts germline defects in telomerase. Blood. 2011 May 26;117(21):5607-11.

[173] Calado RT, Brudno J, Mehta P, Kovacs JJ, Wu C, Zago MA, et al. Constitutional telomerase mutations are genetic risk factors for cirrhosis. Hepatology. 2011 May;53(5): 1600-7.

[174] Fogarty PF, Yamaguchi H, Wiestner A, Baerlocher GM, Sloand E, Zeng WS, et al. Late presentation of dyskeratosis congenita as apparently acquired aplastic anaemia due to mutations in telomerase RNA. Lancet. 2003 Nov 15;362(9396):1628-30.

[175] Gadalla SM, Sales-Bonfim C, Carreras J, Alter BP, Antin JH, Ayas M, et al. Outcomes of allogeneic hematopoietic cell transplantation in patients with dyskeratosis congenita. Biol Blood Marrow Transplant. 2013 Aug;19(8):1238-43.

[176] Ayas M, Nassar A, Hamidieh AA, Kharfan-Dabaja M, Othman TB, Elhaddad A, et al. Reduced intensity conditioning is effective for hematopoietic SCT in dyskeratosis congenita-related BM failure. Bone Marrow Transplant. 2013 Sep;48(9):1168-72.

[177] Islam A, Rafiq S, Kirwan M, Walne A, Cavenagh J, Vulliamy T, et al. Haematological recovery in dyskeratosis congenita patients treated with danazol. Br J Haematol. 2013 Sep;162(6):854-6.

[178] Calado RT, Yewdell WT, Wilkerson KL, Regal JA, Kajigaya S, Stratakis CA, et al. Sex hormones, acting on the TERT gene, increase telomerase activity in human primary hematopoietic cells. Blood. 2009 Sep 10;114(11):2236-43.

[179] Khincha PP, Wentzensen IM, Giri N, Alter BP, Savage SA. Response to androgen therapy in patients with dyskeratosis congenita. Br J Haematol. 2014 May;165(3): 349-57.

[180] Ziegler P, Schrezenmeier H, Akkad J, Brassat U, Vankann L, Panse J, et al. Telomere elongation and clinical response to androgen treatment in a patient with aplastic anemia and a heterozygous hTERT gene mutation. Ann Hematol. 2012 Jul;91(7):1115-20.

[181] Giri N, Pitel PA, Green D, Alter BP. Splenic peliosis and rupture in patients with dyskeratosis congenita on androgens and granulocyte colony-stimulating factor. Br J Haematol. 2007 Sep;138(6):815-7.

[182] Zlateska B, Ciccolini A, Dror Y. Treatment of dyskeratosis congenita-associated pulmonary fibrosis with danazol. Pediatr Pulmonol. 2015 50(12):48-51.

[183] Noble PW, Albera C, Bradford WZ, Costabel U, du Bois RM, Fagan EA, et al. Pirfenidone for idiopathic pulmonary fibrosis: analysis of pooled data from three multinational phase 3 trials. Eur Respir J. 2015 Jan;47(1):243-53.

[184] Richeldi L, du Bois RM, Raghu G, Azuma A, Brown KK, Costabel U, et al. Efficacy and safety of nintedanib in idiopathic pulmonary fibrosis. N Engl J Med. 2014 May 29;370(22):2071-82.

[185] Giri N, Lee R, Faro A, Huddleston CB, White FV, Alter BP, et al. Lung transplantation for pulmonary fibrosis in dyskeratosis congenita: Case Report and systematic literature review. BMC Blood Disord. 2011;11:3.

[186] Silhan LL, Shah PD, Chambers DC, Snyder LD, Riise GC, Wagner CL, et al. Lung transplantation in telomerase mutation carriers with pulmonary fibrosis. Eur Respir J. 2014 Jul;44(1):178-87.

[187] Blasco MA, Lee HW, Hande MP, Samper E, Lansdorp PM, DePinho RA, et al. Telomere shortening and tumor formation by mouse cells lacking telomerase RNA. Cell. 1997 Oct 3;91(1):25-34.

[188] Lee HW, Blasco MA, Gottlieb GJ, Horner JW, 2nd, Greider CW, DePinho RA. Essential role of mouse telomerase in highly proliferative organs. Nature. 1998 Apr 9;392(6676):569-74.

[189] Raval A, Behbehani GK, Nguyen le XT, Thomas D, Kusler B, Garbuzov A, et al. Reversibility of Defective Hematopoiesis Caused by Telomere Shortening in Telomerase Knockout Mice. PLoS One. 2015;10(7):e0131722.

[190] Herrera E, Samper E, Martin-Caballero J, Flores JM, Lee HW, Blasco MA. Disease states associated with telomerase deficiency appear earlier in mice with short telomeres. EMBO J. 1999 Jun 1;18(11):2950-60.

[191] Gu BW, Bessler M, Mason PJ. A pathogenic dyskerin mutation impairs proliferation and activates a DNA damage response independent of telomere length in mice. Proc Natl Acad Sci U S A. 2008 Jul 22;105(29):10173-8.

[192] Beier F, Foronda M, Martinez P, Blasco MA. Conditional TRF1 knockout in the hematopoietic compartment leads to bone marrow failure and recapitulates clinical features of dyskeratosis congenita. Blood. 2012 Oct 11;120(15):2990-3000.

[193] Simeonova I, Jaber S, Draskovic I, Bardot B, Fang M, Bouarich-Bourimi R, et al. Mutant mice lacking the p53 C-terminal domain model telomere syndromes. Cell Rep. 2013 Jun 27;3(6):2046-58.

[194] Garcia-Cao I, Garcia-Cao M, Martin-Caballero J, Criado LM, Klatt P, Flores JM, et al. "Super p53" mice exhibit enhanced DNA damage response, are tumor resistant and age normally. EMBO J. 2002 Nov 15;21(22):6225-35.

[195] Ramunas J, Yakubov E, Brady JJ, Corbel SY, Holbrook C, Brandt M, et al. Transient delivery of modified mRNA encoding TERT rapidly extends telomeres in human cells. FASEB J. 2015 May;29(5):1930-9.

[196] Maida Y, Masutomi K. Telomerase reverse transcriptase moonlights: Therapeutic targets beyond telomerase. Cancer Sci. 2015 106(11):1486-92.

[197] Gu BW, Fan JM, Bessler M, Mason PJ. Accelerated hematopoietic stem cell aging in a mouse model of dyskeratosis congenita responds to antioxidant treatment. Aging Cell. 2011 Apr;10(2):338-48.

[198] Machado-Pinilla R, Sanchez-Perez I, Murguia JR, Sastre L, Perona R. A dyskerin motif reactivates telomerase activity in X-linked dyskeratosis congenita and in telomerase-deficient human cells. Blood. 2008 Mar 1;111(5):2606-14.

[199] Machado-Pinilla R, Carrillo J, Manguan-Garcia C, Sastre L, Mentzer A, Gu BW, et al. Defects in mTR stability and telomerase activity produced by the Dkc1 A353V mutation in dyskeratosis congenita are rescued by a peptide from the dyskerin TruB domain. Clin Transl Oncol. 2012 Oct;14(10):755-63.

[200] Manguan-Garcia C, Pintado-Berninches L, Carrillo J, Machado-Pinilla R, Sastre L, Perez-Quilis C, et al. Expression of the genetic suppressor element 24.2 (GSE24.2) decreases DNA damage and oxidative stress in X-linked dyskeratosis congenita cells. PLoS One. 2014;9(7):e101424.

[201] Iarriccio L, Manguan-Garcia C, Pintado-Berninches L, Mancheno JM, Molina A, Perona R, et al. GSE4, a Small Dyskerin- and GSE24.2-Related Peptide, Induces Telomerase Activity, Cell Proliferation and Reduces DNA Damage, Oxidative Stress and Cell Senescence in Dyskerin Mutant Cells. PLoS One. 2015;10(11):e0142980.

http://dx.doi.org/10.5772/65353

[202] Egusquiaguirre SP, Manguan-Garcia C, Pintado-Berninches L, Iarriccio L, Carbajo D, Albericio F, et al. Development of surface modified biodegradable polymeric nanoparticles to deliver GSE24.2 peptide to cells: a promising approach for the treatment of defective telomerase disorders. Eur J Pharm Biopharm. 2015 Apr;91:91-102.

# Chapter 6

# Telomere Instability Induced by Anticancer Drugs in Mammalian Cells

Alejandro D. Bolzán

Additional information is available at the end of the chapter

http://dx.doi.org/10.5772/64928

**Abstract**

Telomere instability results from chromosome end loss (due to chromosome breakage at one or both ends) or, more frequently, telomere dysfunction. Dysfunctional telomeres arise when they lose their end-capping function or become critically short, which causes chromosomal termini to behave like a DNA double-strand break. At the chromosomal level, this phenomenon is visualized by using Fluorescence In Situ Hybridization (FISH), as chromosomal aberrations directly involving terminal telomeric repeats: loss or duplication of telomeric signals, association or fusion of telomeres of different chromosomes, telomere sister chromatid exchanges, translocation or amplification of telomeric sequences, and extrachromosomal telomeric signals. At the molecular level, telomere instability arises due to the loss or modification of any of the components of the telomere (telomere DNA, telomere-associated proteins or telomere RNA). Since telomeres play a fundamental role in maintaining genomic stability, the study of telomere instability in cells exposed to anticancer drugs is of great importance to understand the genomic instability associated with chemotherapy regimens. In this chapter, we will summarize our current knowledge about telomere instability induced by anticancer drugs on mammalian cells.

**Keywords:** Telomere, telomere instability, telomere loss, telomere dysfunction, telomere erosion, chemotherapy, anticancer drugs

## 1. Introduction

### 1.1. What are telomeres?

Classically defined as the chromosome ends, telomeres (from the Greek, *telo* = end, and *mere* = part) [1] are nowadays defined as specialized nucleoprotein complexes localized at the physical ends of linear eukaryotic chromosomes, that maintain their stability and integrity [2, 3]. They protect chromosomes from degradation, recombination or fusion, by preventing the ends of linear chromosomes from being recognized as DNA double-strand breaks (DSB) by the DNA repair machinery, i.e., they distinguish natural DNA ends from DNA ends resulting from breakage events [2, 3].

In all vertebrates, telomeres are composed of tandem arrays of short, repetitive G-rich sequences (TTAGGG)n, oriented 5′ → 3′ towards the end of the chromosome, ending in an essential 3′ single-stranded overhang that ranges in length from ~50 to 400 nt [4-6], bound by a specialised multiprotein complex known as "shelterin" or telosome [7-9]. The length of the double-stranded telomeric repeat varies greatly among species [2]. In normal human cells, the DNA at each chromosome terminus spans 5-20 kb in length [6, 10, 11], terminating in a 3" single-stranded overhang 100-400 nt in length [10], whereas in human tumor cells, telomere length varies from 1 to 20 kb [12-14].

The telosome is constituted by 6 proteins (POT1, TPP1. TIN2, TRF1, TRF2 and RAP1) and is charged with protecting chromosome ends from activating a DNA damage response, inhibiting inappropriate repair mechanisms, and maintaining telomeric length and structure [7-9]. Besides telomeric repeats and shelterin, telomeres also comprise (UUAGGG)n-containing RNA molecules (telomeric repeat-containing RNA or TERRA), a novel class of RNA for which several functions have been suggested [15-18]. TERRA transcription occurs at most or all chromosome ends and it is regulated by RNA surveillance factors and in response to changes in telomere length. Therefore, telomeres are composed of DNA, proteins, and RNA. In addition to the shelterin complex, many proteins involved in DNA repair are also associated with telomeres [19].

Telomere length is maintained by a dynamic process of telomere shortening and lengthening. Usually, telomere shortening occurs due to nucleolytic degradation and incomplete DNA replication, due to the inability of lagging strand synthesis to completely replicate chromosomal ends (i.e., the so-called "end replication problem") [9]. Telomere shortening is usually prevented by telomerase, a reverse transcriptase-like enzyme containing an RNA subunit (TERC, "Telomere RNA Component") and a catalytic protein subunit called "Telomerase Reverse Transcriptase" (TERT, "Telomere Reverse Transcriptase") which works via an RNA template -using exclusively single-strand 3" telomeric overhangs as primers- [9], by adding telomeric repeats to the chromosome ends. Although repressed in the majority of normal somatic cells (with the exception of a transient S phase activity thought to maintain the single-stranded overhang]), telomerase is present in immortal cell lines, germline cells, stem cells, activated lymphocytes, and most of the tumor cells analyzed so far [20, 21]. Telomerase activity favors 3" overhangs over blunt DNA ends for an addition of telomere sequence, at least *in vitro* [22, 23]. Loss of telomerase enzymatic function leads to progressive telomere shortening over time, eventually resulting in the disappearance of detectable telomeric DNA and the formation of end-to-end chromosome fusions, followed by growth arrest or cell death [24].

It has been suggested that TERRA may be involved in the regulation of telomerase activity and that the accumulation of TERRA at telomeres can interfere with telomere replication, leading to telomere loss [15-18]. Telomere elongation can also occur in the absence of telomerase through the so-called ALT (for 'Alternative Lengthening of Telomeres') mechanism, which

http://dx.doi.org/10.5772/64928

involves homologous recombination between telomeres and has been described in several tumor cells and immortalized cell lines [25].

The analysis of the short- and long-term chromosomal instability produced by anticancer drugs is of great importance to understand the genomic instability associated with chemotherapy regimens. Since telomeres play a fundamental role in maintaining chromosomal/genomic stability, the study of telomere instability induced by antineoplastic drugs is of clinical interest. Therefore, in this chapter, we will consider in detail the phenomenon of telomere instability and summarize our current knowledge concerning the main data available about telomere instability induced by anticancer drugs on mammalian cells. In the next section, we will see what is telomere instability and how it can be generated in the cells.

## 2. What is telomere instability? Telomere loss, dysfunction and erosion

Telomere instability refers to the chromosomal instability caused either by the loss of the chromosome ends (one or both) or the dysfunction of telomeres [26, 27]. These phenomena can take place in the short (at first cell división after the induction of chromosome damage by a given mutagen) or in the long term (in the progeny of the exposed cells). Once telomere instability arises, the involved chromosomes tend to associate or fuse with each other [26, 27].

Chromosomal instability is usually defined as a delayed increase in the production of new aberrations or a delayed appearance of excessive levels of aberrations in the clonal surviving cells after exposure to a given mutagen [28]. However, whenever a chromosome lacks one or both of its ends or suffers telomere dysfunction it becomes unstable, so we can refer to chromosome -or more properly, telomere- instability to the one that arises since the first cell division after the chromosome damage event at the telomeric region occurs.

Telomeric instability may arise when a chromosome, due to a break in one or both of its ends, loses one or both telomeres (ie, becomes an "incomplete chromosome") and, therefore, the chromosome end is exposed to enzymatic degradation or fuses with another chromosome end or enters to what is called a breakage-fusion-bridge (BFB) cycle (see below for details). We refer to this type of instability as telomere instability by telomere or chromosome end loss [26, 27, 29]. Alternatively, if one or both telomeres of the chromosome are excessively shortened, the chromosome tends to associate or fuse with other damaged chromosomes. This shortening can affect any of the four telomeres of a (metaphase) chromosome, resulting in duplication or loss of telomeric signals (after Fluorescence In Situ Hybridization or FISH, each FISH signal representing a block or specific set of telomeric sequences) [26, 29]. It may also be the case that any of the telomeric proteins (the shelterin complex) or telomeric RNA be altered or lost. In all these cases, we refer to telomeric instability by telomere dysfunction because the telomere has lost its protective function, either by excessive shortening (termed "telomere erosion or attrition") or by loss or alteration of the proteins or RNA associated with the telomeric DNA [26]. This phenomenon can be studied at the cytogenetic level by telomere FISH and is visible through telomeric chromosomal aberrations such as telomeric fusions, associations or loss or duplication of telomeric signal [26, 29, 30].

### 2.1. Telomere or chromosome end loss

As previously noted, true telomere loss is due to chromosome breakage at one or both ends of the chromosome, and can generate chromosome instability, both by allowing degradation of the ends of chromosomes and promoting chromosome fusions. Fusion can occur between sister chromatids, or between different chromosomes if telomeres are lost in more than one of the chromosomes of a given cell. Chromosome fusion results in chromosome instability through the abovementioned BFB cycles [26, 27, 29], when chromosomes, after telomere loss, repeatedly fuse and break for many cell generations. BFB cycles can continue for multiple cell generations, leading to extensive chromosomal rearrangements, and terminate when the unstable chromosome eventually acquires a new telomere and so becomes stable [26, 27, 29]. BFB cycles involving sister chromatid fusions result in several types of chromosome rearrangements, including terminal deletions, inverted duplications, DNA amplification, duplicative and nonreciprocal translocations, and dicentric chromosomes, all of which have been associated with human cancer. Chromosomes lacking one telomere remain unstable until they are capped, and lost telomeres after a BFB cycle can be acquired by several mechanisms, including nonreciprocal translocation, duplication/translocation, subtelomeric duplication, or direct telomere addition [26, 27, 29]. For a detailed description of BFB cycles see [26, 27].

### 2.2. Telomere dysfunction and erosion

As previously stated, dysfunctional telomeres arise when they lose their end-capping function or become critically short (a phenomenon called telomere erosion or attrition), which causes chromosomal termini to behave like a DSB [9, 31]. In effect, dysfunctional (uncapped or shorten) telomeres are sensed as true DSB, according to the presence of DNA damage response proteins at telomeres in senescent cells or shelterin deficient cells [32]. Therefore, dysfunctional telomeres act as DSB, interfering with the correct rejoining of broken ends. Both telomeres and DSB are DNA ends, and as such, both recruit many of the same proteins. As previously mentioned, proteins governing the DNA damage response are intimately involved in the regulation of telomeres, which undergo processing and structural changes that elicit a transient DNA damage response [19]. Chromosomes with dysfunctional telomeres tend to fuse with one another, producing dicentrics, which can give rise to the abovementioned BFB cycles [26, 27]. It must be taken into account that telomere shortening does not always mean telomere dysfunction. Only when telomeric repeats loss gives rise to a defective telomere structure a dysfunctional telomere appears. Thus, telomere erosion refers to a dysfunctional telomere which became critically short, so it cannot function properly.

Telomere dysfunction at the chromosomal level is commonly assessed applying the telomere FISH technique to metaphase chromosomes [26, 29, 30]. A normal metaphase chromosome exhibits four telomeric signals, two at each end (one per chromatid). When the telomere becomes dysfunctional, one or more of these telomeric signals are lost or duplicated [26, 29, 30]. The presence of chromosome ends with undetectable telomeric hybridization signals has been shown to be a good indicator of critically short and probably dysfunctional telomeres in mammalian cells [33-36]. It is important to mention that not all telomere involving chromosomal aberrations imply telomere dysfunction, but only those ones directly involving terminal telomeric repeats (see [26, 29] for details).

http://dx.doi.org/10.5772/64928

Telomeres suppress the DNA damaging response, so dysfunctional telomeres activate DNA damage checkpoints [19, 32]. In addition, dysfunctional telomeres induce metabolic and mitochondrial compromise [37], promote carcinogenesis [38, 39], induce chromosome instability [27], and triggers cellular senescence [40].

## 3. Factors promoting telomere instability

Several factors can promote telomere instability. Telomere instability due to true telomere loss can be generated by any mutagen which breaks the chromosome and induces terminal deletions, as shown by several studies (see [26] for review). This kind of instability gives rise to the so-called "incomplete chromosome elements", which comprise chromosomes without one or both telomeres (incomplete chromosomes) and the acentric fragments resulting from the breakage event (termed "terminal fragments") [26, 29, 30].

Telomere instability due to telomere dysfunction can be generated in several ways [26]. Alterations in the shelterin complex or other telomere-binding proteins [7, 8, 41], some DNA damage response proteins required for proper telomere protection [42], the structure of telomeric DNA (loss of telomeric sequences, see below), the structure or activity of telomerase [43], TERRA [15-18] or the enzymes helicases [44, 45] can give rise to dysfunctional telomeres. All these factors are involved in the production of telomere-related chromosomal aberrations. These aberrations have been described in detail elsewhere [26, 29, 30] and thus they will not be considered in the present chapter. Moreover, dysfunctional telomeres may result as a consequence of mutagen-induced telomeric DNA damage [26].

Referring to the relationship between telomere shortening and dysfunction, we must bear in mind that, as previously mentioned, telomere length is maintained by a dynamic process of telomere shortening and lengthening. Telomeres lose approximately 20-300 bp of repeat sequences every cell division mainly due to the "end replication problem" [9]. This is the most obvious mechanism for the loss of telomeric repeat sequences, i.e., attrition due to the failure to compensate for the gradual loss of these repeats during cell division, and is termed replicative erosion or replicative shortening, which leads to replicative senescence of cells. Thus, telomeres regulate the replicative life span of somatic cells, acting as a "mitotic clock". There is another kind of telomere shortening, termed "stress dependant shortening", which is produced by stress-inducing factors like radiation, oncogenes, oxidative damage within telomeric DNA, chromosome end-specific exonuclease activity, and the lack of telomerase activity [46-49]. Stress dependant shortening can lead to the loss of large blocks of telomeric repeat sequences through different mechanisms, including recombination, problems encountered during DNA synthesis or inefficient DNA repair. In addition, telomere shortening is accelerated by active oxygen species and ultraviolet radiation, which are thought to be major environmental causes of human telomere shortening [46]. In the next section, we will summarize our current knowledge concerning the main data available about telomere instability induced by anticancer drugs on mammalian cells.

## 4. Telomere instability produced by anticancer drugs in mammalian cells

In the next sections, we will consider the main data available concerning the short- and long-term telomere instability induced by anticancer drugs in mammalian cells. Firstly, we will refer to those drugs whose effects on telomeres have been intensively investigated: bleomycin, streptonigrin, streptozotocin, paclitaxel, cisplatin, doxorubicin, etoposide and 5-azacytidine. Afterwards, we will shortly refer to other anticancer drugs whose effects on telomeres are barely known, such as gemcitabine, C-1027, ICRF-193, melphalan and 5-fluorouracil. It is important to bear in mind that, in this chapter, when we refer to telomeres, we refer to the very end of the chromosomes (which, at the molecular level is constituted by TTAGGG repeats and the associated RNA and proteins), not the subtelomeric region of them (constituted by telomere-specific sequences located near the telomere). Therefore, we will not refer to those studies involving the effects of anticancer drugs on the subtelomeric regions of the chromosomes.

### 4.1. Bleomycin (BLM), Streptonigrin (SN) and Streptozotocin (STZ)

Several years ago, we carried out in our laboratory a series of experiments to determine the short-term effects of three antibiotics with anticancer properties, bleomycin (BLM), streptonigrin (SN) and streptozotocin (STZ) on mammalian telomeres and telomeric sequences (see [26] for review).

BLM (CAS No. 11056-06-7) is a chemotherapeutic drug isolated from *Streptomyces verticillus* which is commonly used to treat testicular cancer, lymphoma, lung cancer, cervical cancer and cancers of the head and neck [50]. This antibiotic is an S-independent clastogen and a radiomimetic agent that generates free radicals and induces single- and double-strand breaks in DNA [50, 51]. SN (CAS No. 3930-19-6) is an aminoquinone antitumor antibiotic isolated from cultures of *Streptomyces flocculus*, which shows antitumor activity against a broad range of tumors, including breast, lung, head and neck cancer, lymphoma and melanoma [52], although its use in cancer therapy is very limited because it induces severe and prolonged bone marrow depression [52]. Despite of being considered a radiomimetic compound, SN is capable of producing chromosome damage both by S-independent and S-dependent mechanisms [52]. Moreover, SN causes inhibition of topoisomerase II by stabilizing the transesterification intermediate of the enzyme (called cleavable complex) [52]. STZ (CAS No. 18883-66-4) is is an antibiotic isolated from *Streptomyces achromogenes* [53, 54], usually used to experimentally induce diabetes mellitus in laboratory animals, and it has been considered a potential compound for the clinical treatment of some malignant diseases, including advanced pancreatic neuroendocrine tumors and colon cancer. STZ is a potent alkylating agent that directly methylates DNA, giving rise to chromosome and DNA damage [53, 54]. STZ exerts its clastogenic effect mainly in an S-dependent manner, inducing both chromatid- and chromosome-type aberrations [53, 54].

The abovementioned studies, perfomed using FISH with a Peptide Nucleic Acid telomere probe (telomere PNA-FISH) in Chinese hamster cells (CHE cell line), showed that all the above drugs can induce the formation of incomplete chromosomes and terminal fragments [55-58].

http://dx.doi.org/10.5772/64928

These observations were made on metaphase cells obtained 18 h after treatment (i.e., in cells in their first mitosis after treatment) and indicated that, despite of the fact that BLM, SN, and STZ act on chromosomes in a different way, these drugs can induce short-term telomere instability by chromosome end loss in mammalian cells. The induction of short-term telomere instability by BLM was also demonstrated by Benkhaled et al. [59] in human lymphocytes. More recently, our studies were focused on the effects of these antibiotics on the progeny of the exposed cells, to determine if telomeres play some role in the long-term chromosomal instability induced by these drugs and if telomere instability can persist in the exposed cells for several generations after treatment. To accomplish our goal, we exposed rat cells (ADIPO-P2 cell line) to a single pulse of BLM, SN or STZ, and determined the type and frequency of chromosomal aberrations at 18 h (first mitosis after exposure), 10 days and 15 days after treatment by using PNA-FISH with a telomeric probe.

We found that BLM induces persistent telomere instability in mammalian cells, cytogenetically manifested as incomplete chromosome elements (i.e., chromosome end loss) and telomere FISH signal loss and duplication (i.e., telomere dysfunction) ([60] and Paviolo, unpublished data). In addition, our results suggested that BLM can induce delayed telomere instability in the form of telomere (end-to-end) fusions. Therefore, we concluded that BLM induces telomere instability at the chromosome level both by chromosome end loss and telomere dysfunction [60]. The delayed appearance of dicentric chromosomes and telomere fusions (which produces dicentric chromosomes without accompanying fragment) that we observed in ADIPO-P2 cells exposed to BLM suggests that the BFB cycles [27] might play a significant role in the maintenance of the long-term telomere instability induced by this compound. In effect, by inducing breakage at terminal regions of chromosomes, resulting in incomplete chromosomes, BLM could promote genome instability through BFB cycles, which can continue for multiple cell generations, leading to extensive chromosomal rearrangements in the progeny of the cells exposed to this compound. According to our data, the persistent telomere instability induced by BLM in rat cells is neither related to telomerase activity nor telomere length variations ([60] and Paviolo, unpublished data).

In the case of SN, we found that this drug induces persistent (i.e., up to 15 days after treatment) telomere dysfunction in ADIPO-P2 cells in the form of additional telomeric FISH signals, extrachromosomal telomeric FISH signals, and telomere FISH signal loss and duplications [61]. Several studies have provided a large body of evidence indicating that SN directly interacts with DNA, binding covalently but not interacting into the double helix (see [52] for review). Therefore, the persistence of the clastogenic action of SN in terms of telomere-associated aberrations could be due to the formation of a stable complex between SN and the DNA molecule, which may induce chromosome damage through a persistent cyclic redox process and the resulting generation of active oxygen species [52]. Moreover, we found that SN causes persistent inhibition of telomerase activity in rat cells [61]. A decreased telomerase activity could promote extensive telomere shortening, cytogenetically detected as telomere FISH signal loss. However, using the Flow-FISH technique, we were able to determine that SN does not have a persistent effect on telomere length in rat cells, since we observed a transient telomere lengthening in these cells only at 10 days after treatment (Paviolo, unpublished data). Therefore, the precise relationship between telomerase activity, telomere length and telomere instability in SN-exposed cells remains to be determined.

It is interesting to note that despite of the fact that both BLM and SN are radiomimetic compounds, they exhibit some important differences in their long-term effects on telomeres [60, 61]. First, BLM induces persistent chromosome end loss and telomere dysfunction, whereas SN induces persistent telomere dysfunction but not persistent chromosome end loss. Second, BLM induces telomere fusions, whereas SN not. Finally, BLM induces delayed increase of telomerase activity in mammalian cells, while SN decreases telomerase activity. Although these discrepancies could be due to differences between SN and BLM in their mode of action [50-52], further studies will be needed to confirm this assumption.

Finally, we found that also STZ induces persistent telomere dysfunction in rat cells, cytogenetically detected mainly as telomere FISH signal loss and duplications, most of them being chromatid-type aberrations [62]. We observed that STZ induces significantly more signal loss than duplications, telomere loss thus being the most significant effect of STZ on telomere function at the chromosome level in ADIPO-P2 cells. As previously mentioned, telomere FISH signal loss and duplication were also observed in BLM- [60] and SN-exposed ADIPO-P2 cells [61]. Therefore, these types of aberrations seem to be the predominant chromosome aberrations directly related to telomere dysfunction induced by anticancer drugs. In addition, our experiments with rat cells exposed to STZ showed that this compound also induces long-term telomere instability in the form of incomplete chromosome elements, as previously observed in the short-term in Chinese hamster cells [57]. We found that STZ induces a transient increase in telomere length in ADIPO-P2 cells at 10 days after treatment, a delayed effect not related with telomerase activity, which remained unchanged in both treated and untreated cells [62]. Therefore, the persistence of chromosomal aberrations related to telomere dysfunction in rat cells exposed to STZ seems to be unrelated to telomerase activity or telomere length.

Besides the abovementioned studies, other researchers reported additional data on the effect of BLM on telomeres. No further studies have been made concerning the effects of SN and STZ on telomeres so far. The most important finding with regard to BLM was that human telomeric DNA sequences are a major target for this anticancer drug [63, 64]. In effect, these authors examined the DNA sequence specificity of BLM in a target DNA sequence containing 17 repeats of the human telomeric sequence and other primary sites of BLM cleavage and found that BLM cleaved primarily at 5′-GT in the telomeric sequence 5′-GGGTTA [63, 64]. The telomeric region constituted 57% of the 30 most intense BLM damage sites in the DNA sequence examined, these data indicating that telomeric DNA sequences are a major target for BLM damage. Previously, by using the Comet-FISH technique (i.e., single cell gel electrophoresis or Comet assay in combination with Fluorescent in situ hybridization), with a telomere-specific PNA probe, Arutyunyan et al. [65] found that BLM and Mitomycin C (MMC, CAS No. 50-07-7) induce breaks in telomere-associated DNA in human lymphocytes. The breakage frequency for telomeric DNA was found to be proportional to that of the total DNA, which suggests random induction of DNA breaks by these drugs. A year later, these authors using the same technique showed that, in human lymphocytes, BLM and also the anticancer drug cisplatin induce telomere DNA damage [66]. The action of cisplatin on telomeres will be considered in detail later in this chapter.

The induction of telomere DNA damage by BLM (and also MMC) in mammalian cells was confirmed by Hovhannisyan et al. [67], who analyzed the effect of these drugs in normal human leukocytes and three transformed cell lines (HT1080, CCRF-CEM and CHO) using the Comet-

FISH assay. They found significant differences between these cells with respect to quantitative head/tail distribution of telomeric signals after BLM exposure, which indicates that the extent of the telomere DNA damage induced by this compound depends on the cell type. Recently, Liu et al., studied the effect of BLM and other anticancer drugs on telomeres of a mouse spermatogonial cell line and found that BLM damages telomeric DNA (as seen by the co-localization of telomere and gamma-H2AX signals after FISH and immunofluorescence) [68].

### 4.2. Paclitaxel

Paclitaxel or Taxol (CAS No. 33069-62-4) is an anticancer drug, isolated from the bark of the Pacific yew *Taxus brevifolia*, that has been shown to be clinically effective against a wide range of human cancers, including ovarian, breast, lung and pancreatic cancers [69]. The anticancer effect of paclitaxel is attributable principally to irreversible promotion of microtubule stabilization and is hampered upon development of chemoresistance by tumor cells [70, 71].

It has been shown that paclitaxel and water-soluble poly (L-glutamic acid)-paclitaxel induce telomeric associations in a murine metastatic melanoma cell line (K1735, clone X-21), being the effect of the water-soluble form of paclitaxel more pronounced than the effect of paclitaxel alone [72]. Two years later, these authors analyzed the effects of the above compounds and two other water-soluble forms of paclitaxel (sodium-pentetic acid-paclitaxel and polyethylene glycol-paclitaxel) in the same murine cell line and found that these drugs induce the formation of telomeric associations [73]. In addition, they found that paclitaxel and its water-soluble conjugates induce extensive telomere erosion (visualized as reduced telomeric signal intensity after telomere FISH) but do not change telomerase activity [73]. Therefore, these drugs induce telomere dysfunction in mammalian cells by producing telomeric associations and telomere erosion (which means loss of telomeric repeats). Telomeric associations and reduction of telomeric signal intensity were also observed in Tax-18 and Tax-2-4, two paclitaxel-requiring mutant Chinese hamster ovary (CHO) cell lines [74]. Moreover, in these cells, cell death was driven by the loss of telomeric DNA repeats, as shown by the analysis of terminal telomeric restriction fragments [74]. Telomere erosion induced by paclitaxel can be enhanced by telomerase inhibitors, such as 3'-azido-3'-deoxythymidine (AZT) [75, 76]. More recently, using telomerase-deficient cells derived from mTERC−/− (mouse telomerase RNA component-minus) mice, Park et al. demonstrated that, upon telomere erosion, paclitaxel stimulates chromosomal fusion and instability in cells with dysfunctional telomeres [77]. Chromosomal fusions promoted by paclitaxel involve both q- and p-chromosome arms, being the q-arm fusions both unstable and lethal [77]. These chromosomal fusions occur in response to microtubule disruption induced by paclitaxel in cells with dysfunctional telomeres [77]. Thus, telomere dysfunction, rather than telomerase inhibition seems to be essential to sensitize transformed cells to paclitaxel.

### 4.3. Cisplatin

Cisplatin (CAS No. 15663-27-1), another well-known anticancer drug, was also found to interact with telomeric DNA sequences. Ishibashi and Lippard [78] showed that cisplatin can bind to telomeric repeats: Duplex DNA containing five telomeric repeats treated with cisplatin at formal platinum/strand ratios of 5 or 10 in water was platinated with efficiencies of 91.0% and 76.4%, respectively. More recently, Paul and Murray, using an automated capillary DNA sequencer investigated the interaction of cisplatin with purified telomeric DNA sequences and found that cisplatin strongly formed adducts with telomeric DNA sequences [79]. A similar result was obtained by Murray and Kandasamy, using a plasmid clone containing seven telomeric repeats and a sequence of ten consecutive guanine bases [80]. Although cisplatin preferentially damaged the guanine sequence, the telomeric DNA was also a major site of cisplatin adduct formation [80]. Furthermore, Nguyen et al. analyzed the DNA sequence specificity of cisplatin in a long telomeric tandem repeat (a human telomeric DNA sequence containing 17 tandem repeats) and found that the 3'-end of the G-rich strand of the telomeric repeat was preferentially damaged by this compound [81].

Even though several studies showed that cisplatin inhibits telomerase activity in a specific and concentration-dependent manner in several types of cancer cells (see [82, 83] for example), little is known about whether this compound induces telomere instability. Ishibashi and Lippard [78] by using Analysis of Terminal Restriction Fragment (TRF) Length (by Southern blot) showed that cisplatin induces telomere loss (shortening) and degradation in HeLa cells. A recent study from Liu et al. in a mouse spermatogonial cell line, showed that the alkylating compounds cisplatin and 4-hydroperoxycyclophosphamide (4OOH-CPA, a preactivated analog of cyclophosphamide, CAS No. 50-18-0) induce telomere dysfunction in mouse cells [68]. These authors found that these compounds decrease telomerase activity and shorten telomere length, thus causing telomere dysfunction [68]. Thus, cisplatin and 4OOH-CPA could induce long-term telomeric loss in mammalian cells, resulting from the inhibition of the enzyme telomerase.

### 4.4. Doxorubicin and etoposide

Doxorubicin (also called Adriamycin, CAS No. 23214-92-8) and etoposide (CAS No. 33419-42-0) are both topoisomerase II inhibitors with anticancer properties. As is the case with BLM and cisplatin, doxorubicin can also bind to human telomeric repeats. In effect, it was demonstrated that this drug binds to the human telomeric sequence 5'-d[GGG(TTAGGG)(3)]-3' (21-mer), assuming a G-quadruplex structure in the presence of K(+) [84]. It has been found that doxorubicin inhibits telomerase activity and shortens mean telomere length in human hepatoma cells [85]. Thus, it has been proposed that telomerase inhibition and telomere shortening by doxorubicin may contribute to its efficiency in the treatment of hepatocellular carcinoma. However, doxorubicin showed no effect on telomerase or telomere length in human ovarian cancer cells [86], induces telomere dysfunction (as determined by the presence of end-to-end chromosome fusions and end breaks by conventional staining with Giemsa, not telomere FISH) and decreases telomerase activity but has no effect on telomere length in breast tumor cells [87], and decreases telomerase activity in several human breast and stomach cancer cell lines [88]. Thus, the effect of doxorubicin on telomeres depends on the cell type. Moreover, it has been shown that doxorubicin induces senescence or apoptosis in rat neonatal cardio-myocites by regulating the expression levels of the telomere binding factors 1 and 2: High-dose doxorubicin strongly reduces TRF2 expression while enhancing TRF1 expression, and it

http://dx.doi.org/10.5772/64928

determines early apoptosis, whereas low-dose doxorubicin induces downregulation of both TRF2 and TRF1 [89]. The exposed cells maintain telomere dysfunction and a senescent phenotype over time and undergo late death. Therefore, this study suggests that doxorubicin induces telomere dysfunction at the molecular level by regulating the expression levels of TRF1 and TRF2, both of them being part of the shelterin complex. A few years ago, it was reported that doxorubicin and etoposide induce progressive telomere shortening (assessed by flow-fluorescence in situ hybridization and Southern blotting) in human mesenchymal stem cells (MSCs), obtained from bone marrow (BM) cells from normal adults and grown in the presence of platelet lysates [90]. A year later, Li et al. reported that the treatment of normal human T lymphocytes and fibroblasts with doxorubicin or etoposide led to significant shortening of telomeres, down-regulation of telomerase activity, diminished expression of telomerase reverse transcriptase (hTERT) and the telomere binding proteins TPP1 and POT1 and telomere dysfunction in these cells [91]. Therefore, both topoisomerase II poisons doxorubicin and etoposide, induce telomere dysfunction. However, recent data reported by Liu et al. showed that etoposide alone does not specifically affects telomeres of a mouse spermatogonial cell line and that this drug did not induce telomere dysfunction in these cells [68], but in combination with BLM and cisplatinum, etoposide produces telomere shortening in rat male germ cells [92]. In addition, it was demonstrated that etoposide did not affect telomere length in the neuroblastoma cell line SHSY5Y, with very short telomeres and the acute lymphoblastic T cell line 1301, which displays extremely long telomeres [93]. Thus, the effect of etoposide on telomeres depends on the cell type.

### 4.5. 5-azacytidine (5-AZA)

5-azacytidine (5-AZA, Ladakamycin, CAS No. 320-67-2) and its deoxy derivative 5-aza-2'deoxycytidine (Decitabine, CAS No. 2353-33-5) are demethylating compounds (inhibit DNA methyltransferases) with anticancer properties, usually employed against myelodysplastic syndrome and acute myeloid leukemia [94]. It has been shown that 5-aza-2'deoxycytidine, either alone or in combination with trichostatin A, induces up-regulation of shelterin genes, which leads to telomere elongation in breast cancer cell lines [95]. In addition, 5-AZA was found to induce DNA damage at telomeres and telomere dysfunction in acute myeloid leukemia cell lines [96]. Telomere dysfunction was coupled with telomere shortening, diminished TERT expression and apoptosis in the exposed cells [96]. Thus, these authors suggested that another mechanism (besides DNA demethylation) by which 5-AZA exerts its anticancer activity is telomere dysfunction [96]. On the contrary, Choudhury et al., using the glioblastoma cell line SF-767, found that 5-AZA caused significant changes in DNA methylation of subtelomeric regions of chromosomes but did not modify the telomere length in these cells [97]. Thus, further studies will be needed to clarify the effect of this compound on telomeres.

### 4.6. Gemcitabine

It has been recently reported that the cytidine analog gemcitabine (2′, 2′-diflurodeoxycytidine) (CAS No. 95058-81-4), an effective anticancer drug against several types of solid tumors, including colorectal, breast, pancreatic, renal and lung cancer [98], causes telomere attrition or shortening in Hela cells, by increasing the level and stability of TRF2 [99], that is required for the Xeroderma pigmentosum group F protein (XPF)-dependent telomere loss or degradation. By increasing TRF2 expression, gemcitabine enhances XPF activity, and because XPF is a nuclease, binding of the nuclease to telomeres may lead to inappropriate excision of telomeric DNA. The anticancer effect of gemcitabine is due to the incorporation of the active derivative compound dFdCTP into DNA in proliferating cells, leading to inhibition of DNA synthesis and repair. Thus, the above findings by Su et al. [99] suggest that the promotion of telomere attrition by induction of TRF2 is a new mechanism of action of gemcitabine against cancer. This effect of gemcitabine seems to be independent of telomerase, since this drug had no effect on telomerase activity in Hela cells 3 days after treatment. No further studies have been made to analyze the effect of gemcitabine on mammalian telomeres.

### 4.7. C-1027

The enediyne antibiotic C-1027 or Lidamycin (CAS No. 120177-69-7) is a new kind of macromolecular antitumor antibiotics, produced by *Streptomyces globisporus* in soil, consisting of a noncovalently bound apoprotein and a labile chromophore which is responsible for most of the biological activities [100-102]. This drug is a potent anticancer drug with radiomimetic properties, which is being currently evaluated in Phase II clinical trials [103]. Several years ago, it was demonstrated in cultured human colon carcinoma HCT116 cells exposed to C-1027 that this drug induces telomere fusions (i.e., chromosomes joined end to end at their telomeres or fused together after complete loss of telomere sequences) in these cells [104]. Therefore, C-1027 induces short-term telomere dysfunction in human cells. No further studies on the effects of C-1027 on telomere stability have been performed so far.

### 4.8. ICRF-193

ICRF-193 ([meso-2, 3-bis (2, 6-dioxopiperazin-4-yl) butane], CAS No. 21416-68-2) is a topoisomerase II catalytic inhibitor [105]. Two recent publications deal with the effect of ICRF-193 on telomeres [106, 107]. These studies show that this drug induces DNA damage at telomeres (as assessed by colocalization of telomere PNA-FISH signals and immunofluorescence of 53BP1 foci) [106] and telomere dysfunction in the HT1080 fibrosarcoma cell lines [106] and telomere shortening in mice cells [107]. In particular, it was found that ICRF-193 induces damage at telomeres properly capped by TRF2 but not by POT1 [106]. Moreover, ICRF-193 treatment blocks ALT-associated phenotypes in vitro and inhibits ALT cell proliferation in mice [107], which suggests that this drug could be used to prevent cell proliferation in cancer cells with an ALT mechanism of telomere elongation. No further studies on the effects of ICRF-193 on telomere stability have been performed so far.

### 4.9. Melphalan

Melphalan, L-phenylalanine mustard, L-PAM, Alkeran or L-Sarcolysine (CAS No. 148-82-3) is a chemotherapeutic drug belonging to the class of nitrogen mustard alkylating agents [108]. It has been reported that melphalan has no effect on telomerase activity in human testicular cancer cells [82]. More recently, by studying the induction and persistence of chromosome aberrations in bone marrow and spleen cells of p53+/- (and wild type) mice exposed for 4, 13, or 26 weeks to 2 mg/kg melphalan (MLP), Sgura et al. [109] were able to demonstrate that this drug induces telomere shortening in bone marrow cells of wild-type mice, while in p53+/- mice the exposure to this compound induces telomere elongation. No further studies on the effect of melphalan on telomeres have been reported so far.

### 4.10. 5-fluorouracil (5-FU)

In the case of 5-fluorouracil (CAS No. 51-21-8), a thymine analog with anticancer properties commonly used against several types of solid tumors, including breast, colorectal, pancreatic, skin and cervical carcinoma [110], there is no information about its effects on telomeres as a single drug, since this compound is usually employed in chemotherapy in combination with several drugs. Thus, for example, it has been reported that, combined with cisplatin, 5-FU increases telomerase activity and causes long-term telomere elongation in colorectal carcinoma cells (LoVo and DLD-1 cell lines) [111]. It is interesting to mention that it has been recently demonstrated that overexpression of a human telomerase reverse transcriptase polypeptide (hTERT)C27, which induces telomere dysfunction by promoting end-to-end chromosome fusions, sensitizes HeLa cells and nasopharyngeal carcinoma cells to 5-FU cytotoxic effects [112, 113]. Thus, despite the fact that 5-FU does not induce telomere dysfunction, these recent studies suggest that combinational therapy of this drug with hTERTC27 may provide a novel approach to treat cancer.

## 5. Telomere instability induced by anticancer drugs: Conclusions and future prospects

Even though the studies performed so far demonstrate that a lot of work needs to be done in order to fully understand the effects of anticancer drugs on telomere stability and function, some important conclusions can be drawn from these studies.

1. For some drugs (BLM, SN. STZ, paclitaxel, 5-azacytidine, etc.) it is clearly established that they induce telomere instability (either by chromosome end loss or telomere dysfunction) in the short- and/or the long-term in mammalian cells, whereas for most of the anticancer drugs this effect remains to be determined. In fact, the literature reviewed in this chapter clearly shows that there are very few studies concerning the long-term effect of anticancer drugs on telomeres. Most of these studies were performed in the last few years. Moreover, little is currently known about the effect of several chemotherapeutic agents (for example, cyclophosphamide, mitomycin C and melphalan) on mammalian telomere dynamics, including potential effects on telomere length, structure, function, telomerase activity, and telomere shelterin proteins.

2. For some drugs (for example, 5-fluorouracil) it remains to be determined if they induce telomere instability per se, since the studies performed so far were carried out using these drugs in combination with other drugs, but not in a single form.

3. For several anticancer drugs (i.e., doxorubicin, etoposide, 5-azacytidine), published data on the effects of telomeres are contradictory. Thus, additional studies will be needed to clarify this issue.

4. Some drugs (i.e., 5-azacytidine and trichostatin A) could exert its anticancer effect by inducing telomere lengthening instead of shorthening or erosion. Telomere elongation induced by these drugs may have the effect of stabilizing the telomere thus reducing the amount of genetic damage the cell will undergo, thereby stopping the clonal evolution of the cancer cell population. As a result, these tumors may be more susceptible to further treatment. Alternatively, the elongation of telomeres in cancer cells may give rise to chemoresistant tumors.

5. Some anticancer drugs -like paclitaxel- could exert their anticancer effect by inducing telomere fusions. Thus, this drug could be used to enhance chemosensitivity in cells with dysfunctional telomeres.

6. Finally, regardless of the underlying mechanism involved in the long-term telomere instability induced by some anticancer drugs, the data available raise concern about the potential risks of a long-term chemotherapy based on these drugs. Damage to telomeres induced by cytostatic therapy theoretically could generate telomere shortening and, subsequently, induce an additional genomic instability in neoplastic cells, this effect causing undesirable side effects, including secondary malignancies in long-term survivors of cancer.

In summary, further studies will be needed to fully elucidate the effects of anticancer drugs on telomere stability. Depending on the drug, these studies should be aimed at determining whether it induces short- and long-term telomere instability or not, and if this telomere instability is due to chromosome breakage or telomere dysfunction. Undoubtedly, these studies will contribute to a better understanding of the effects of the anticancer drugs on mammalian telomeres. This information will be of great importance to understand the genomic instability associated with chemotherapy regimens.

## Acknowledgements

The author acknowledges the financial support of the Consejo Nacional de Investigaciones Científicas y Técnicas (CONICET, grant PIP No. 0182), Comisión de Investigaciones Científicas de la Provincia de Buenos Aires (CICPBA), and University of La Plata (UNLP) from Argentina.

## Author details

Alejandro D. Bolzán*

Address all correspondence to: abolzan@imbice.gov.ar; adbolzan64@gmail.com

Laboratorio de Citogenética y Mutagénesis, Instituto Multidisciplinario de Biología Celular (IMBICE, CCT-CONICET La Plata – CICPBA-UNLP), La Plata, Argentina

## References

[1] Muller HJ: The remaking of chromosomes. Collecting Net. 1938;13:181-198.

[2] Zakian VA: Telomeres: beginning to understand the end. Science 1995;270(5242): 1601-1607. DOI: 10.1126/science.270.5242.1601

[3] Blackburn EH: Switching and signaling at the telomere. Cell 2001;106(6):661-673. DOI:10.1016/S0092-8674(01)00492-5

[4] Meyne J, Ratliff RL, Moyzis RK: Conservation of the human telomere sequence (TTAGGG)n among vertebrates. Proc. Natl. Acad. Sci. USA 1989;86(18):7049-7053

[5] Meyne J, Baker RJ, Hobart HH, Hsu TC, Ryder OA, Ward OG et al.: Distribution of nontelomeric sites of (TTAGGG)n telomeric sequences in vertebrate chromosomes. Chromosoma 1990;99(1):3-10.

[6] Moyzis RK, Buckingham JM, Cram LS, Dani M, Deaven LL, Jones MD et al.: A highly conserved repetitive DNA sequence, (TTAGGG)n, present at the telomeres of human chromosomes. Proc. Natl. Acad. Sci. USA 1988;85(18):6622-6626.

[7] Schmutz I, de Lange, T: Shelterin. Current Biology 2016; 26(10):R397-399. DOI: 10.1016/j.cub.2016.01.056

[8] Palm W, de Lange T: How shelterin protects mammalian telomeres. Annu. Rev. Genet. 2008;42:301-334. DOI: 10.1146/annurev.genet.41.110306.130350

[9] O'Sullivan RJ, Karlseder J: Telomeres: protecting chromosomes against genome instability. Nat. Rev. Mol. Cell Biol. 2010;11(3):171-181. DOI: 10.1038/nrm2848

[10] Wright WE, Tesmer VM, Huffman KE, Levene SD, Shay JW: Normal human chromosomes have long G-rich telomeric overhangs at one end. Genes Dev. 1997;11(21): 2801-2809.

[11] Allsopp RC, Vaziri H, Patterson C, Goldstein S, Younglai EV, Futcher AB et al.: Telomere length predicts replicative capacity of human fibroblasts. Proc. Natl. Acad. Sci. U S A. 1992;89(21):10114-10118.

[12] Schmitt H, Blin N, Zankl H, Scherthan H: Telomere length variation in normal and malignant human tissues. Genes Chromosom. Cancer 1994;11(3):171-177.

[13] Bolzán AD, Páez GL, Bianchi MS, Bianchi NO: Analysis of telomeric repeats and telomerase activity in human colon carcinoma cells with gene amplification. Cancer Genet. Cytogenet. 2000;120(2):166-170. DOI: 10.1016/S0165-4608(00)00209-0

[14] Kim NW, Piatyszek MA, Prowse KR, Harley CB, West MD, Ho PL et al.: Specific association of human telomerase activity with immortal cells and cancer. Science 1994;266(5193):2011-2015. DOI: 10.1126/science.7605428

[15] Azzalin CM, Lingner J: Telomeres: the silence is broken. Cell Cycle 2008;7(9): 1161-1165. DOI:10.4161/cc.7.9.5836

[16] Luke B, Lingner J: TERRA: telomeric repeat-containing RNA. EMBO J. 2009;28(17): 2503-2510. DOI: 10.1038/emboj

[17] Feuerhahn S, Iglesias N, Panza A, Porro A, Lingner J: TERRA biogenesis, turnover and implications for function. FEBS Lett. 2010;584(17):3812-3818. DOI: 10.1016/j.febslet

[18] Cusanelli E, Chartrand P: Telomeric repeat-containing RNA TERRA: a noncoding RNA connecting telomere biology to genome integrity. Front. Genet. 2015;6(143):1-9. DOI: 10.3389/fgene

[19] Arnoult N, Karlseder J: Complex interactions between the DNA-damage response and mammalian telomeres. Nat. Struct. Mol. Biol. 2015;22(11):859-866. DOI: 10.1038/nsmb.3092

[20] Artandi SE, DePinho RA:Telomeres and telomerase in cancer. Carcinogenesis 2010;31(1):9-18. DOI: 10.1093/carcin/bgp268

[21] Chiodi I, Belgiovine C, Mondello C: Telomerase and telomeric proteins: A life beyond telomeres. In A.N. Gagnon, editor. Telomerase: Composition, Functions and Clinical Implications. 1st ed. New York: Nova Science; 2010 p. 35-58

[22] Blackburn EH: Telomeres and telomerase: their mechanisms of action and the effects of altering their functions. FEBS Lett. 2005;579(4):859-862. DOI: 10.1016/j.febslet.2004.11.036

[23] Chan SR, Blackburn EH: Telomeres and telomerase. Philos. Trans. R. Soc. Lond. B. Biol. Sci. 2004;359(1441):109-121. DOI: 10.1098/rstb.2003.1370

[24] Masutomi K, Yu EY, Khurts S, Ben-Porath I, Currier JL, Metz GB et al.: Telomerase maintains telomere structure in normal human cells. Cell 2003;114(2):241-253. DOI: 10.1016/S0092-8674(03)00550-6

[25] Draskovic I, Londono-Vallejo A: Telomere recombination and the ALT pathway: a therapeutic perspective for cancer. Curr Pharm Des. 2014;20(41):6466-6471. DOI: 10.2174/1381612820666140630085857

[26] Bolzán AD: Chromosomal aberrations involving telomeres and interstitial telomeric sequences. Mutagenesis 2012;27(1):1-15. DOI: 10.1093/mutage/ger052

[27] Murnane JP: Telomere dysfunction and chromosome instability. Mutat. Res. 2012;730(1-2):28-36. DOI: 10.1016/j.mrfmmm.2011.04.008

[28] Bouffler SD, Morgan WF, Pandita TK, Slijepcevic P: The involvement of telomeric sequences in chromosomal aberrations. Mutat. Res. 1996;366(2):129-135. DOI: 10.1016/S0165-1110(96)90033-0

[29] Bolzán AD: Cytogenetic evaluation of telomere dysfunction: Chromosomal aberrations involving telomeres and interstitial telomeric sequences. In: L. Mancini, editor. Telomeres: Function, Shortening and Lengthening. 1st ed. New York: Nova Science Publishers Inc.; 2009 p. 133-185.

[30] Bolzán AD, Bianchi MS: Telomeres, interstitial telomeric repeat sequences, and chromosomal aberrations. Mutat. Res. 2006;612(3):189-214. DOI: 10.1016/j.mrrev.2005.12.003

[31] Bailey SM, Cornforth MN: Telomeres and DNA double-strand breaks: ever the twain shall meet? Cell. Mol. Life Sci. 2007;64(22):2956-2964. DOI: 10.1007/s00018-007-7242-4

[32] Denchi EL: Give me a break: How telomeres suppress the DNA damage response. DNA Repair 2009; 8(9):1118-1126. DOI: 10.1016/j.dnarep.2009.04.013

[33] Hemann MT, Strong MA, Hao LY, Greider CW: The shortest telomere, not average telomere length, is critical for cell viability and chromosome stability. Cell 2001;107(1):67-77. DOI: 10.1016/S0092-8674(01)00504-9

[34] Espejel S, Franco S, Rodríguez-Perales S, Bouffler SD, Cigudosa JC, Blasco MA: Mammalian Ku86 mediates chromosomal fusions and apoptosis caused by critically short telomeres. EMBO J. 2002;21(9): 2207-2219. DOI: 10.1093/emboj/21.9.2207

[35] Deng W, Tsao SW, Guan XY, Lucas JN, Si HX, Leung CS et al.: Distinct profiles of critically short telomeres are a key determinant of different chromosome aberrations in immortalized human cells: whole-genome evidence from multiple cell lines. Oncogene 2004;23(56):9090-9101. DOI: 10.1038/sj.onc.1208119

[36] Soler D, Genesca A, Arnedo G, Egozcue J, Tusell L: Telomere dysfunction drives chromosomal instability in human mammary epithelial cells. Genes Chromosomes Cancer 2005;44(4):339-350. DOI: 10.1002/gcc.20244

[37] Sahin E, Colla S, Liesa M, Moslehi J, Müller FL, Guo M et al.: Telomere dysfunction induces metabolic and mitochondrial compromise. Nature 2011;470(7334):359-365. DOI: 10.1038/nature09787

[38] Bojovic B, Crowe DL: Telomere dysfuction promotes metastasis in a TERC null mouse model of head and neck cancer. Mol. Cancer Res. 2011;9(7):901-913. DOI: 10.1158/1541-7786.MCR-10-0345

[39] Ma H, Zhou Z, Wei S, Liu Z, Pooley KA, Dunning AM et al.: Shortened telomere length is associated with increased risk of cancer: a meta-analysis. PLoS One 2011;6(6):e20466. DOI: 10.1371/journal.pone.0020466

[40] Cao K, Blair CD, Faddah DA, Kieckhaefer JE, Olive M, Erdos MR et al.: Progerin and telomere dysfunction collaborate to trigger cellular senescence in normal human fibroblasts. J. Clin. Invest. 2011; 121(7):2833-2844. DOI: 10.1172/JCI43578

[41] Donate LE, Blasco MA: Telomeres in cancer and ageing. Philos. Trans. R. Soc. Lond. B Biol. Sci. 2011; 366(1561):76-84. DOI: 10.1098/rstb.2010.0291

[42] Raynaud CM, Sabatier L, Philipot O, Olaussen KA, Soria JC: Telomere length, telomeric proteins and genomic instability during the multistep carcinogenic process. Critical Rev. Oncol. Hematol. 2008;66(2):99-117. DOI: 10.1016/j.critrevonc.2007.11.006

[43] Stohr BA, Xu L, Blackburn EH: The terminal telomeric DNA sequence determines the mechanism of dysfunctional telomere fusion. Mol. Cell 2010;39(2):307-314. DOI: 10.1016/j.molcel.2010.06.020.

[44] Chavez A, Tsou AM, Johnson FB: Telomeres do the (un)twist: helicase actions at chromosome termini. Biochim. Biophys. Acta 2009;1792(4):329-340. DOI: 10.1016/j.bbadis.2009.02.008

[45] Paeschke K, McDonald KR, Zakian VA: Telomeres: structures in need of unwinding. FEBS Lett. 2010; 584(17):3760-3772. DOI: 10.1016/j.febslet.2010.07.007

[46] von Zglinicki T, Saretzki G, Docke W, Lotze C: Mild hyperoxia shortens telomeres and inhibits proliferation of fibroblasts: a model for senescence? Exp. Cell Res. 1995;220(1):186-193. DOI: 10.1006/excr.1995.1305

[47] Kawanishi S, Oikawa S: Mechanism of telomere shortening by oxidative stress. Ann. N. Y. Acad. Sci. 2004;1019:278-284. DOI: 10.1196/annals.1297.047

[48] Blasco MA, Lee HW, Hande MP, Samper E, Lansdorp PM, DePinho RA et al.: Telomere shortening and tumor formation by mouse cells lacking telomerase RNA. Cell 1997;91(1):25-34. DOI: 10.1016/S0092-8674(01)80006-4

[49] Ayouaz A, Raynaud C, Heride C, Revaud D, Sabatier L: Telomeres: Hallmarks of radiosensitivity. Biochimie 2008;90(1):60-72. DOI: 10.1016/j.biochi.2007.09.011

[50] Chen J, Stubbe J: Bleomycins: towards better therapeutics. Nat. Rev. Cancer 2005;5(2): 102-112. DOI: 10.1038/nrc1547

[51] Povirk LF, Austin MJ: Genotoxicity of bleomycin. Mutat. Res. 1991;257(2):127-143. DOI: 10.1016/0165-1110(91)90022-N

[52] Bolzán AD, Bianchi MS: Genotoxicity of streptonigrin: a review. Mutat. Res. 2001;488(1):25-37. DOI: 10.1016/S1383-5742(00)00062-4

[53] Bolzán AD, Bianchi MS: Genotoxicity of streptozotocin. Mutat. Res. 2002;512(2-3): 121-134. DOI: 10.1016/S1383-5742(02)00044-3

[54] Bolzán AD: Genotoxic effects of Streptozotocin. In: Gauthier EL, editor. Streptozotocin: Uses, Mechanism of Action and Side Effects. 1st ed. New York: Nova Science Publishers Inc.; 2014. p. 99-120.

[55] Bolzán AD, Bianchi MS: Detection of incomplete chromosome elements and interstitial fragments induced by bleomycin in hamster cells using a telomeric PNA probe. Mutat. Res. 2004;554(1-2):1-8. DOI: 10.1016/j.mrfmmm.2004.02.016

[56] Bolzán AD, Bianchi MS: Analysis of streptonigrin-induced incomplete chromosome elements and interstitial fragments in Chinese hamster cells using a telomeric PNA probe. Environ. Mol. Mutagen. 2004;44(4):277-282. DOI: 10.1002/em.20051

[57] Bolzán AD, Bianchi MS: Analysis of streptozotocin-induced incomplete chromosome elements and excess acentric fragments in Chinese hamster cells using a telomeric PNA probe. Mutat. Res. 2005;570(2):237-244. DOI: 10.1016/j.mrfmmm.2004.11.008

[58] Díaz-Flaqué MC, Bianchi MS, Bolzán AD: A comparative analysis of bleomycin-induced incomplete chromosome elements in two mammalian cell lines using a telomeric PNA probe. Environ. Mol. Mutagen. 2006;47(9):674-681. DOI: 10.1002/em.20254

[59] Benkhaled L, Xunclá M, Caballín MR, Barrios L, Barquinero JF: Induction of complete and incomplete chromosome aberrations by bleomycin in human lymphocytes. Mutat. Res. 2008;637(1-2):134-141. DOI: 10.1016/j.mrfmmm.2007.07.013

[60] Paviolo NS, Quiroga IY, Castrogiovanni DC, Bianchi MS, Bolzán AD: Telomere instability is present in the progeny of mammalian cells exposed to bleomycin. Mutat. Res. 2012;734(1-2):5-11. DOI: 10.1016/j.mrfmmm.2012.04.008

[61] Paviolo NS, Castrogiovanni DC, Bolzán AD: The radiomimetic compound streptonigrin induces persistent telomere dysfunction in mammalian cells. Mutat. Res. 2014;760:16-23. DOI: 10.1016/j.mrfmmm.2013.11.009

[62] Paviolo NS, Santiñaque FF, Castrogiovanni DC, Folle GA, Bolzán AD: The methylating agent streptozotocin induces persistent telomere dysfunction in mammalian cells. Mutat. Res. 2015;794:17-24. DOI: 10.1016/j.mrgentox.2015.09.007

[63] Nguyen TV, Murray VA: Human telomeric DNA sequences are a major target for the antitumour drug bleomycin. J. Biol. Inorg. Chem. 2012;17(1):1-9. DOI: 10.1007/s00775-011-0818-3.

[64] Nguyen HT, Murray V: The DNA sequence specificity of bleomycin cleavage in telomeric sequences in human cells. J. Biol. Inorg. Chem. 2012;17(8):1209-1215. DOI: 10.1007/s00775-012-0934-8.

[65] Arutyunyan R, Gebhart E, Hovhannisyan G, Greulich KO, Rapp A: Comet-FISH using peptide nucleic acid probes detects telomeric repeats in DNA damaged by bleomycin and mitomycin C proportional to general DNA damage. Mutagenesis 2004;19(5):403-408. DOI: 10.1093/mutage/geh049

[66] Arutyunyan R, Rapp A, Greulich KO, Hovhannisyan G, Haroutiunian S, Gebhart E: Fragility of telomeres after bleomycin and cisplatin combined treatment measured in human leukocytes with the Comet-FISH technique. Exp Oncol. 2005;27(1):38-42.

[67] Hovhannisyan G, Rapp A, Arutyunyan R, Greulich KO, Gebhart E: Comet-assay in combination with PNA-FISH detects mutagen-induced DNA damage and specific repeat sequences in the damaged DNA of transformed cells. Int. J. Mol. Med. 2005;15(3):437-442 DOI: 10.3892/ijmm.15.3.437

[68] Liu M, Hales BF, Robaire B: Effects of four chemotherapeutic agents, bleomycin, etoposide, cisplatin, and cyclophosphamide, on DNA damage and telomeres in a mouse spermatogonial cell line. Biol. Reprod. 2014;90(4):1-10. DOI: 10.1095/biolreprod.114.117754

[69] Mekhail TM, Markman M: Paclitaxel in cancer therapy. Expert. Opin. Pharmacother. 2002;3(6):755-766. DOI: 10.1517/14656566.3.6.755

[70] Schiff PB, Fant J, Horwitz SB: Promotion of microtubule assembly in vitro by taxol. Nature 1979;277(5698):665-667.

[71] Schiff PB, Horwitz SB: Taxol stabilizes microtubules in mouse fibroblast cells. Proc. Natl. Acad. Sci. USA 1980;77(3):1561-1565.

[72] Multani AS, Li C, Ozen M, Yadav M, Yu DF, Wallace S et al.: Paclitaxel and water-soluble poly (L-glutamic acid)-paclitaxel, induce direct chromosomal abnormalities and cell death in a murine metastatic melanoma cell line. Anticancer Res. 1997;17(6D):4269-4274.

[73] Multani AS, Li C, Ozen M, Imam AS, Wallace S, Pathak S: Cell-killing by paclitaxel in a metastatic murine melanoma cell line is mediated by extensive telomere erosion with no decrease in telomerase activity. Oncol. Rep. 1999;6(1):39-44. DOI: 10.3892/or.6.1.39

[74] Multani AS, Chandra J, Mcconker J, Sen S, Cabral TF, Pathak S: Cell death in paclitaxel-dependent chinese hamster ovary cells is initiated by the loss of telomeric DNA repeats. Oncol. Res. 1999;11(10):455-460. DOI:

[75] Mo Y, Gan Y, Song S, Johnston J, Xiao X, Wientjes MG et al.: Simultaneous targeting of telomeres and telomerase as a cancer therapeutic approach. Cancer Res. 2003;63(3):579-585.

[76] Johnston JS, Johnson A, Gan Y, Wientjes MG, Au JL: Synergy between 3'-azido-3'-deoxythymidine and paclitaxel in human pharynx FaDu cells. Pharm. Res. 2003 ;20(7):957-961.

[77] Park JE, Woo SR, Kang CM, Juhn KM, Ju YJ, Shin HJ et al.: Paclitaxel stimulates chromosomal fusion and instability in cells with dysfunctional telomeres: implication in multinucleation and chemosensitization. Biochem. Biophys. Res. Commun. 2011;404(2):615-621. DOI: 10.1016/j.bbrc.2010.12.018

[78] Ishibashi T, Lippard SJ: Telomere loss in cells treated with cisplatin. Proc. Natl. Acad. Sci. U.S.A. 1998;95(8):4219-4223.

[79] Paul M, Murray V: Use of an automated capillary DNA sequencer to investigate the interaction of cisplatin with telomeric DNA sequences. Biomed. Chromatogr. 2012;26(3):350-354. DOI: 10.1002/bmc.1664

[80] Murray V, Kandasamy N: The sequence specificity of the anti-tumour drug, cisplatin, in telomeric DNA sequences compared with consecutive guanine DNA sequences. Anticancer Agents Med. Chem. 2012;12(3):177-181. DOI: 10.2174/187152012800228742

[81] Nguyen HT, Galea AM, Murray V. The interaction of cisplatin with a human telomeric DNA sequence containing seventeen tandem repeats. Bioorg. Med. Chem. Lett. 2013;23(4):1041-1045. DOI: 10.1016/j.bmcl.2012.12.021

[82] Burger AM, Double JA, Newell DR: Inhibition of telomerase activity by cisplatin in human testicular cancer cells. Eur. J. Cancer. 1997;33(4):638-644. DOI: 10.1016/S0959-8049(96)00521-7

[83] Błasiak J, Kadłubek M, Kowalik J, Romanowicz-Makowska H, Pertyński T: Inhibition of telomerase activity in endometrial cancer cells by selenium-cisplatin conjugate despite suppression of its DNA-damaging activity by sodium ascorbate. Teratog. Carcinog. Mutagen. 2002;22(1):73-82.

[84] Manet I, Manoli F, Zambelli B, Andreano G, Masi A, Cellai L et al.: Affinity of the anthracycline antitumor drugs Doxorubicin and Sabarubicin for human telomeric G-quadruplex structures. Phys. Chem. Chem. Phys. 2011;13(2):540-551. DOI: 10.1039/c0cp00898b

[85] Zhang RG, Guo LX, Wang XW, Xie H: Telomerase inhibition and telomere loss in BEL-7404 human hepatoma cells treated with doxorubicin. World J. Gastroenterol. 2002;8(5):827-831. DOI: 10.3748/wjg.v8.i5.827

[86] Kiyozuka Y, Yamamoto D, Yang J, Uemura Y, Senzaki H, Adachi S et al.: Correlation of chemosensitivity to anticancer drugs and telomere length, telomerase activity and telomerase RNA expression in human ovarian cancer cells. Anticancer Res. 2000;20(1A):203-212.

[87] Elmore LW, Rehder CW, Di X, McChesney PA, Jackson-Cook CK, Gewirtz DA et al.: Adriamycin-induced senescence in breast tumor cells involves functional p53 and telomere dysfunction. J. Biol. Chem. 2002;277(38):35509-35515. DOI: 10.1074/jbc.M205477200

[88] Park KH, Rha SY, Kim CH, Kim TS, Yoo NC, Kim JH et al.: Telomerase activity and telomere lengths in various cell lines: changes of telomerase activity can be another method for chemosensitivity evaluation. Int. J. Oncol. 1998;13(3):489-495. DOI: 10.3892/ijo.13.3.489

[89] Spallarossa P, Altieri P, Aloi C, Garibaldi S, Barisione C, Ghigliotti G et al.: Doxorubicin induces senescence or apoptosis in rat neonatal cardiomyocytes by regulating the

expression levels of the telomere binding factors 1 and 2. Am. J. Physiol. Heart Circ. Physiol. 2009;297(6):H2169-2181. DOI: 10.1152/ajpheart.00068

[90] Buttiglieri S, Ruella M, Risso A, Spatola T, Silengo L, Avvedimento EV et al.: The aging effect of chemotherapy on cultured human mesenchymal stem cells. Exp. Hematol. 2011;39(12):1171-1181. DOI: 10.1016/j.exphem.2011.08.009

[91] Li P, Hou M, Lou F, Björkholm M, Xu D: Telomere dysfunction induced by chemotherapeutic agents and radiation in normal human cells. Int. J. Biochem. Cell Biol. 2012;44(9):1531-1540. DOI: 10.1016/j.biocel.2012.06.020

[92] Liu M, Maselli J, Hales BF, Robaire B: The effects of chemotherapy with bleomycin, etoposide, and cis-platinum on telomeres in rat male germ cells. Andrology 2015;3(6):1104-1112. DOI: 10.1111/andr.12102

[93] Jeyapalan J, Leake A, Ahmed S, Saretzki G, Tilby M, von Zglinicki T: The role of telomeres in Etoposide induced tumor cell death. Cell Cycle 2004;3(9):1169-1176.

[94] Christman JK: 5-Azacytidine and 5-aza-2'-deoxycytidine as inhibitors of DNA methylation: mechanistic studies and their implications for cancer therapy. Oncogene 2002;21(35):5483-5495. DOI: 10.1038/sj.onc.1205699

[95] Motevalli A, Yasaei H, Virmouni SA, Slijepcevic P, Roberts T: The effect of chemotherapeutic agents on telomere length maintenance in breast cancer cell lines. Breast Cancer Res. Treat. 2014;145(3):581-591. DOI: 10.1007/s10549-014-2975-x

[96] Zhang X, Li B, de Jonge N, Björkholm M, Xu D: The DNA methylation inhibitor induces telomere dysfunction and apoptosis of leukemia cells that is attenuated by telomerase over-expression. Oncotarget 2015;6(7):4888-4900. DOI: 10.18632/oncotarget.2917

[97] Choudhury SR, Cui Y, Milton JR, Li J, Irudayaraj J: Selective increase in subtelomeric DNA methylation: an epigenetic biomarker for malignant glioma. Clin. Epigenetics. 2015;7:107. DOI: 10.1186/s13148-015-0140-y.

[98] Grindey GB, Hertel LW, Plunkett W: Cytotoxicity and antitumor activity of 2', 2'-difluorodeoxycytidine (Gemcitabine). Cancer Invest. 1990;8(2):313.

[99] Su CH, Chu WC, Lan KH, Li CP, Chao Y, Lin HC et al.: Gemcitabine causes telomere attrition by stabilizing TRF2. Eur. J. Cancer. 2012;48(18):3465-3474. DOI: 10.1016/j.ejca.2012.04.015

[100] Hu JL, Xue YC, Xie MY, Zhang R, Otani T, Minami Y et al.: A new macromolecular antitumor antibiotic, C-1027. I. Discovery, taxonomy of producing organism, fermentation and biological activity. J. Antibiot. (Tokyo) 1988;41:1575-1579.

[101] Otani T, Minami Y, Marunaka T, Zhang R, Xie MY: A new macromolecular antitumor antibiotic, C-1027. II. Isolation and physico-chemical properties. J. Antibiot. (Tokyo) 1988;41:1580-1585.

[102] Zhen YS, Ming XY, Yu B, Otani T, Saito H, Yamada Y. A new macromolecular antitumor antibiotic, C-1027. III. Antitumor activity. J. Antibiot. (Tokyo) 1989;42:1294-1298.

[103] Chen Y, Yu D, Zhang C, Shang B, He H, Chen J et al.: Lidamycin inhibits tumor initiating cells of hepatocellular carcinoma Huh7 through GSK3β/β-catenin pathway. Mol. Carcinog. 2015;54(1):1-8. DOI: 10.1002/mc.22069

[104] McHugh MM, Gawron LS, Matsui S, Beerman TA: The antitumor enediyne C-1027 alters cell cycle progression and induces chromosomal aberrations and telomere dysfunction. Cancer Res. 2005;65(12):5344-5351. DOI: 10.1158/0008-5472.CAN-05-0015

[105] Downes CS, Clarke DJ, Mullinger AM, Giménez-Abián JF, Creighton AM, Johnson RT: A topoisomerase II-dependent G2 cycle checkpoint in mammalian cells. Nature 1994;372(6505):467-470. DOI: 10.1038/372467a0

[106] Chen L, Zhu X, Zou Y, Xing J, Gilson E, Lu Y et al.: The topoisomerase II catalytic inhibitor ICRF-193 preferentially targets telomeres that are capped by TRF2. Am. J. Physiol. Cell. Physiol. 2015;308(5):C372-377. DOI: 10.1152/ajpcell.00321.2014

[107] Hsieh MH, Tsai CH, Lin CC, Li TK, Hung TW, Chang LT et al.: Topoisomerase II inhibition suppresses the proliferation of telomerase-negative cancers. Cell. Mol. Life Sci. 2015;72(9):1825-1837. DOI: 10.1007/s00018-014-1783-0

[108] Dronkert ML, Kanaar R: Repair of DNA interstrand cross-links. Mutat. Res. 2001;486(4):217-247. DOI:10.1016/S0921-8777(01)00092-1

[109] Sgura A, De Amicis A, Stronati L, Cinelli S, Pacchierotti F, Tanzarella C: Chromosome aberrations and telomere length modulation in bone marrow and spleen cells of melphalan-treated p53+/- mice. Environ. Mol. Mutagen. 2008;49(6):467-475. DOI: 10.1002/em.20405

[110] Malet-Martino M, Martino R: Clinical studies of three oral prodrugs of 5-fluorouracil (capecitabine, UFT, S-1): a review. Oncologist 2002;7(4):288-323. DOI: 10.1634/theoncologist.7-4-288

[111] Kuranaga N, Shinomiya N, Mochizuki H: Long-term cultivation of colorectal carcinoma cells with anti-cancer drugs induces drug resistance and telomere elongation: an in vitro study. BMC Cancer 2001;1:10. DOI: 10.1186/1471-2407-1-10

[112] Lin G, Lin MC, Lin S, Yao H, Yu S, Yi W et al.: Early growth response protein-1 promoter-mediated synergistic antitumor effect of hTERTC27 gene therapy and 5-Flurorouracil on nasopharyngeal carcinoma. Cancer Biother. Radiopharm. 2012;27(7): 434-441. DOI: 10.1089/cbr.2011.1153

[113] Lin G, Chen Q, Yu S, Lin S, Yao H, Ding Z et al.: Overexpression of human telomerase reverse transcriptase C-terminal polypeptide sensitizes HeLa cells to 5-fluorouracil-induced growth inhibition and apoptosis. Mol. Med. Rep. 2014;9(1):279-284. DOI: 10.3892/mmr.2013.1777

Chapter 7

# Telomeres and Cellular Senescence in Metabolic and Endocrine Diseases

Ryusaku Matsumoto and Yutaka Takahashi

Additional information is available at the end of the chapter

http://dx.doi.org/10.5772/64759

**Abstract**

A number of observations suggest a close connection between telomere length and mortality and age-related disease, suggesting that telomere length is a useful marker of individual biological aging and the shortening of telomere length is causally related with the pathogenesis in age-related diseases. To date, the significance of telomere length in metabolic and endocrine diseases has also been clarified. It has been reported that obesity, type 2 diabetes mellitus (T2DM), NAFLD, and hypertension were associated with shortened telomere length. In endocrine diseases, polycystic ovary syndrome (PCOS), Cushing's syndrome, and acromegaly were associated with shortened telomere length. In these conditions, an increased oxidative stress associated with the metabolic and hormonal abnormalities appears to play a pivotal role in the shortened telomere length. Recently, a large population-based study demonstrated that shortened telomeres at baseline were associated with an increased risk of metabolic diseases, suggesting that the shortened telomere itself plays a causal role for the onset or development of the metabolic diseases. In this chapter, the pathophysiological role of shortened telomere length in metabolic and endocrine diseases and the significance of cellular senescence are discussed.

**Keywords:** metabolic disease, endocrine disease, telomere, oxidative stress, cellular senescence

## 1. Introduction

Telomeres consist of repetitive DNA sequences, thousands of "TTAGGG" tandem repeats, which are located at the ends of linear chromosomes in most somatic cells [1]. Telomere ends form a cap-like structure to protect the ends of chromosomes from degeneration and fusion. However, telomeres shorten during each cell division, and when they reach a critically short length, cell cycle arrest and cellular senescence occur in the cellular level. In the body, telomeres gradually shorten with aging [2]. A number of observations suggest a close connection between telomere length, generally assessed in leukocytes, and mortality or age-related disease, suggesting telomere length as a "mitotic clock," a marker for individual biological aging [3]. In this regard, to date, telomere length in various diseases has been investigated, including cancers, immune insufficiency, and cardiovascular disease. In addition, metabolic diseases, such as obesity and diabetes mellitus (DM), have shown a strong association with telomere shortening. Several endocrine disorders, such as polycystic ovary syndrome (PCOS), Cushing's syndrome, and acromegaly, are also reportedly associated with telomere shortening (**Figure 1**).

Furthermore, several recent studies have focused on the pathophysiological role of telomeres for metabolic or endocrine diseases. Telomere shortening is one of the important causes of cellular senescence, and recently, it has emerged that cellular senescence plays a pivotal role in the aging and pathogenesis of age-related disease [4]. Actually, several clinical studies have shown that shortened telomeres at baseline are associated with an increased risk for development of age-related diseases.

Here, we review the association and pathophysiological role of telomere length in metabolic and endocrine diseases. Furthermore, we discuss the mechanistic insight and significance of shortened telomeres and associated cellular senescence. Finally, we discuss a possible therapeutic approach for these diseases in the aspect of telomere shortening.

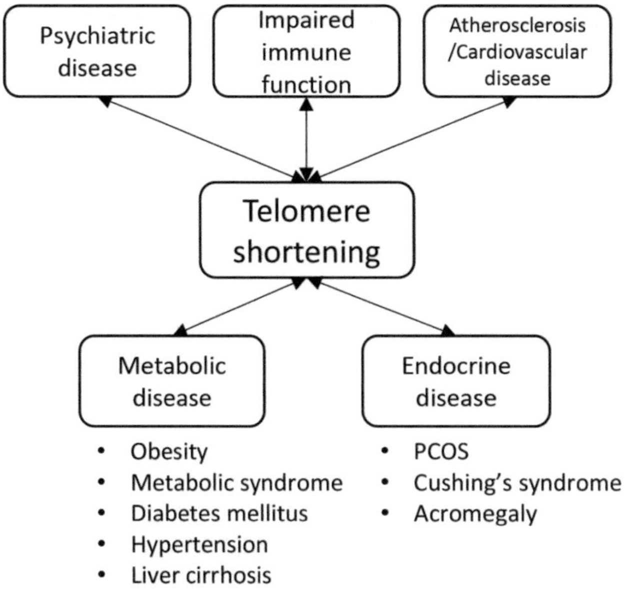


**Figure 1.** Telomere shortening and human diseases. Shortened telomere length is associated with various disorders, including psychiatric disease, impaired immune function, and atherosclerotic disease as well as metabolic and endocrine diseases.

http://dx.doi.org/10.5772/64759

## 2. Telomeres and cellular senescence

### 2.1. Telomeres

Telomere is a dynamic complex at chromosome ends, which consists of repetitive DNA sequences [1,5]. In human cells, telomeres consist of thousands of "TTAGGG" tandem repeats. This base sequence is universal and consistent among most species. Human telomere complex consists of chromosomal-terminal tract of telomeric repeats bound by protective shelterin component proteins, with additional protective proteins. This complex, which binds specifically to telomeres, forms a cap-like structure and prevents end-to-end fusion or damage of the chromosome ends.

The general chromosomal DNA replication cannot completely copy the DNA sequence in the ends of the linear chromosomes, which is called "end replication problem." During the course of cell divisions, this leads to attrition of chromosome ends. Therefore, normal telomere maintenance requires the ribonucleoprotein enzyme named telomerase, which can add telomeric repeat sequences to the end of the chromosomes [6]. However, in most of the human somatic cells, the levels of telomerase are limited and telomeres shorten throughout the life span. Other genetic or environmental factors can also contribute to telomere shortening; defects of telomere maintenance system, DNA replication stress, increased oxidative stress, chemical damage, and inflammatory status are involved in telomere shortening [1].

### 2.2. Cellular senescence and senescence-associated secretary phenotype (SASP)

Cellular senescence refers to the irreversible growth arrest that occurs when cells experience potentially oncogenic insults [7]. Telomere shortening is one of the most important causes of cellular senescence. Telomere shortening causes DNA damage response (DDR), a signaling pathway, in which cell cycle progression is blocked through an increased production of p53 and cyclin-dependent kinase (Cdk) inhibitor p21 protein. DDR subsequently induces cellular senescence. Recently, accumulating evidences suggest that senescent cells are also important for age-related pathologies, including metabolic diseases such as obesity and DM [8,9]. Elimination of senescent cells can delay age-related dysfunctions in mouse model [10], indicating that a presence of senescent cells itself plays a causal role in the process of aging. Aging tissues, in which senescent cells are increased, show a low-level chronic inflammation, termed "sterile inflammation" [11]. Sterile inflammation is, at least in part, derived from senescent cells, which secrete proinflammatory cytokines, chemokines, and proteases, which is called "senescence-associated secretary phenotype (SASP)" [12]. Proteins that are associated with SASP, such as tumor necrosis factor (TNF)-$\alpha$, interleukin (IL)-6, matrix metalloproteinases (MMPs), and monocyte chemoattractant protein (MCP)-1, increase in multiple tissues with chronological aging in conjunction with sterile inflammation [13]. These SASP-related cytokines, such as TNF-$\alpha$ and IL-6, are reportedly associated with insulin resistance and the development of DM [14,15]. Although whether the SASP actually causes age-related diseases including metabolic diseases *in vivo* is still unclear, at least, telomere shortening and subsequent cellular senescence have revealed a strong association with age-related diseases including metabolic diseases that are discussed in the following sections.

## 3. Telomeres in metabolic diseases

### 3.1. Obesity

Obesity is a leading preventable cause of death and growing health problem worldwide with increasing rate in both adults and children. A number of studies have reported the association of telomere length with obesity. Although the results were inconsistent and the relationship of telomere shortening and obesity is still inconclusive, several large population-based studies showed telomere shortening in obesity. In cross-sectional epidemiological studies, shortened telomeres were associated with body mass index (BMI), waist-to-hip ratio, visceral fat, and weight gain [3,16,17]. Consistently, calorie-restricted diets and subsequent weight loss were associated with the increased telomere length in obese men [18]. These results indicated the relationship between obesity and shortened telomeres. As an underlying mechanism of telomere shortening in obesity, leptin might be involved. Leptin plays an essential role in the regulation of body fat mass, and it has some proinflammatory properties with increasing oxidative stress [19]. Valdes et al. reported that age, smoking, and serum leptin concentration were independently associated with telomere length, but BMI did not, suggesting that leptin may directly contribute the telomere shortening.

### 3.2. Diabetes mellitus

The number of patients with type 2 DM has drastically been increasing worldwide in association with the changes in lifestyle and increased prevalence of obesity. DM is categorized into several clinical types: type 1 DM (T1DM), type 2 DM (T2DM), gestational DM, and others. In particular, T2DM accounts for the majority of DM patients and the pathophysiology of T2DM has an age-related aspect. DM increases the risk of cardiovascular and cerebrovascular events, and cognitive dysfunction, which are known as age-related diseases. Telomere length in patients with DM has been examined in many studies [20]. In 1998, Jeanclos et al. [21] showed that patients with insulin-dependent DM (IDDM) had shorter telomeres in peripheral leukocytes than non-DM individuals. Patients with T2DM also showed shortened telomeres [22,23]. Furthermore, it has been reported that telomere shortening rate increased with the duration of T2DM [24]. As an underlying mechanism of the telomere shortening in DM, increased production of reactive oxygen species (ROS) caused by hyperglycemia and hyperinsulinemia is supposed. Polyol pathway activation, protein kinase C pathway activation, and increased production of advanced glycation end products (AGEs) also play a pathological role in increased levels of oxidative stress [25]. In fact, Sampson et al. [23] showed an inverse correlation between the level of oxidative stress marker, 8-hydroxy-deoxyguanosine, and the telomere length. These results suggest that the increased oxidative stress in DM may accelerate the telomere shortening.

To date, several studies have focused on the relationship between telomere length and the mortality and progression of DM complications. In a prospective follow-up study, telomere length in T1DM was associated with all cause of mortality [26]. However, the association of telomere length with DM complication has been controversial. Several studies exhibited that DM patients with shorter telomeres has tended to show severer complications of DM [27,28].

On the other hand, Astrup et al. [26] reported that telomere length did not differ between patients with and without nephropathy. Although further studies are needed, these results suggest that telomere length could be used as a surrogate marker for mortality and some of the morbidity in patients with DM.

### 3.3. Hypertension

Hypertension can develop with various genetic and environmental factors, which is considered to be an essential risk factor for cardiovascular or cerebrovascular diseases. However, most of the pathogenesis remains unclear. Recent evidence suggests that telomere length may be, at least in part, involved in the pathogenesis of hypertension [29]. Jeanclos et al. [30] reported the results of a twin study, in which 49 twin pairs were assessed their relation of blood pressure parameters with telomere length in leukocytes. They showed that telomere length were highly familial and negatively correlated with pulse pressure, implying that telomere shortening might be genetically regulated and associated with vascular aging. The Framingham Heart Study also demonstrated that hypertensive individuals exhibited shorter telomere length in leukocytes compared with normotensive individuals [31]. Furthermore, telomere shortening is associated with an increased atherosclerosis and cardiovascular risk [32–34]. These results suggest a close connection of telomeres and hypertension and its complications.

The underlying mechanism of telomere shortening in hypertension is still unclear. Mice lacking telomerase activity showed hypertension as a result of increased plasma endothelin-1 levels [35]. Telomerase activity was decreased in endothelial progenitor cells from both hypertensive rats and patients with essential hypertension [36]. These data suggest that endothelial cells play a key role in the association of telomere length and premature vascular aging.

### 3.4. Nonalcoholic fatty liver disease/nonalcoholic steatohepatitis

The role of telomeres in chronic liver diseases, such as viral hepatitis, nonalcoholic fatty liver disease (NAFLD)/nonalcoholic steatohepatitis (NASH), and liver cirrhosis, has been investigated [37]. It is well known that in these conditions, fibrosis generally determines the severity and prognosis of the disease. Older age and duration of chronic liver disease are the major risk factors for fibrosis [38].

Kitada et al. [39] first reported that telomere shortening was accelerated in hepatocyte of chronic liver disease, including chronic viral hepatitis or liver cirrhosis. Aikata et al. [40] also confirmed that telomere length was significantly shorter in the liver with chronic viral hepatitis or cirrhosis. Telomere length was significantly shorter in cirrhotic liver induced by broad etiologies compared with noncirrhotic liver [41]. Furthermore, telomerase-deficient mice showed impaired hepatic regenerative potential and developed liver cirrhosis. The regenerative potential of organ depends on the amount of the cells with sufficient telomere length, which reserves the potential for cell proliferation. Telomere shortening restricts the replicative capacity of these cells. Interestingly, adenoviral telomerase gene delivery inhibited the progression of liver cirrhosis [42]. These data indicate that telomere shortening in hepatocytes might impair the regenerative capacity in response to liver injury, which might result in liver fibrosis.

## 4. Telomeres in endocrine diseases

### 4.1. Polycystic ovary syndrome (PCOS)

To the best of our knowledge, the first endocrine disease, in which telomere length was investigated, was polycystic ovary syndrome (PCOS) [43]. PCOS is characterized by polycystic ovaries, irregular menstrual cycles, androgen excess, and insulin resistance [44]. PCOS is a complex and multigenetic disorder, in which single nucleotide polymorphisms (SNPs) in several genes have been found to be associated. Phenotypes of the disease vary according to the ethnic origin, race, genetic factors, and other environmental factors [45,46]. In addition, no single etiologic factor was able to fully account for the pathogenesis of this disorder. Interestingly, patients with PCOS exhibited a significantly shorter telomere length than the controls after adjusting for age [43]. In addition, significant negative correlation between telomere length and dehydroepiandrosterone sulfate (DHEA-S) was observed. There are several lines of evidences, which suggest that oxidative stress plays a role in the pathogenesis of PCOS [47, 48]. Telomere shortening can cause dysregulation of the insulin sensitivity, mitochondrial function, and $Ca^{2+}$ metabolism [49,50], suggesting a causal role of shortened telomere length in the development of PCOS. Conversely, an elevated oxidative stress associated with the androgen excess, abdominal adiposity, insulin resistance, and obesity might play a role in telomere shortening.

### 4.2. Cushing's syndrome

Cushing's syndrome is characterized by excessive secretion of cortisol, which leads to increased mortality and severe morbidity, including cardiovascular risk, obesity, fatigability, osteopenia, and impaired quality of life [51]. These comorbidities are not completely reversible after the biochemical control [52]. Hyperstimulation of hypothalamus-pituitary-adrenal (HPA) axis and subsequent hypercortisolemia may also occur in several kinds of psychiatric disorders or life stressors [53]. Interestingly, these situations are reportedly associated with shortened telomeres, in which chronic stress and enhanced HPA axis are observed. For example, patients with depression exhibited shorter telomere length than healthy controls [54]. Telomere length of newborn baby was shorter in proportion to the stress levels experienced by the mother during her pregnancy [55]. The exposure to violence or neglect in childhood was associated with shorter telomere length either in children or retrospectively in adults [56]. *In vitro* analysis has revealed that high levels of glucocorticoid reduce a 50% of telomerase activity in lymphocytes [57]. In this aspect, to elucidate the reason why comorbidities of Cushing's syndrome are not completely recover after a biochemical control, Aulinas et al. [58] hypothesized that shortening of telomere might occur in Cushing's syndrome and evaluated the telomere length in patients with Cushing's syndrome. They evaluated 77 patients with Cushing's syndrome (59 pituitary adenoma, 17 adrenal adenoma, and 1 ectopic; 21 with active disease). Although mean telomere length in patients with Cushing's syndrome and age-, sex-, and smoking-matched controls were comparable, in the longitudinal evaluation, telomere length was shorter in active disease than controlled disease after adjustment for age. They also showed that dyslipidemic patients with Cushing's syndrome had shorter telomere length than non-dyslipidemic patients with Cushing's syndrome and total cholesterol and triglycerides negatively correlated with telomere length. In addition, inflammatory markers and serum levels of CRP and IL-6 were also negatively correlated with telomere length in patients with Cushing's syndrome [59]. These observations suggested that hypercortisolism might negatively regulate telomere maintenance through the production of inflammatory cytokines or lipids.

### 4.3. Acromegaly

Patients with acromegaly exhibit reduced life expectancy and increased comorbidities, such as DM, hypertension, cardiovascular and cerebrovascular diseases, and malignant diseases, which are also known as age-related diseases. Underlying mechanisms of these increased age-related diseases are mainly explained by over secretion of GH and IGF-I; however, precise mechanisms have not been fully elucidated. Therefore, we investigated the telomere length of peripheral leukocytes in patients with acromegaly [60]. Intriguingly, patients with acromegaly exhibited shorter telomere length compared with patients with nonfunctioning pituitary adenoma or healthy control subjects. In addition, telomere length in acromegaly was negatively correlated with the disease duration, suggesting that exposure to increased serum GH or IGF-I levels may reduce telomere length. *In vitro* analysis revealed that not GH but IGF-I increased the telomere shortening rate per one cell division in human skin fibroblasts. Furthermore, IGF-I–treated cells showed cellular senescence and increased expression of SASP-related cytokines (e.g., IL-6). It has been reported that the development of age-related diseases, such as DM and vascular diseases, is associated with cellular senescence and SASP [8]. Together with our data, it is suggested that cellular senescence induced by telomere shortening may be involved in the increased morbidity and mortality in acromegalic patients.

The underlying mechanisms of how excess IGF-I induces telomere shortening and subsequent cellular senescence remain unclarified. It has been reported that various factors, including ROS, defects in the telomere repair system, inflammatory reactions, and increased cellular turn over, cause telomere shortening [61]. Intriguingly, oxidative stress was enhanced both in GH-transgenic rats and patients with acromegaly [62]. In addition, it has been reported that IGF-I enhances ROS-p53 pathway and subsequent cellular senescence in cultured cells with a confluent status [63]. Bayram et al. [64] also reported that patients with acromegaly exhibited increased oxidative stress and DNA damage. Furthermore, the causal role of increased oxidative stress in telomere shortening has been reported. Human fibroblasts cultured under 40% oxygen, in which oxidative stress is increased, exhibited an accelerated rate of telomere shortening [33] and inhibition of the glutathione-dependent antioxidant system results in telomere shortening and senescence in human endothelial cells [65]. Taken together, although further investigations are needed, we speculate that the increased oxidative stress associated with the increased serum levels of IGF-I may lead to the telomere shortening in patients with acromegaly.

## 5. Telomere shortening as a risk for onset of metabolic diseases

Telomere length is closely associated with morbidity and mortality [66,67]. Therefore, telomere length has been thought as a marker for individual cellular aging [68,69]. However, several recent studies have focused on the possibility of causal role of shortened telomeres as a risk for the development of several age-related diseases, including metabolic diseases [70–72].

### 5.1. Diabetes mellitus

Telomere length is already reduced in pre-diabetic stage; impaired glucose tolerance and this is recognized as a risk factor for the onset of T2DM [73]. To date, several prospective studies have focused on the telomere shortening as a risk factor for the onset of T2DM [74–76]. Although these results have been inconsistent, some studies showed positive results. You et al. [76] conducted a large-scale prospective study of healthy postmenopausal women with 6-year follow-up. However, there was no relationship between telomere shortening and the onset of DM. Recently, Zhao et al. [75] also reported the results of a large-scale cohort study of American Indians. Among 2328 participants who were free of DM at baseline, 292 subjects developed DM during an average 5.5 years of follow-up. Subjects in the lowest quartile of telomere length showed approximately twofold-increased risk of DM incidence compared with the highest quartile. Willeit et al. [74] also reported the similar results of prospective cohort study of healthy subjects. Over 15 years of follow-up, 44 of 606 participants developed DM. The adjusted hazard ratio for DM comparing the lowest and highest quartile of baseline telomere length was 2.0. These results may indicate that telomere shortening is not only a mere marker of biological aging but also plays a causal role in the development of DM.

### 5.2. Metabolic syndrome

As shown above, many studies have demonstrated that the components of metabolic syndrome individually exhibited a significant association with shortened telomeres [21,30,33]. Very recently, Revesz et al. [70] reported the result of a large population-based study with 6 years of follow-up, which included 2981 adult individuals (age: 18–65 years); the subject consists of 1701 persons with a diagnosis of depression and/or anxiety disorder, 907 persons with subthreshold depressive or anxiety symptoms, and 373 healthy controls. They assessed that whether shorter telomere length at baseline was associated with a worse metabolic profile. This study demonstrated that shorter telomere length at baseline was not only cross-sectionally associated with metabolic syndrome components (decreased HDL and increased waist circumference, triglycerides, and fasting glucose) but also associated with an increased risk of having an abnormal metabolic profile, which continues to be unfavorable even after a follow-up period of 6 years. Based on the results, they advocated that cellular aging assessed by telomere length might play a role in the metabolic alterations.

### 5.3. Liver cirrhosis

Liver cirrhosis is the end-stage complication of chronic liver disease, which leads to impairment of liver function and increased risk of hepatocellular carcinoma. In particular, viral hepatitis, fatty liver disease, and alcohol consumption have been reportedly associated with an increased risk of cirrhosis, and the majority of the patients have these risks. However, even in the same condition, a part of the patients progress to cirrhosis, whereas others do not. The reason that determines the progression remains still unclear. Several SNPs have been reportedly associated with the development of cirrhosis. Interestingly, it has been recently reported that telomere shortening might be a risk factor for the liver cirrhosis [77]. In the liver tissue with chronic liver injury, because a high cellular turnover was required for the regeneration and repair process, telomere shortening was accelerated. Telomerase-deficient mice were prone to develop cirrhosis in response to chronic liver injury, and restoration of telomerase activity was able to improve fibrosis and liver function [42]. Furthermore, patients with telomere diseases, in which telomerase complex gene mutation was identified, such as dyskeratosis congenita showed a shortened telomeres and increased prevalence of liver disease including fibrosis and cirrhosis [61]. These data suggest that shortened telomeres are causally involved in the development of liver cirrhosis.

## 6. Telomere as therapeutic targets

The analysis of mouse genetic models demonstrated the causal role of shortened telomeres in aging. Mice deficient for *TERC* show accelerated telomere shortening, chromosome instability, premature aging phenotype, and premature death [78,79]. Another mouse model, *TERT*-deficient mice also showed a shorter telomere length and genome instability [80,81]. In contrast, mice with increased transgenic telomerase expression were able to maintain longer telomeres through their lifespan and showed decreased appearance of age-related disorders and increased longevity. These results indicate that the maintenance of telomere length, at least in mice, plays an essential role in the regulation of aging and longevity [82]. In this regard, to prevent the onset of age-related diseases, telomere and telomerase as a potential therapeutic target have been emerged [83].

### 6.1. Telomerase activator

Small molecule named TA-65 derived from an extract of a plant used in traditional Chinese medicine, *Astragalus membranaceus*, upregulates telomerase activity *in vivo* [84]. TA-65 has been shown a mild increase in telomere length in mice [85] and humans [84]. However, there was no increase in longevity in mice [85]. Recently, the result of a randomized control study conducted on 117 healthy subjects using TA-65 has been reported [86]. Low dose oral administration of TA-65 significantly increased telomere length over the 12-month period, whereas subjects in the placebo group significantly lost telomere length. The high dose administration of TA-65 showed a trend of improvement in telomere length; however, it did not reach statistical significance. Although it remains elusive that telomerase activator can increase life span and delay the onset of age-related diseases, these findings suggest a possibility of telomere/telomerase as a therapeutic target for preventing aging.

### 6.2. Danazol

Androgen has been used to treat bone mallow failure and aplastic anemia with the anabolic effect on bone marrow [87], although precise mechanisms have not been fully understood. It has been reported that telomere diseases with mutations in genes responsible for telomere maintenance and repair lead to bone mallow failure [88]. Interestingly, considerable evidence suggests that androgen directly regulates telomerase activity [89]. Recently, it has been reported that the treatment with androgen leads to telomere elongation in a mouse model of telomerase dysfunction [90]. In addition, serum dihydrotestosterone and estradiol levels and aromatase gene polymorphisms were associated with telomere length [91]. Very recently, Townsley et al. reported that danazol, the synthetic sex hormone, which has androgen activity, was efficacious to elongate the telomere length in bone marrow cells [92]. Patients with mutations in the genes related to the telomere maintenance or repairment, such as *TERT*, *TERC*, and *DKC1*, were enrolled and orally administered danazol at a dose of 800 mg/day for a total of 24 months. Surprisingly, almost all the patients (11 of 12) had a substantial gain in telomere length at 24 months when compared with baseline. Hematologic responses were also observed in 10 of 12 patients at 24 months. As an underlying mechanism, *in vitro* study showed a direct effect of androgen on telomerase activity by upregulation of *TERT* expression [93]. Although whether androgen is also effective to subjects without gene mutations in telomere-related genes is still unclear, there is a possibility that pharmacological intervention for telomere elongation may be applicable for the treatment of age-related disease.

## 7. Conclusion

In summary, telomere length assessed in peripheral leukocytes is associated with various metabolic and endocrine diseases **Figure 2A**. In addition, recent studies suggest that shortened telomeres may have a causal role in the pathophysiology of age-related diseases, such as T2DM, metabolic syndrome, and cardiovascular disease **Figure 2B** [70,94]. However, it has not yet been elucidated that how shortened telomeres cause these age-related diseases. One possible explanation is SASP. Shortened telomeres activate DDR pathway, which results in apoptosis and/or cell cycle arrest, and cellular senescence. Recently, it has emerged that cellular senescence and the related SASP play important roles in the development of age-related diseases [8,9,95,96]. In conclusion, although there is a strong association between telomere shortening and metabolic and endocrine diseases, further studies are needed to understand the mechanisms underlying these associations. Also, it is suggested that interventions that restore telomere length may be a potential therapeutic target for age-related disease **Figure 2C**.

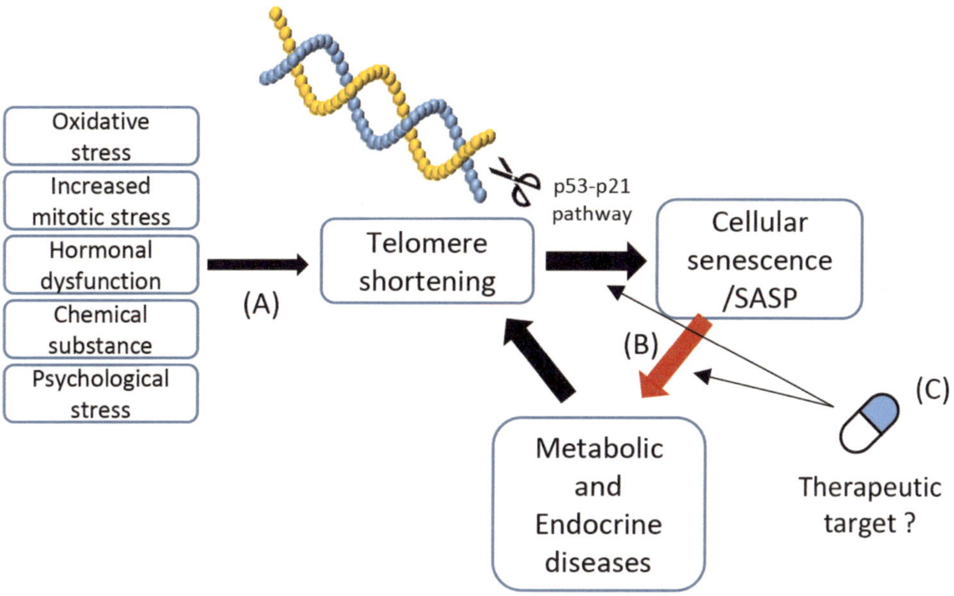


**Figure 2.** Schematic summary. A) Various factors such as oxidative stress, mitotic stress, and hormonal dysfunction can shorten telomere length. B) Shortened telomeres are not a mere marker for individual aging but a pathological contributor to the development of age-related disease, including metabolic and endocrine diseases. As the underlying mechanism, cellular senescence and/or SASP might be involved. C) These pathways might be potential therapeutic targets for prevention of these age-related disorders.

## Author details

Ryusaku Matsumoto and Yutaka Takahashi*

*Address all correspondence to: takahash@med.kobe-u.ac.jp

Division of Diabetes Endocrinology, Kobe University Graduate School of Medicine, Kobe, Japan

## References

[1] Blackburn EH, Epel ES, Lin J. Human telomere biology: a contributory and interactive factor in aging, disease risks, and protection. Science. 2015;350(6265):1193-1198. DOI: 10.1126/science.aab3389

[2] Frenck RW, Jr., Blackburn EH, Shannon KM. The rate of telomere sequence loss in human leukocytes varies with age. Proc Natl Acad Sci U S A. 1998;95(10):5607-5610.

[3] Valdes AM, Andrew T, Gardner JP, Kimura M, Oelsner E, Cherkas LF, et al. Obesity, cigarette smoking, and telomere length in women. Lancet. 2005;366(9486):662-664. DOI: 10.1016/S0140-6736(05)66630-5

[4] Childs BG, Durik M, Baker DJ, van Deursen JM. Cellular senescence in aging and age-related disease: from mechanisms to therapy. Nat Med. 2015;21(12):1424-1435. DOI: 10.1038/nm.4000

[5] Sfeir A, de Lange T. Removal of shelterin reveals the telomere end-protection problem. Science. 2012;336(6081):593-597. DOI: 10.1126/science.1218498

[6] Blackburn EH, Greider CW, Szostak JW. Telomeres and telomerase: the path from maize, Tetrahymena and yeast to human cancer and aging. Nat Med. 2006;12(10): 1133-1138. DOI: 10.1038/nm1006-1133

[7] Campisi J, d'Adda di Fagagna F. Cellular senescence: when bad things happen to good cells. Nat Rev Mol Cell Biol. 2007;8(9):729-740. DOI: 10.1038/nrm2233

[8] Tchkonia T, Zhu Y, van Deursen J, Campisi J, Kirkland JL. Cellular senescence and the senescent secretory phenotype: therapeutic opportunities. J Clin Invest. 2013;123(3): 966-972. DOI: 10.1172/JCI64098

[9] van Deursen JM. The role of senescent cells in ageing. Nature. 2014;509(7501):439-446. DOI: 10.1038/nature13193

[10] Baker DJ, Wijshake T, Tchkonia T, LeBrasseur NK, Childs BG, van de Sluis B, et al. Clearance of p16Ink4a-positive senescent cells delays ageing-associated disorders. Nature. 2011;479(7372):232-236. DOI: 10.1038/nature10600

[11] Vasto S, Candore G, Balistreri CR, Caruso M, Colonna-Romano G, Grimaldi MP, et al. Inflammatory networks in ageing, age-related diseases and longevity. Mech Ageing Dev. 2007;128(1):83-91. DOI: 10.1016/j.mad.2006.11.015

[12] Coppe JP, Patil CK, Rodier F, Sun Y, Munoz DP, Goldstein J, et al. Senescence-associated secretory phenotypes reveal cell-nonautonomous functions of oncogenic RAS and the p53 tumor suppressor. PLoS Biol. 2008;6(12):2853-2868. DOI: 10.1371/journal.pbio.0060301

[13] Freund A, Orjalo AV, Desprez PY, Campisi J. Inflammatory networks during cellular senescence: causes and consequences. Trends Mol Med. 2010;16(5):238-246. DOI: 10.1016/j.molmed.2010.03.003

[14] Spranger J, Kroke A, Mohlig M, Hoffmann K, Bergmann MM, Ristow M, et al. Inflammatory cytokines and the risk to develop type 2 diabetes: results of the prospective population-based European Prospective Investigation into Cancer and Nutrition (EPIC)-Potsdam Study. Diabetes. 2003;52(3):812-817. DOI: 10.2337/diabetes.52.3.812

[15] Hu FB, Meigs JB, Li TY, Rifai N, Manson JE. Inflammatory markers and risk of developing type 2 diabetes in women. Diabetes. 2004;53(3):693-700. DOI: 10.2337/diabetes.53.3.693

[16] Kim S, Parks CG, DeRoo LA, Chen H, Taylor JA, Cawthon RM, et al. Obesity and weight gain in adulthood and telomere length. Cancer Epidemiol Biomarkers Prev. 2009;18(3): 816-820. DOI: 10.1158/1055-9965.EPI-08-0935

[17] Zannolli R, Mohn A, Buoni S, Pietrobelli A, Messina M, Chiarelli F, et al. Telomere length and obesity. Acta Paediatr. 2008;97(7):952-954. DOI: 10.1111/j.1651-2227.2008.00783.x

[18] O'Callaghan NJ, Clifton PM, Noakes M, Fenech M. Weight loss in obese men is associated with increased telomere length and decreased abasic sites in rectal mucosa. Rejuvenation Res. 2009;12(3):169-176. DOI: 10.1089/rej.2008.0819

[19] Beltowski J, Wojcicka G, Jamroz A. Leptin decreases plasma paraoxonase 1 (PON1) activity and induces oxidative stress: the possible novel mechanism for proatherogenic effect of chronic hyperleptinemia. Atherosclerosis. 2003;170(1):21-29. DOI: 10.1016/S0021-9150(03)00236-3

[20] Tamura Y, Takubo K, Aida J, Araki A, Ito H. Telomere attrition and diabetes mellitus. Geriatr Gerontol Int. 2016;16 Suppl 1:66-74. DOI: 10.1111/ggi.12738

[21] Jeanclos E, Krolewski A, Skurnick J, Kimura M, Aviv H, Warram JH, et al. Shortened telomere length in white blood cells of patients with IDDM. Diabetes. 1998;47(3): 482-486. DOI: 10.2337/diabetes.47.3.482

[22] Zee RY, Castonguay AJ, Barton NS, Germer S, Martin M. Mean leukocyte telomere length shortening and type 2 diabetes mellitus: a case-control study. Transl Res. 2010;155(4):166-169. DOI: 10.1016/j.trsl.2009.09.012

[23] Sampson MJ, Winterbone MS, Hughes JC, Dozio N, Hughes DA. Monocyte telomere shortening and oxidative DNA damage in type 2 diabetes. Diabetes Care. 2006;29(2): 283-289. DOI: 10.2337/diacare.29.02.06.dc05-1715

[24] Murillo-Ortiz B, Albarran-Tamayo F, Arenas-Aranda D, Benitez-Bribiesca L, Malacara-Hernandez JM, Martinez-Garza S, et al. Telomere length and type 2 diabetes in males, a premature aging syndrome. Aging Male. 2012;15(1):54-58. DOI: 10.3109/13685538.2011.593658

[25] Araki E, Nishikawa T. Oxidative stress: a cause and therapeutic target of diabetic complications. J Diabetes Investig. 2010;1(3):90-96. DOI: 10.1111/j.2040-1124.2010.00013.x

[26] Astrup AS, Tarnow L, Jorsal A, Lajer M, Nzietchueng R, Benetos A, et al. Telomere length predicts all-cause mortality in patients with type 1 diabetes. Diabetologia. 2010;53(1):45-48. DOI: 10.1007/s00125-009-1542-1

[27] Fyhrquist F, Tiitu A, Saijonmaa O, Forsblom C, Groop PH, FinnDiane Study G. Telomere length and progression of diabetic nephropathy in patients with type 1 diabetes. J Intern Med. 2010;267(3):278-286. DOI: 10.1111/j.1365-2796.2009.02139.x

[28] Testa R, Olivieri F, Sirolla C, Spazzafumo L, Rippo MR, Marra M, et al. Leukocyte telomere length is associated with complications of type 2 diabetes mellitus. Diabet Med. 2011;28(11):1388-1394. DOI: 10.1111/j.1464-5491.2011.03370.x

[29] Ma L, Li Y, Wang J. Telomeres and essential hypertension. Clin Biochem. 2015;48(16-17):1195-1199. DOI: 10.1016/j.clinbiochem.2015.07.013

[30] Jeanclos E, Schork NJ, Kyvik KO, Kimura M, Skurnick JH, Aviv A. Telomere length inversely correlates with pulse pressure and is highly familial. Hypertension. 2000;36(2):195-200. DOI: 10.1161/01.hyp.36.2.195

[31] Demissie S, Levy D, Benjamin EJ, Cupples LA, Gardner JP, Herbert A, et al. Insulin resistance, oxidative stress, hypertension, and leukocyte telomere length in men from the Framingham Heart Study. Aging Cell. 2006;5(4):325-330. DOI: 10.1111/j.1474-9726.2006.00224.x

[32] Fuster JJ, Andres V. Telomere biology and cardiovascular disease. Circ Res. 2006;99(11):1167-1180. DOI: 10.1161/01.RES.0000251281.00845.18

[33] Nilsson PM, Tufvesson H, Leosdottir M, Melander O. Telomeres and cardiovascular disease risk: an update 2013. Transl Res. 2013;162(6):371-380. DOI: 10.1016/j.trsl.2013.05.004

[34] Samani NJ, Boultby R, Butler R, Thompson JR, Goodall AH. Telomere shortening in atherosclerosis. Lancet. 2001;358(9280):472-473. DOI: 10.1016/S0140-6736(01)05633-1

[35] Perez-Rivero G, Ruiz-Torres MP, Rivas-Elena JV, Jerkic M, Diez-Marques ML, Lopez-Novoa JM, et al. Mice deficient in telomerase activity develop hypertension because of an excess of endothelin production. Circulation. 2006;114(4):309-317. DOI: 10.1161/CIRCULATIONAHA.105.611111

[36] Imanishi T, Moriwaki C, Hano T, Nishio I. Endothelial progenitor cell senescence is accelerated in both experimental hypertensive rats and patients with essential hypertension. J Hypertens. 2005;23(10):1831-1837.

[37] Donati B, Valenti L. Telomeres, NAFLD and chronic liver disease. Int J Mol Sci. 2016;17(3):383. DOI: 10.3390/ijms17030383

[38] Pinzani M. Pathophysiology of liver fibrosis. Dig Dis. 2015;33(4):492-497. DOI: 10.1159/000374096

[39] Kitada T, Seki S, Kawakita N, Kuroki T, Monna T. Telomere shortening in chronic liver diseases. Biochem Biophys Res Commun. 1995;211(1):33-39. DOI: 10.1006/bbrc.1995.1774

[40] Aikata H, Takaishi H, Kawakami Y, Takahashi S, Kitamoto M, Nakanishi T, et al. Telomere reduction in human liver tissues with age and chronic inflammation. Exp Cell Res. 2000;256(2):578-582. DOI: 10.1006/excr.2000.4862

[41] Wiemann SU, Satyanarayana A, Tsahuridu M, Tillmann HL, Zender L, Klempnauer J, et al. Hepatocyte telomere shortening and senescence are general markers of human liver cirrhosis. FASEB J. 2002;16(9):935-942. DOI: 10.1096/fj.01-0977com

[42] Rudolph KL, Chang S, Millard M, Schreiber-Agus N, DePinho RA. Inhibition of experimental liver cirrhosis in mice by telomerase gene delivery. Science. 2000;287(5456):1253-1258. DOI: 10.1126/science.287.5456.1253

[43] Li Q, Du J, Feng R, Xu Y, Wang H, Sang Q, et al. A possible new mechanism in the pathophysiology of polycystic ovary syndrome (PCOS): the discovery that leukocyte telomere length is strongly associated with PCOS. J Clin Endocrinol Metab. 2014;99(2):E234-E240. DOI: 10.1210/jc.2013-3685

[44] Ehrmann DA. Polycystic ovary syndrome. N Engl J Med. 2005;352(12):1223-1236. DOI: 10.1056/NEJMra041536

[45] Kauffman RP, Baker VM, Dimarino P, Gimpel T, Castracane VD. Polycystic ovarian syndrome and insulin resistance in white and Mexican American women: a comparison of two distinct populations. Am J Obstet Gynecol. 2002;187(5):1362-1369.

[46] Williamson K, Gunn AJ, Johnson N, Milsom SR. The impact of ethnicity on the presentation of polycystic ovarian syndrome. Aust N Z J Obstet Gynaecol. 2001;41(2): 202-206.

[47] Murri M, Luque-Ramirez M, Insenser M, Ojeda-Ojeda M, Escobar-Morreale HF. Circulating markers of oxidative stress and polycystic ovary syndrome (PCOS): a systematic review and meta-analysis. Hum Reprod Update. 2013;19(3):268-288. DOI: 10.1093/humupd/dms059

[48] Hyderali BN, Mala K. Oxidative stress and cardiovascular complications in polycystic ovarian syndrome. Eur J Obstet Gynecol Reprod Biol. 2015;191:15-22. DOI: 10.1016/j.ejogrb.2015.05.005

[49] Guo N, Parry EM, Li LS, Kembou F, Lauder N, Hussain MA, et al. Short telomeres compromise beta-cell signaling and survival. PLoS One. 2011;6(3):e17858. DOI: 10.1371/journal.pone.0017858

[50] Sahin E, Colla S, Liesa M, Moslehi J, Muller FL, Guo M, et al. Telomere dysfunction induces metabolic and mitochondrial compromise. Nature. 2011;470(7334):359-365. DOI: 10.1038/nature09787

[51] Nieman LK. Cushing's syndrome: update on signs, symptoms and biochemical screening. Eur J Endocrinol. 2015;173(4):M33-M38. DOI: 10.1530/EJE-15-0464

[52] Valassi E, Crespo I, Santos A, Webb SM. Clinical consequences of Cushing's syndrome. Pituitary. 2012;15(3):319-329. DOI: 10.1007/s11102-012-0394-8

[53] Pariante CM, Miller AH. Glucocorticoid receptors in major depression: relevance to pathophysiology and treatment. Biol Psychiatry. 2001;49(5):391-404. DOI: 10.1016/S0006-3223(00)01088-X

[54] Lin PY, Huang YC, Hung CF. Shortened telomere length in patients with depression: a meta-analytic study. J Psychiatr Res. 2016;76:84-93. DOI: 10.1016/j.jpsychires.2016.01.015

[55] Entringer S, Epel ES, Kumsta R, Lin J, Hellhammer DH, Blackburn EH, et al. Stress exposure in intrauterine life is associated with shorter telomere length in young adulthood. Proc Natl Acad Sci U S A. 2011;108(33):E513-E518. DOI: 10.1073/pnas.1107759108

[56] Price LH, Kao HT, Burgers DE, Carpenter LL, Tyrka AR. Telomeres and early-life stress: an overview. Biol Psychiatry. 2013;73(1):15-23. DOI: 10.1016/j.biopsych.2012.06.025

[57] Choi J, Fauce SR, Effros RB. Reduced telomerase activity in human T lymphocytes exposed to cortisol. Brain Behav Immun. 2008;22(4):600-605. DOI: 10.1016/j.bbi.2007.12.004

[58] Aulinas A, Ramirez MJ, Barahona MJ, Valassi E, Resmini E, Mato E, et al. Telomere length analysis in Cushing's syndrome. Eur J Endocrinol. 2014;171(1):21-29. DOI: 10.1530/EJE-14-0098

[59] Aulinas A, Ramirez MJ, Barahona MJ, Valassi E, Resmini E, Mato E, et al. Dyslipidemia and chronic inflammation markers are correlated with telomere length shortening in Cushing's syndrome. PLoS One. 2015;10(3):e0120185. DOI: 10.1371/journal.pone.0120185

[60] Matsumoto R, Fukuoka H, Iguchi G, Odake Y, Yoshida K, Bando H, et al. Accelerated telomere shortening in acromegaly; IGF-I induces telomere shortening and cellular senescence. PLoS One. 2015;10(10):e0140189. DOI: 10.1371/journal.pone.0140189

[61] Calado RT, Young NS. Telomere diseases. N Engl J Med. 2009;361(24):2353-2365. DOI: 10.1056/NEJMra0903373

[62] Nishizawa H, Handayaningsih AE, Iguchi G, Cho Y, Takahashi M, Yamamoto M, et al. Enhanced oxidative stress in GH-transgenic rat and acromegaly in humans. Growth Horm IGF Res. 2012;22(2):64-68. DOI: 10.1016/j.ghir.2012.02.001

[63] Handayaningsih AE, Takahashi M, Fukuoka H, Iguchi G, Nishizawa H, Yamamoto M, et al. IGF-I enhances cellular senescence via the reactive oxygen species-p53 pathway. Biochem Biophys Res Commun. 2012;425(2):478-484. DOI: 10.1016/j.bbrc.2012.07.140

[64] Bayram F, Bitgen N, Donmez-Altuntas H, Cakir I, Hamurcu Z, Sahin F, et al. Increased genome instability and oxidative DNA damage and their association with IGF-1 levels

in patients with active acromegaly. Growth Horm IGF Res. 2014;24(1):29-34. DOI: 10.1016/j.ghir.2013.12.002

[65] Kurz DJ, Decary S, Hong Y, Trivier E, Akhmedov A, Erusalimsky JD. Chronic oxidative stress compromises telomere integrity and accelerates the onset of senescence in human endothelial cells. J Cell Sci. 2004;117(11):2417-2426. DOI: 10.1242/jcs.01097

[66] Cawthon RM, Smith KR, O'Brien E, Sivatchenko A, Kerber RA. Association between telomere length in blood and mortality in people aged 60 years or older. Lancet. 2003;361(9355):393-395. DOI: 10.1016/S0140-6736(03)12384-7

[67] Brouilette SW, Moore JS, McMahon AD, Thompson JR, Ford I, Shepherd J, et al. Telomere length, risk of coronary heart disease, and statin treatment in the West of Scotland Primary Prevention Study: a nested case-control study. Lancet. 2007;369(9556):107-114. DOI: 10.1016/S0140-6736(07)60071-3

[68] Olovnikov AM. Telomeres, telomerase, and aging: origin of the theory. Exp Gerontol. 1996;31(4):443-448. DOI: 10.1016/0531-5565(96)00005-8

[69] Blackburn EH. Switching and signaling at the telomere. Cell. 2001;106(6):661-673. DOI: 10.1016/S0092-8674(01)00492-5

[70] Revesz D, Milaneschi Y, Verhoeven JE, Penninx BW. Telomere length as a marker of cellular aging is associated with prevalence and progression of metabolic syndrome. J Clin Endocrinol Metab. 2014;99(12):4607-4615. DOI: 10.1210/jc.2014-1851

[71] Nilsson PM. Genetics: telomere length and the metabolic syndrome-a causal link? Nat Rev Endocrinol. 2014;10(12):706-707. DOI: 10.1038/nrendo.2014.182

[72] Fyhrquist F, Saijonmaa O, Strandberg T. The roles of senescence and telomere shortening in cardiovascular disease. Nat Rev Cardiol. 2013;10(5):274-283. DOI: 10.1038/nrcardio.2013.30

[73] Adaikalakoteswari A, Balasubramanyam M, Ravikumar R, Deepa R, Mohan V. Association of telomere shortening with impaired glucose tolerance and diabetic macroangiopathy. Atherosclerosis. 2007;195(1):83-89. DOI: 10.1016/j.atherosclerosis.2006.12.003

[74] Willeit P, Raschenberger J, Heydon EE, Tsimikas S, Haun M, Mayr A, et al. Leucocyte telomere length and risk of type 2 diabetes mellitus: new prospective cohort study and literature-based meta-analysis. PLoS One. 2014;9(11):e112483. DOI: 10.1371/journal.pone.0112483

[75] Zhao J, Zhu Y, Lin J, Matsuguchi T, Blackburn E, Zhang Y, et al. Short leukocyte telomere length predicts risk of diabetes in american indians: the strong heart family study. Diabetes. 2014;63(1):354-362. DOI: 10.2337/db13-0744

[76] You NC, Chen BH, Song Y, Lu X, Chen Y, Manson JE, et al. A prospective study of leukocyte telomere length and risk of type 2 diabetes in postmenopausal women. Diabetes. 2012;61(11):2998-3004. DOI: 10.2337/db12-0241

[77] Carulli L. Telomere shortening as genetic risk factor of liver cirrhosis. World J Gastroenterol. 2015;21(2):379-383. DOI: 10.3748/wjg.v21.i2.379

[78] Blasco MA, Lee HW, Hande MP, Samper E, Lansdorp PM, DePinho RA, et al. Telomere shortening and tumor formation by mouse cells lacking telomerase RNA. Cell. 1997;91(1):25-34. DOI: 10.1016/S0092-8674(01)80006-4

[79] Lee HW, Blasco MA, Gottlieb GJ, Horner JW, 2nd, Greider CW, DePinho RA. Essential role of mouse telomerase in highly proliferative organs. Nature. 1998;392(6676): 569-574. DOI: 10.1038/33345

[80] Erdmann N, Liu Y, Harrington L. Distinct dosage requirements for the maintenance of long and short telomeres in mTert heterozygous mice. Proc Natl Acad Sci U S A. 2004;101(16):6080-6085. DOI: 10.1073/pnas.0401580101

[81] Liu Y, Snow BE, Hande MP, Yeung D, Erdmann NJ, Wakeham A, et al. The telomerase reverse transcriptase is limiting and necessary for telomerase function in vivo. Curr Biol. 2000;10(22):1459-1462. DOI: 10.1016/S0960-9822(00)00805-8

[82] Tomas-Loba A, Flores I, Fernandez-Marcos PJ, Cayuela ML, Maraver A, Tejera A, et al. Telomerase reverse transcriptase delays aging in cancer-resistant mice. Cell. 2008;135(4):609-622. DOI: 10.1016/j.cell.2008.09.034

[83] Bär C, Blasco M. Telomeres and telomerase as therapeutic targets to prevent and treat age-related diseases. F1000Res;5(F1000 Faculty Rev):89. DOI: 10.12688/f1000research.7020.1

[84] Harley CB, Liu W, Blasco M, Vera E, Andrews WH, Briggs LA, et al. A natural product telomerase activator as part of a health maintenance program. Rejuvenation Res. 2011;14(1):45-56. DOI: 10.1089/rej.2010.1085

[85] Bernardes de Jesus B, Schneeberger K, Vera E, Tejera A, Harley CB, Blasco MA. The telomerase activator TA-65 elongates short telomeres and increases health span of adult/old mice without increasing cancer incidence. Aging Cell. 2011;10(4):604-621. DOI: 10.1111/j.1474-9726.2011.00700.x

[86] Salvador L, Singaravelu G, Harley CB, Flom P, Suram A, Raffaele JM. A natural product telomerase activator lengthens telomeres in humans: a randomized, double blind, and placebo controlled study. Rejuvenation Res. 2016. DOI: 10.1089/rej.2015.1793

[87] Camitta BM, Thomas ED, Nathan DG, Gale RP, Kopecky KJ, Rappeport JM, et al. A prospective study of androgens and bone marrow transplantation for treatment of severe aplastic anemia. Blood. 1979;53(3):504-514.

[88] Townsley DM, Dumitriu B, Young NS. Bone marrow failure and the telomeropathies. Blood. 2014;124(18):2775-2783. DOI: 10.1182/blood-2014-05-526285

[89] Bayne S, Liu JP. Hormones and growth factors regulate telomerase activity in ageing and cancer. Mol Cell Endocrinol. 2005;240(1-2):11-22. DOI: 10.1016/j.mce.2005.05.009

[90] Bar C, Huber N, Beier F, Blasco MA. Therapeutic effect of androgen therapy in a mouse model of aplastic anemia produced by short telomeres. Haematologica. 2015;100(10): 1267-1274. DOI: 10.3324/haematol.2015.129239

[91] Yeap BB, Knuiman MW, Divitini ML, Hui J, Arscott GM, Handelsman DJ, et al. Epidemiological and Mendelian randomization studies of dihydrotestosterone and estradiol and leukocyte telomere length in men. J Clin Endocrinol Metab. 2016;101(3): 1299-1306. DOI: 10.1210/jc.2015-4139

[92] Townsley DM, Dumitriu B, Liu D, Biancotto A, Weinstein B, Chen C, et al. Danazol treatment for telomere diseases. N Engl J Med. 2016;374(20):1922-1931. DOI: 10.1056/NEJMoa1515319

[93] Calado RT, Yewdell WT, Wilkerson KL, Regal JA, Kajigaya S, Stratakis CA, et al. Sex hormones, acting on the TERT gene, increase telomerase activity in human primary hematopoietic cells. Blood. 2009;114(11):2236-2243. DOI: 10.1182/blood-2008-09-178871

[94] Haycock PC, Heydon EE, Kaptoge S, Butterworth AS, Thompson A, Willeit P. Leucocyte telomere length and risk of cardiovascular disease: systematic review and meta-analysis. BMJ. 2014;349:g4227. DOI: 10.1136/bmj.g4227

[95] Tyner SD, Venkatachalam S, Choi J, Jones S, Ghebranious N, Igelmann H, et al. p53 mutant mice that display early ageing-associated phenotypes. Nature. 2002;415(6867): 45-53. DOI: 10.1038/415045a

[96] Minamino T, Orimo M, Shimizu I, Kunieda T, Yokoyama M, Ito T, et al. A crucial role for adipose tissue p53 in the regulation of insulin resistance. Nat Med. 2009;15(9): 1082-1087. DOI: 10.1038/nm.2014

# Chapter 8

# Telomere Length and Its Relation to Human Health

Vivian F. S. Kahl and Juliana da Silva

Additional information is available at the end of the chapter

http://dx.doi.org/10.5772/64713

**Abstract**

Telomeres are complex nucleotide sequences that cap the end of chromosomes from degradation, unwanted recombination-fusion, inappropriate activation of DNA damage response and play a critical role in cell division and chromosome stability. There is growing evidence that telomere stability can be affected by occupational and environmental exposure, as some of these factors have been correlated with increase in inflammation, oxidative stress, DNA damage, chromosome aberration, and epigenetic alterations. Both extremely short and long telomeres have been associated with neurodegenerative, cardiovascular diseases (CVD) and cancer risk. Occupational and environmental exposure to several synthetic and natural chemicals has been found to be associated with changes in telomere length, although the molecular mechanism is not fully understood. Telomeric DNA is relatively less capable of repair, resulting in accelerated shortening during the cell cycle and replicative senescence. It is recognized that diet plays an important role in telomere maintenance. Prevention of exposure to environmental and occupational hazards as well as psychological stressors can reduce the risk of telomere instability. This review provides a broad evaluation of the associated mechanism between human health and environmental and occupational exposure with telomere length, including recent findings and future perspectives.

**Keywords:** telomere length, biomarkers, human health, occupational exposure, environmental exposure

## 1. Introduction

The telomere structure is essential for maintaining chromosomal stability. It prevents the chromosome ends from being identified as damaged DNA and, therefore, nucleolytic degradation, chromosome end-to-end fusion, and break-fusion-bridge cycle (reviewed by Kahl et al. [1]). Human telomeres are nucleoprotein structures that consist of a repeat TTAGGG sequence, located at the end of chromosomes. Along with its complementary sequence, AATCCC, telomeres form a t-loop structure at the terminal ends of chromosomes [2]. A single-strand 3′ G-rich overhang, several DNA-binding proteins and specific telomerase-binding proteins, named "shelterin" complex, also comprise telomeres. The shelterin complex is formed by six proteins: TRF1, TRF2, and POT1 that directly recognize TTAGGG repeats; and TIN2, TPP1, and Rap1 that interlink the first three proteins. Even though telomeres and double-strand breaks (DSBs) are processed in the same manner, the DNA repair system clearly distinguishes the telomere region from sites of damaged DNA because of shelterin [3]. Telomere length (TL) is balanced by telomerase, a riboenzyme that synthesizes telomeric DNA *de novo* using its own RNA component as template. Even in complex organisms, telomerase-dependent telomere elongation occurs, although it is difficult to access this *in vivo*, as this happens in leukocytes, which means moving cells [4]. Telomeres shorten in each cell division due to incomplete replication of the lagging strand, the so-called "end replication problem". In most normal somatic cells of human adults, telomere length decreases with age, suggesting that telomere attrition contributes to the organismal senescence by reducing cell proliferation. So far, it is not yet understood how telomere length is set in an organism [5], but it is known that they are dynamic structures, especially when examined during short periods [4]. Because of their close relationship to lifespan and cellular senescence, telomeres have been widely studied with regard to human health and the development of diseases. One of the topics most often associated with telomere length dysfunction is, for example, how human cancers are invariably related to activation of some mechanisms to maintain telomere length [6]. Telomerase is commonly expressed in human cancer cells, mainly in 85–90% of cancers. Recent studies suggest that telomerase is implicated in tumor progression in several manners, most of them unexpected and new to science [7]. Yet, some reports have shown the reactivation of telomerase, resulting in cell immortalization, without chromosome aberrations, tumorigenic parameters or oncogenic activation (reviewed by Cech [6]). Although normal cells have some active telomerase, telomere dynamics is still unclear with regard to several pathologies. Further, whether telomeres shorten or elongate in different human everyday life situations, and by which mechanism this occurs, are still under investigation. What is known is that telomere length is strongly influenced by many other factors such as genetics, diseases, occupational and environmental exposures, and diet (reviewed by Kahl et al. [1]). Optimum telomere function and length are important for cell proliferation and apoptosis. Critically short telomeres initiate senescence resulting either in apoptosis or cell cycle arrest, through proteins such as BUB1, CENP-E, CENP-A, Chk2, among others [8]. Therefore, it is relevant to identify yielding factors that are responsible for accelerated telomere shortening.

## 2. Earlier telomere shortening: why?

Due to its high content of guanine, telomeric DNA is highly susceptible to accumulation of oxidative stress through induction of a wide range of DNA lesions, including base modifications, such as 8-oxo-guanine and $O^6$-methylguanine. In the first case, guanine oxidation converts it into 8-oxo-7,8-dihydroguanine (8-oxo-G), a tautomeric form of guanine nucleotide. Thereby, 8-oxo-G erroneously pairs with adenine instead of cytosine, causing a mutation

http://dx.doi.org/10.5772/64713

through transversion G-C→T-A [9]. This damage is not easily repaired by DNA repair mechanism and may lead to reduction of TRF1 and TRF2 linking, generating telomeric dysfunction [10, 11]. Moreover, accumulation of single-strand breaks (SSBs), as a result of the hydroxyl radical attacks on the DNA strand throughout telomere and subtelomeric regions, leads to accelerated telomere shortening or to complete loss of telomeres [12]. Telomere integrity appears to be a critical element in chromosomal stability and telomere shortening, which is induced by an increase in oxidative stress and can also be influenced by DNA repair mechanisms and polymorphisms, epigenetic status, and lifestyle habits.

Reactive oxygen species (ROS) are generated in aerobic organisms by cellular metabolism and by exogenous sources such as ionizing radiations, UV radiation, redox cycling drugs, carcinogenic compounds, and environmental toxins. DNA lesions resulting from this type of damage are mutagenic and cytotoxic and, if not repaired, can cause genetic instability, cell proliferation problems, oxidative enzyme imbalance, cell death, apoptosis, and angiogenesis. Consequences of DNA damages depend on their severity and cell type. DNA effects may lead to the development of diseases, including carcinogenesis [13].

Living organisms evolved to possess DNA repair mechanisms to repair DNA damage and thus to protect the genetic stability for survival [13, 14]. Telomeric DNA is less capable of repair, resulting in accelerated telomere attrition during the cell cycle and replicative senescence [15]. Telomeres seem to be very sensitive for both single-strand breaks (SSBs) and double-strand breaks (DSBs). As a mechanism to prevent end-to-end fusions, telomeric repeats have been shown to inhibit non-homologous end joining (NHEJ) repair mechanism. NHEJ is a major pathway to repair DSBs and has been reported to be inhibited *in vitro* by TRF2, which could be a main contributor to a persistent DNA damage response (reviewed by Hewitt et al. [15]). Furthermore, ROS produce SSBs and in contrast to the majority of genomic DNA, telomeric DNA may be deficient in repairing this type of damage [16, 17]. Single-strand breaks caused by hydrogen peroxide and an alkylating agent in human fibroblasts took at least 19 days to be repaired in telomeres, but it was repaired in 24 h in the bulk of genome and minisatellite regions (reviewed by Coluzzi et al. [17]). Failure to repair DNA damage may lead to detrimental biological consequences for organisms.

Mutations and polymorphisms also occur in DNA repair genes adversely affecting DNA repair systems. An example of DNA damage influenced by repair polymorphisms was recently shown by Borghini et al. [18], in which authors demonstrated that individuals exposed to higher levels of arsenic combined with the hOGG1 allele were associated with significantly lower TL in leukocytes [18]. As OGG1 is a protein part of the base excision repair mechanism and catalyzes the excision of oxidized purines, mainly 8-oxo-dG [13], it is reasonable that it produce some effect on telomeres. Other authors showed that individuals with congenital heart disease had reduced TL when compared to controls, related to XRCC1 194Trp allele [19]. In addition to these polymorphisms, XRCC1 399Gln allele [20] and XRCC4-null cells [21] were already associated with telomere dynamics by different repair routes.

The instable condition of telomeres can lead to activation of molecular cascades evolved in response to cellular stress, such as p53 and p16INK4a pathways, resulting in some cases in apoptosis or cellular senescence [21]. Shorter telomeres in peripheral blood lymphocytes have been shown to predict cancer risk [22, 23]. It is also relevant that p16 methylation is found in several types of cancer such as melanoma, oropharynx, and esophagus [24-26]. In addition, increasing evidence indicates that epigenetic modifications are important regulators of mammalian telomeres [27]. Epigenetic regulators, such as histone methyltransferases and DNA methyltransferases, correlate with loss of telomere-length control, thus telomere shortening affects the epigenetic status of telomeres and subtelomeres. It has been shown that such oxidative lesions interfere with the DNA's ability to function as a substrate for DNA methyltransferases, resulting in global hypomethylation [28]. Thus, genomic DNA, including the subtelomeric region, may become hypomethylated. Methylation in subtelomeric regions of the chromosomes is associated with telomere length and hence could be an important region for epigenetic regulation of the biology of telomere length maintenance [29]. A number of studies also indicate the posttranslational ubiquitination in TL proteins, albeit this modification effect on telomeres has not been directly demonstrated. The ubiquitinated telomere unbound form of TRF1 induces telomere elongation [30], while the *MKRN1* gene that encodes a portion of ubiquitin promotes the degradation of hTERT [31]. A progressive loss of DNA methylation in repetitive elements was recently shown [32], providing evidence that methylation can decrease over time as individuals age. Therefore, the association of aging with telomere epigenetic regulation is an important factor. Links between epigenetic status and telomere-length regulation provide important new avenues for understanding processes such as cancer development, which are characterized by telomere-length defects.

Several studies suggest that telomere dynamics can be challenged according to lifestyle factors. Recent studies showed that smokers had shortened telomere length when compared to never smokers [33, 34]. A cohort study found shorter telomeres for active smokers in a dose-dependent manner [34]. Other publications reported that smokers presented shorter telomere length, and irrespective of the number of cigarettes smoked per year, the lifetime accumulating exposure to smoking was more important to this outcome [35]. The main mechanisms related to reduction of telomere length by cigarette smoking are increased oxidative stress levels and inflammation [36]. Exercise and a balanced diet can also influence telomere maintenance, in a positive manner, attempting to support a healthier life.

## 3. Telomere length and human health

Aging starts even before birth, that is why is necessary not only to study telomere length at birth, as a prerequisite to understand its dynamics throughout life, but also to investigate several exposures, and genetic and epigenetic factors that may contribute to accelerate this process [37]. Aging is defined as the time-dependent event that results in a progressive functional decline that affects most living organisms. This process is the subject of several scientific studies, including mutagenesis, as the accumulation of DNA damage throughout life is a common denominator of aging [38].

Much attention has been given to the relationship of telomeres with human health in the last few decades. The natural telomere shortening can be accelerated by unhealthy lifestyle habits

http://dx.doi.org/10.5772/64713

and a poor diet [39, 40] and also due to occupational and environmental exposures [1, 41]. Exogenous physical, biological, and chemical stressors, such as environmental pollutants, medicines, chemotherapeutics, continuously challenge DNA stability. In addition, endogenous agents such as DNA replication errors, ROS, and spontaneous hydrolytic reactions can have the same effect on DNA. Different lesions arise from this damage and may include chromosomal aberrations, translocations, point mutations, gene disruption, and telomere shortening. There are various causes of ROS overexpression and exacerbated oxidative stress increases telomere shortening [9–12, 15–17]. One example is hyperglycemia, which increases ROS from the mitochondrial electron transport chain and increased glucose auto-oxidation, production of advanced glycation end-products, and activation of polyol pathway and kinase K pathway [42].

Critical telomere shortening induces cellular senescence or even the definitive inability of cells to divide. Telomere attrition in stem cells results in the depletion of their tissue and self-renewal ability. In both cases, telomere shortening can lead to different age-related pathologies [43]. The average difference of telomere length between proliferative and minimally proliferative tissues was constant in a study performed with patients whose ages ranged from 19 to 77 years old suggesting that the first 20 years are a crucial period in establishing some differences [44]. The telomere shortening in somatic cells results in changes on telomere structure that may induce replicate senescence depending on p53 and p16/retinoblastoma proteins [45].

A wide range of studies have shown that dysfunctional telomere length in biological human samples is usually related to increased risk of degenerative diseases of aging, diabetes, cardiovascular diseases (CVD), dementia, cognitive impairments, and cancer [46–51]. Ultimately, cancer and aging can be considered two different expressions of the same process: the accumulation of DNA damage. Specific location of shelterin complex is what lastly enables chromosome end protection. It is also known that within shelterin, certain components are responsible for preventing specific aspects of DNA damage repair mechanism [5]. The great challenge is to understand what signal triggers checkpoint activation at dysfunctional telomeres [5, 52].

Telomere length in pancreatic β-cells is reduced in individuals with type 2 diabetes mellitus (DM) [49] as a pathophysiology of diabetes shows an age-related aspect. The authors propose that shorter telomeres in type 2 DM could lead to an impaired ability for proliferation and insulin secretion, accelerating cell death. Obesity, which is also associated with shortened telomere length [53], is frequently associated with type 2 DM. In both cases, it is considered that excessive oxidative stress induces telomere damage, together with hyperglycemia in DM patients. In cancer biology, telomere dysfunction has been linked to tissue decrease on mitochondrial DNA copy number, while mitochondrial oxidative stress appears to be required to maintain cellular senescence [54]. A recent review suggests the hypothesis that heterogeneity of mitochondria uncoupling proteins may affect oxidative stress that imbalance telomere and cell cycle regulation, further diabetes risk and metabolic disease progression [55]. In diabetes mellitus, oxidative stress is higher in leukocytes, but also in pancreatic β-cells, which could result in shortening of β-cell telomeres, subsequently causing dysfunction of insulin secretion [49]. Results show that obesity can be associated with shortened telomeres [53], as the excessive accumulation of adipose tissue and the associated metabolic imbalance increases oxidative stress and may deregulate inflammatory cytokines. Chronic heart failure and coronary disease are strongly associated with inflammatory processes, and as expected, have also been linked to telomere shortening [41].

Cardiovascular diseases (CVD) are the main reason for heart failure, the leading cause of mortality worldwide. Two different studies have shown that telomere biology plays a role in CVD [56, 57]. The first study found an association of risk factors for CVD and telomere length, mainly with interleukin-6, an inflammatory factor. Burnett-Hartman et al. [56] observed that two single nucleotide polymorphisms in *OBCF1* and *TERC* genes (both related to leukocyte telomere length) were similarly associated with CVD mortality in women. CVD is strongly linked to the inflammation process, which may lead to increased oxidative stress. In both cases, telomere attrition may be attributed to increased oxidative stress and inflammation [56, 57].

Telomeres are related to several other humans diseases in which some mutations of TERC are reported, such as dyskeratosis congenita, several hereditary, several hereditary syndromes of bone marrow failure, and idiopathic pulmonary fibrosis (reviewed by Armanios [58]). Although the presentation of these diseases is different, shortened telomeres are present in all patients with dyskeratosis congenita, in some with bone marrow failure syndromes, and in an unknown proportion of idiopathic pulmonary fibrosis patients [59]. Shortened telomeres were also observed in patients with aplastic anemia. Some studies suggest that baseline TL is associated with late events of hematologic relapse in aplastic anemia patients treated with immunosuppressant therapy [60]. Valdes et al. [61] showed that clinical osteoporosis is related to shorter telomeres in over 2000 women, in whom leukocyte telomere length was significantly correlated with bone mineral density. This result was corroborated by Tang et al. [62], who analyzed women and men regarding telomere length and bone marrow density, and a positive correlation was found for females. These studies even suggest that TL could be a new bone aging biomarker, but these conclusions should be carefully observed as other reports did not find the same correlations [63, 64]. Both short and long telomeres have been associated with neurodegenerative and cardiovascular diseases, cancer risk [46, 59], and some human polymorphisms [65]. Indeed, several loci were identified by linkage analysis of modulators supposedly linked to telomeres and through genome global association studies. *DDX11* [66], *SIRT1*, and *XRCC6* [67] genes, as chromosome 14 and loci 10q26.13 and 3p26.1 [68], seem to be involved in telomeric dynamics. Mostly, loci near the RNA component of telomerase (TERC) are more evident in studies that correlate genetic heritage and telomere length [59]. Some polymorphisms of *OBCF1* [56] and *MEN1* [65] genes, as the $^{-1327}$C/T hTERT polymorphism [69], were associated with critically shorter and longer telomeres. However, two studies showed a greater influence of environmental effect than the genetic one on telomere length (reviewed by Andrew et al. [68]).

Another study analyzed telomere length in white blood cells and buccal cells in patients with Alzheimer's disease (AD). The researchers observed reduced telomere length in both cell types for individuals with AD. More than that, telomeres with less than 115 kb per diploid genome in white blood cells showed an odds ratio of 10.8 for a diagnosis of AD, while telomeres shorter than 40 kb per diploid genome had an odds ratio of 4.6 for AD diagnosis [48]. In concordance with this study, Hochstrasser et al. [70] also suggests that AD may contribute to telomere shortening. They found shorter telomeres on monocytes of AD patients compared to healthy subjects. In fact, a recent work found out that telomere length is significantly shorter in AD patients with alipoprotein E (ApoE) homozygote than in those with ApoE heterozygote and noncarriers. ApoE is a strong genetic risk factor for developing Alzheimer's, and seems to be associated with shorter TL when in homozygosis [71].

Telomere dynamic has been also correlated with psychological and psychosocial effects. Some authors observed telomere shortening associated with severe and/or chronic diseases in childhood, besides adverse events, such as anxiety disorders and mistreatment in childhood [39, 72]. Children aged 4-14 from over 80 neighborhoods in Louisiana, USA, were evaluated with regard to the influence of social stress on telomere length. Children living in highly disturbed neighborhoods showed shorter salivary telomere length when compared with less disturbed environments [73]. These data may indicate that childhood adversities have an impact on wellbeing throughout life. High levels of stress related to psychosocial facts and high levels of depressive symptoms were observed in caregivers of individuals with Alzheimer's, and shortened telomeres were associated with those stress factors (reviewed by Lin et al. [39]). A recent review of telomerase activity and its associations with psychological and mental factors observed a mixture of results, but some consistent findings reported decreased telomerase activity in individuals under chronic stress and increased telomerase activity in individuals with depressive disorders [74]. Oxidative stress has been suggested to play a role in the etiology of anxiety disorders and psychological distress, supporting the involvement of oxidative stress in the regulation of telomere length in psychological and psychosocial adverse effects.

Telomere shortening is a risk factor for several types of cancer [46]. A recent review investigated telomere length in several types of cancer in surrogate tissues and observed only longer telomeres in melanoma skin and hepatocellular carcinoma. No effect on telomere length was seen for colorectal, prostate, and endometrial cancers and squamous-cell carcinoma. For breast cancer, although longer and shorter telomeres were found in nine different studies, no effect on telomere length was prevalent among the findings. Two kinds of cancer were linked to both longer and shorter telomeres: lung and kidney [46]. Up to now, reduced telomere length has been prevalently found in patients with these cancers. As regards lung cancer, a study included 122 Chinese with clinical symptoms [22]. In general, telomere length was not associated with lung cancer. Nevertheless, three SNPs in telomere length maintenance genes were linked to risk of lung cancer. The *G* variant at *POT1* rs10244817 and the *A* variant of *TERT* rs2075786 were associated with decreased risk of developing lung cancer; while the G variant of *TERT* rs251796 was associated with increased risk. The *POT1* SNP interacted significantly with telomere length and lung cancer risk, showing the close relation between shelterin proteins and cancer [22]. In the review, for most types of cancers evaluated, only shorter telomeres were found: bladder, head/neck, ovarian, gastric, skin (basal cell carcinoma), osteosarcoma, and esophagus [46]. It is interesting to observe that for different types of skin cancer, the cancer etiology has a different telomere dynamic, which only shows that telomere dynamic is heterogeneous according to tissues and even with their differentiation process.

In another meta-analysis with regard to telomere length and cancer risk population studies, authors reviewed more than 50 publications [50]. Their results revealed heterogeneous association between different cancer types. In opposition to other reviews, they did not observe a significant association of short telomeres with the overall risk of cancer. Still, shorter telomeres were found associated with increased risk of gastrointestinal and head and neck cancers, similar to prior review [46]. Both are mainly cases of epithelial malignancies, which mostly appear to develop from morphologically defined precursor lesions termed intraepithelial neoplasia. The meta-analyses also revealed a significant dose-response association of gastrointestinal tumor and head and neck cancer with telomere length. The authors also highlight that telomere length is critically shortened in more than 90% of intraepithelial neoplasias. It is accepted that telomeres have different roles in different types of cancer, but again, this review indicates that short telomeres may be risk factors for tumors, especially of the digestive system [50]. A shorter TL in individuals with cancer when compared to healthy controls is biologically plausible. The accumulated mutations from critically shortened telomeres, genetic lesions, and inactivated tumor suppressor checkpoints may ultimately result in cancer [6, 7, 47, 52].

For many years, oncogenesis has been linked to telomerase activity in somatic cells [6, 7]. In fact, overexpression of telomerase is enough to neutralize the natural telomere shortening and to indefinitely extend the replicative lifespan of cultured cells when genomic instability is lacking, turning them into cancerous cells. The active telomerase complex may be more necessary to cancerous cells than to normal somatic cells due to its chromosomal aneuploidy and rapid cell division cycle [47, 75]. Thus, it seems conflicting that shortened telomeres are linked to several types of cancer. However, the mechanism of the shortened telomere relationship with cancer is through genomic instability. In the oncogenesis process, the inactivation of senescence pathways by some viral oncogenes, mutations on key-genes or chemical substances allows cells to bypass replicative checkpoints. This enables the propagation of cells with damaged telomere leading to end-to-end fusions and genome instability, and then to age-associated diseases, like cancer [43].

## 4. Occupational and environmental exposures

Different approaches are used to evaluate effects and risks of exposure to chemical, physical, and biological agents during routine work or where an individual lives. Biomarker is a general term for analysis of the interaction of a biological system and an environmental agent. There are three classes of biomarkers: (a) of exposure, that involve exogenous substances or their metabolites, or a product of interaction between a xenobiotic agent and some target cells or molecules; (b) of effect, that are biochemical, physiological or behavioral parameters, or other changes within the body and, depending upon the extent, they can be recognized in association with a disease or as a potential risk for the development of a disease; and (c) of susceptibility, that refers to the inherent or acquired ability of an organism to respond to changes in exposure to xenobiotic specific substances [76–78].

There is growing evidence that telomeric stability may be affected by environmental and/or occupational exposure, as some of those factors have been related to inflammation and chronic diseases. Occupational exposures related to shorter telomeres include polycyclic aromatic hydrocarbons (PAHs), benzene and toluene, particulate matter and long-term exposure to lead (reviewed by Zhang et al. [41]). PAHs are known for generating DNA adducts and, therefore, genomic instability. A recent study has shown the relationship between telomere shortening and pesticide use in workers associated with the agricultural industry [79]. Lead, in turn, induces double-strand breaks in DNA, particularly in lagging strands on telomeres (for a review, see [41]). Working as a hairdresser has been associated with increasing risk of cancer, due to cancer-related DNA alterations. Telomere length was shortened in a group of Sweden hairdressers [80]. The authors suggest that, as hairdressers are exposed to strong oxidative agents, it is likely that oxidative stress is the main reason for telomere shortening in these workers [80].

A study from our group observed shortening telomeres in individuals occupationally chronically exposed to low doses of pesticides at tobacco farms [33], in addition to various kinds of DNA damages already found in those individuals [81–84], corroborated by several other studies [85, 86]. Pesticides are known for inducing oxidative stress [33, 82, 87, 88], and although not all action mechanism of these chemicals are clear, induction of oxidative stress and of ROS seems to be involved. Senescent cells present 30% more modified guanines within their DNA and fourfold more free 8-oxo-dG basis, contributing to telomeric loss through oxidative stress [89]. Recently, our group was able to show two different pathways involving the ubiquitin proteasome system (UPS) by which pesticides and nicotine influence telomere length. Using System Biology approach tools, we evaluated proteins involved in telomere maintenance and their relation to pesticides used in tobacco crops at Brazil, including the natural pesticide of tobacco leaves, nicotine. In this interaction network of proteins related to telomere length and tobacco pesticides, it is important to highlight the ubiquitination bioprocess of proteins involved in some clusters of interaction [90]. The UPS is a highly conserved cell pathway that plays an important role in the selective degradation of proteins that are essential for several cell functions [91]. Some works have shown the role of ubiquitination in maintaining telomeric length [30, 31].

Longer telomeres may also reflect a health problem. Persistent organic pollutant (POPs) was associated with telomere elongation, but the mechanism remains unknown. Increasing telomerase activity and, therefore, longer telomeres were also observed in occupational exposure to arsenic [41]. The Agricultural Health Study (AHS) analyzed farmers with regard to telomere length and both cumulative and recent use of several pesticides [92]. Shorter telomeres were found associated with the lifetime use of two pesticides, and one with recent use, while only alachlor was significantly associated with longer telomeres for both cumulative and recent use [92]. The Chernobyl nuclear power plant accident forced workers to clean up the region. Some studies revealed high occurrence of age-associated degenerative diseases, cardiovascular disorders, and cancer among them (reviewed by Reste et al. [93]). However, when telomere length was analyzed, longer telomeres were found for the workers undertaking excavation and deactivation, and in workers with cancer. The authors suggest that the exposure to ionizing radiation led to longer telomeres through telomerase activation, which could potentiate carcinogenesis [93]. Even so, it is possible to highlight that most occupational exposures induce telomere shortening.

Environmental factors can also trigger epigenetic changes [94], which can also be related to telomere maintenance [67, 95]. Previous studies suggested that DNA methylation plays an important role in maintaining genomic stability, and is highly sensitive to environmental exposure [96, 97]. The impact of adverse exposure on telomere shortening starts at a very early developmental stage. Environmental exposure to lead in children appears to be associated with shorter telomeres [98], as prenatal exposure to toxic agents also seems to be a predictor of telomere imbalance. Neonatal umbilical cord blood showed a positive association between shortened fetal telomere length and smoking during pregnancy [99]. Even with the concept that high variation in telomere length between individuals is already present before birth and could increase due to environmental exposure, 128 Indian newborns from high-level natural background radiation areas showed no evidence of telomere length attrition [100]. On the other hand, placental tissues of over 200 twins were evaluated with regard to telomere length [101]. The aim was to verify if maternal residential traffic exposure was associated with telomere length. Maternal residential proximity to a major road was linked to shortened placental telomere length, while maternal residence closer to more wooded sites increased placental telomere length by 3.6%. As traffic exposure is an important source of free radicals that are known for accelerating aging, the air pollution-related adverse outcomes started early in life [101].

A group of Italian pregnant women living close to waste landfill sites was analyzed with regard to telomere length to investigate if pollution, as an environmental stressor, could affect their health. The authors observed that pollution from illegal waste sites was significantly associated with shorter telomere length, higher oxidative stress levels, and lower telomerase activity, which are known factors of cellular senescence and aging-related meiotic dysfunction in women [102]. Even low levels of cadmium shortened buccal cell telomere length in adolescents environmentally exposed to this metal [103]. Arsenic exposure to drinking water increased telomere length in individuals from West Bengal, India. This effect was telomerase-dependent but did not exhibit an overexpression of alternative lengthening of telomere-associated proteins TRF1 and TRF2 [104]. Some environmental toxic metals can produce epigenetic changes, such as DNA methylation, loss of expression of tumor suppressor gene *p16*, among others [105], eventually leading to telomere dynamics alterations.

## 5. What can be done to help maintain telomere length?

Diet is known to play an important role in telomere maintenance and personalized nutrition is a growing and promising field to prevent DNA damage [40]. A proper diet combined with physical exercises seems to prevent genomic instability, possibly providing a proper intake of antioxidants and reduction of inflammation levels [40, 53, 106, 107]. Several intervention studies have been performed to challenge the common sense that telomeres only shorten during a lifetime. According to literature, dietary patterns and individual micronutrients can influence telomere length and function. A recent review reported that individuals undergoing the following lifestyle interventions presented increased telomerase activity: practice of physical exercise, diet micronutrient supplementation, yoga, and mindfulness meditation [74].

Folate is an important vitamin required for DNA synthesis, one-carbon metabolism and repair. When there is folate deficiency, the incorporation of uracil instead of thymine in DNA is increased [108]. Plasma homocysteine concentration, which is increased when folate and vitamin B12 are deficient, seems to be inversely associated with telomere length. On the other hand, homocysteine and folate are inversely correlated [109]. Low levels of folate were associated with shorter telomeres in an older male cohort, although this effect was not observed either in female subjects or younger adults [108]. Another study showed that the MTHFR C677T polymorphism of the folate metabolism gene, which may raise plasma homocysteine, was weakly associated with increased telomere length at below-median folate levels [110]. A recent study showed that folate deficiency leads to long but dysfunctional telomeres, associated with increased chromosome instability, possible due to DNA hypomethylation [107]. Some molecular mechanisms have been proposed on how folate deficiency induces telomere shortening, such as (a) abnormal epigenetic state of subtelomeric DNA; (b) ineffective binding of shelterin complex proteins to telomeric DNA due to decrease affinity to uracil; (c) the increased excision of uracil in the telomere structure that generates abasic sites and DNA breaks. Therefore, folate status modifies telomere length by affecting DNA integrity and the epigenetic regulation of telomere length through DNA methylation [111].

As discussed earlier in this chapter, DNA damage in adulthood may originate in early life [98, 101], as lifelong dietary patterns are established in childhood. Yet, most studies with regard to telomere length in children are conducted on the effects of environmental exposure and socioeconomic and psychological status [72, 73, 98, 99, 101, 103]. A recently published study analyzed whether nutritional factors are associated with telomere length in children [112]. Between 2009 and 2011, 437 children aged 3, 6, and 9, were sampled and telomere length and micronutrient levels were measured. After adjustment for several parameters, telomere length was inversely associated with plasma levels of zinc. Also, children with the homozygous mutant genotype of the *RFC* G80A (rs1051266) polymorphism presented the shortest telomere. The RFC (reduced folate carrier) gene encodes for an enzyme required for bioavailability and metabolism of folate and vitamin B12. The chosen polymorphism is known to reduce the activity of the enzyme; indeed, the *RFC G80AA* genotype was associated with a 26 kb/diploid genome telomere loss when compared to the *RFC 80GG* genotype. Although the association between zinc levels and telomere length is still not clearly understood, the authors suggest that the inverse relationship between the two parameters may be a result of an increase in telomere sequence deletions by labile zinc induction of oxidative stress [112, 113].

High levels of plasma vitamin D were associated with longer telomeres in women, with evidence of a dose-response relationship [114]. Vitamin D is known for reducing inflammation and cell proliferation. Because both increased inflammation and enhanced cell proliferation accelerate telomere attrition [8, 56, 57], vitamin D seems to improve telomere biology through anti-inflammation and antiproliferative mechanisms [114]. Individuals treated daily with vitamin preparations are characterized by 273 bp longer telomeres than those who are not treated [115]. Vitamins C and E have also shown associations with longer telomeres [115]. It is relevant that both ascorbic acid (vitamin C) and tocopherol (vitamin E) are recognized antioxidants [116–119] that can prevent ROS generation, therefore increasing oxidative stress. For patients with Alzheimer's disease, elevated oxidative stress levels were found, besides shorter telomeres [120]. When vitamin E was administered to these patients, although there was no significant difference in telomere length after 6 months, levels of oxidative stress were lower [120].

Iron is a biologically very important trace element for maintaining metabolic homeostasis and genome stability. Nevertheless, it is required in a relatively narrow range, otherwise iron becomes a high potential generator of ROS [121]. Iron catalyses the Fenton reaction by generating the 8-hydroxy-guanine adduct, one of the most common DNA oxidative damages [13], found also in telomeres [17]. Iron overload induces DNA hypermethylation and can shorten telomere length [122], although the relationship between iron status and telomere dynamics is not totally clear. Shortened telomeres were found in patients with primary hematochromatosis and in patients taking supplements containing iron [123]. In women using iron preparations, telomeres were shortened by 9% when compared to non-users [115].

A low fat diet has also been associated with improvements in telomere dynamics. Men with prostate cancer who changed their lifestyle to a low fat diet, increased activity and stress reduction, presented increased peripheral blood mononuclear cells telomerase activity [124]. Also, polyunsaturated fatty acid intake was inversely associated with telomere length after multivariate adjustment in a group of 2284 American women [125]. The practice of physical exercise is well known as an important resource for a healthier life. Considering its effect on telomere length, some studies have reported no effect at all. One study observed a significant moderating effect of vigorous physical activity in protecting telomeres against cellular stress in women [126]. Endurance exercises were also relevant for older athletes. When compared to individuals of the same age, but low levels of exercise, older athletes had longer telomere length. Yet, among younger athletes, this difference was not observed regardless of endurance or practicing lower levels of exercise [106]. This result suggests that the lifetime practice of exercises might help the slower shortening of telomere length.

## 6. Conclusion

The observed associations reported in this chapter between telomere length and the risk of many different diseases suggest that telomeres play a fundamental role in health both at cells and organism levels. **Figure 1** summarizes some aspects that could influence telomere length. Nevertheless, for several of those diseases it is not clear if telomere length is itself the cause or consequence. For many cancers, though, telomere length shortening seems to be a major cause for triggering oncogenesis through genomic instability. It is recognized that telomeres shorten with age, but also that other factors may accelerate this process, or even reverse it in an unhealthy manner. Both occupational and environmental exposure to toxic agents has been

http://dx.doi.org/10.5772/64713

shown to modify telomere dynamics. At the same time, telomere length has emerged as a biomarker for studies analyzing this kind of exposure. Interventions aimed at increasing telomere length proposing to reverse the ageing process or preventing diseases have obtained strong evidence but are not yet enough. On the other hand, it is clear that dietary factors are associated with telomere maintenance in humans. Considering molecular and cellular mechanisms by which telomere dynamics can be modified, it is evident that epigenetic status, mainly DNA methylation, and oxidative stress are strongly involved. Oxidative damage appears to be the main condition that can destabilize telomere dynamics. We still have a long way to go trying to figure out all the particularities of telomere maintenance. The current challenge for researchers is to include other markers and analysis beyond the telomere length to further understand its mechanism and elucidate telomere biology and its influence on human health.

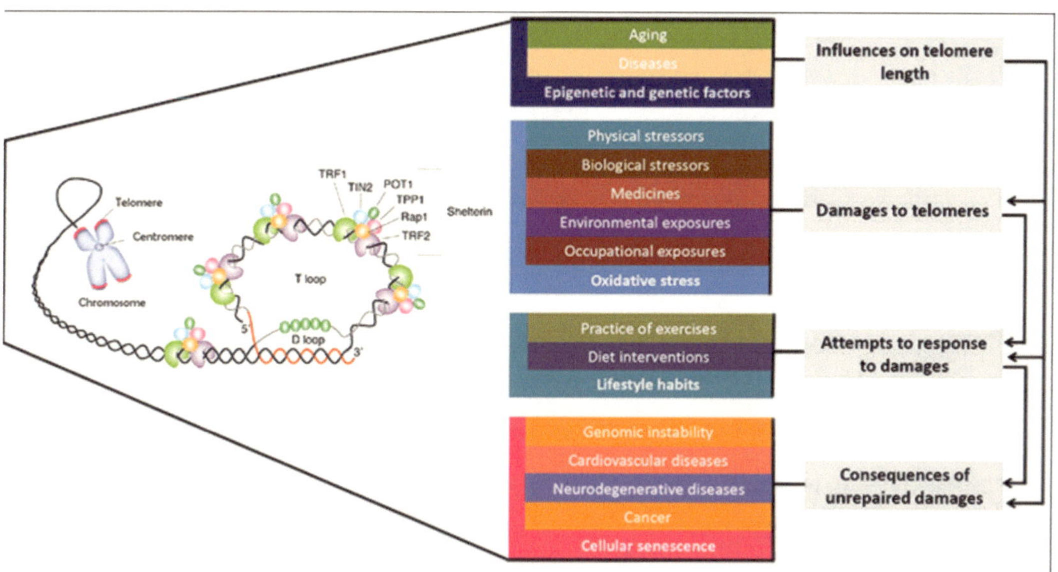


**Figure 1.** Graphical representation of factors that influence telomere length in different aspects.

## Acknowledgements

All our studies involving telomere length and occupational exposure received financial support from CAPES (Coordenação de Aperfeiçoamento de Pessoal de Nível Superior), CNPq (Conselho Nacional de Desenvolvimento Científico e Tecnológico), FAPERGS (Fundação de Amparo à Pesquisa do Estado do Rio Grande do Sul) and ULBRA (Lutheran University of Brazil), Brazil.

## Author details

Vivian F. S. Kahl and Juliana da Silva*

*Address all correspondence to: juliana.silva@ulbra.br

Laboratory of Toxicological Genetics, Postgraduate Program in Cellular and Molecular Biology Applied to Health, Lutheran University of Brazil (ULBRA), Canoas, RS, Brazil

## References

[1] Kahl VFS, Fenech M, Simon D, Da Silva J. Telomere length: What it could tell us? Applied Research in Toxicology. 2015;1(1):46-7.

[2] Zakian VA. Telomeres: The beginnings and ends of eukaryotic chromosomes. Experimental Cell Research. 2012;318(12):1456-60.

[3] de Lange T. Shelterin: The protein complex that shapes and safeguards human telomeres. Genes & Development. 2005;19(18):2100-10.

[4] Epel E. How "Reversible" is telomeric aging? Cancer Prevention Research. 2012;5(10): 1163-8.

[5] Denchi EL. Give me a break: How telomeres suppress the DNA damage response. DNA Repair. 2009;8(9):1118-26.

[6] Cech TR. Beginning to understand the end of the chromosome. Cell. 2004;116(2):273-9.

[7] Blackburn EH. Telomerase and cancer – Kirk A. Landon – AACR prize for basic cancer research lecture. Molecular Cancer Research. 2005;3(9):477-82.

[8] Choi KH, Farrell AS, Lakamp AS, Ouellette MM. Characterization of the DNA binding specificity of Shelterin complexes. Nucleic Acids Research. 2011;39(21):9206-23.

[9] Markkanen E, Huebscher U, van Loon B. Regulation of oxidative DNA damage repair: The adenine: 8-oxo-guanine problem. Cell Cycle. 2012;11(6):1070-5.

[10] Opresko PL, Fan JH, Danzy S, Wilson DM, Bohr VA. Oxidative damage in telomeric DNA disrupts recognition by TRF1 and TRF2. Nucleic Acids Research. 2005;33(4):1230-9.

[11] Rhee DB, Ghosh A, Lu J, Bohr VA, Liu Y. Factors that influence telomeric oxidative base damage and repair by DNA glycosylase OGG1. DNA Repair. 2011;10(1):34-44.

[12] von Zglinicki T. Oxidative stress shortens telomeres. Trends in Biochemical Sciences. 2002;27(7):339-44.

[13] Dizdaroglu M. Oxidatively induced DNA damage and its repair in cancer. Mutation Research. 2015;763:212-45.

[14] Friedberg EC, Walker GC, Siede W, Wood RD, Schultz RA, Ellenberger T. DNA Repair and Mutagenesis. Washington, DC: American Society for Microbiology; 2006. 1118 p.

[15] Hewitt G, Jurk D, Marques FDM, Correia-Melo C, Hardy T, Gackowska A, et al. Telomeres are favoured targets of a persistent DNA damage response in ageing and stress-induced senescence. Nature Communications. 2012;3:1–9.

[16] Houben JMJ, Moonen HJJ, van Schooten FJ, Hageman GJ. Telomere length assessment: Biomarker of chronic oxidative stress? Free Radical Biology and Medicine. 2008;44(3): 235-46.

[17] Coluzzi E, Colamartino M, Cozzi R, Leone S, Meneghini C, O'Callaghan N, et al. Oxidative stress induces persistent telomeric DNA damage responsible for nuclear morphology change in mammalian cells. PLoS One. 2014;9(10):1–12. e110963.

[18] Borghini A, Faita F, Mercuri A, Minichilli F, Bustaffa E, Bianchi F, et al. Arsenic exposure, genetic susceptibility and leukocyte telomere length in an Italian young adult population. Mutagenesis. 2016. Apr 15. pii: gew017. doi: 10.1093/mutage/gew017 [Epub ahead of print].

[19] Vecoli C, Borghini A, Foffa I, Ait-Ali L, Picano E, Andreassi MG. Leukocyte telomere shortening in grown-up patients with congenital heart disease. International Journal of Cardiology. 2016;204:17-22.

[20] Verde Z, Reinoso-Barbero L, Chicharro L, Resano P, Sánchez-Hernández I, Rodríguez González-Moro JM, et al. The effect of polymorphisms in DNA repair genes and carcinogen metabolizers on leukocyte telomere length: A cohort of healthy Spanish smokers. Nicotine & Tobacco Research. 2016;18(4):447-52.

[21] di Fagagna FD, Hande MP, Tong WM, Roth D, Lansdorp PM, Wang ZQ, et al. Effects of DNA nonhomologous end-joining factors on telomere length and chromosomal stability in mammalian cells. Current Biology. 2001;11(15):1192-6.

[22] Hosgood HD, III, Cawthon R, He X, Chanock S, Lan Q. Genetic variation in telomere maintenance genes, telomere length, and lung cancer susceptibility. Lung Cancer. 2009;66(2):157-61.

[23] Wu XF, Amos CI, Zhu Y, Zhao H, Grossman BH, Shay JW, et al. Telomere dysfunction: A potential cancer predisposition factor. Journal of the National Cancer Institute. 2003;95(16):1211-8.

[24] Jonsson A, Tuominen R, Grafstrom E, Hansson J, Egyhazi S. High Frequency of p16 (INK4A) Promoter Methylation in NRAS-Mutated Cutaneous Melanoma. Journal of Investigative Dermatology. 2010;130(12):2809-17.

[25] Ma K, Cao B, Guo M. The detective, prognostic, and predictive value of DNA methylation in human esophaegal squamous cell carcinoma. Clinical Epigenetics. 2016;8:43.

[26] Kawakami H, Okamoto I, Terao K, Sakai K, Suzuki M, Ueda S, et al. Human papillomavirus DNA and p16 expression in Japanese patients with oropharyngeal squamous cell carcinoma. Cancer Medicine. 2013;2(6):933-41.

[27] Blasco MA. The epigenetic regulation of mammalian telomeres. Nature Reviews. Genetics. 2007;8(4):299-309.

[28] Zekry D, Herrmann FR, Irminger-Finger I, Graf C, Genet C, Vitale A-M, et al. Telomere length and ApoE polymorphism in mild cognitive impairment, degenerative and vascular dementia. Journal of the Neurological Sciences. 2010;299(1-2):108-11.

[29] Yehezkel S, Segev Y, Viegas-Pequignot E, Skorecki K, Selig S. Hypomethylation of subtelomeric regions in ICF syndrome is associated with abnormally short telomeres and enhanced transcription from telomeric regions. Human Molecular Genetics. 2008;17(18):2776-89.

[30] Chang W, Dynek JN, Smith S. TRF1 is degraded by ubiquitin-mediated proteolysis after release from telomeres. Genes & Development. 2003;17(11):1328-33.

[31] Kim JH, Park SM, Kang MR, Oh SY, Lee TH, Muller MT, et al. Ubiquitin ligase MKRN1 modulates telomere length homeostasis through a proteolysis of hTERT. Genes & Development. 2005;19(7):776-81.

[32] Bollati V, Schwartz J, Wright R, Litonjua A, Tarantini L, Suh H, et al. Decline in genomic DNA methylation through aging in a cohort of elderly subjects. Mechanisms of Aging and Development. 2009;130(4):234-9.

[33] Silva Kahl VF, Simon D, Salvador M, dos Santos Branco C, Dias JF, da Silva FR, et al. Telomere measurement in individuals occupationally exposed to pesticide mixtures in tobacco fields. Environmental and Molecular Mutagenesis. 2016;57(1):74-84.

[34] Huzen J, Wong LSM, van Veldhuisen DJ, Samani NJ, Zwinderman AH, Codd V, et al. Telomere length loss due to smoking and metabolic traits. Journal of Internal Medicine. 2014;275(2):155-63.

[35] Verde Z, Reinoso-Barbero L, Chicharro L, Garatachea N, Resano P, Sanchez-Hernandez I, et al. Effects of cigarette smoking and nicotine metabolite ratio on leukocyte telomere length. Environmental Research. 2015;140:488-94.

[36] Babizhayev MA, Yegorov YE. Smoking and health: Association between telomere length and factors impacting on human disease, quality of life and life span in a large population-based cohort under the effect of smoking duration. Fundamental & Clinical Pharmacology. 2011;25(4):425-42.

[37] Factor-Litvak P, Susser E, Kezios K, McKeague I, Kark JD, Hoffman M, et al. Leukocyte telomere length in newborns: implications for the role of telomeres in human disease. Pediatrics. 2016;137(4); pii: e20153297. doi: 10.542/peds.2015-3927. Epub 2016 Mar 11.

[38] Moskalev AA, Shaposhnikov MV, Plyusnina EN, Zhavoronkov A, Budovsky A, Yanai H, et al. The role of DNA damage and repair in aging through the prism of Koch-like criteria. Ageing Research Reviews. 2013;12(2):661-84.

[39] Lin J, Epel E, Blackburn E. Telomeres and lifestyle factors: Roles in cellular aging. Mutation Research-Fundamental and Molecular Mechanisms of Mutagenesis. 2012;730(1-2):85-9.

[40] Fenech M. A public health genomics approach to improving well-being based on DNA damage prevention using nutritional, lifestyle, environmental and psychosocial strategies. ACNEM Journal. 2013;32(1):9-16.

[41] Zhang X, Lin S, Funk WE, Hou L. Environmental and occupational exposure to chemicals and telomere length in human studies. Occupational and Environmental Medicine. 2013;70(10):743-9.

[42] Araki E, Nishikawa T. Oxidative stress: A cause and therapeutic target of diabetic complications. Journal of Diabetes Investigation. 2010;1(3):90-6.

[43] Bär C, Blasco MA. Telomeres and telomerase as therapeutic targets to prevent and treat age-related diseases. F1000Research. DOI: 10.12688/f1000research.7020.1.

[44] Daniali L, Benetos A, Susser E, Kark JD, Labat C, Kimura M, et al. Telomeres shorten at equivalent rates in somatic tissues of adults. Nature Communications. 2013;4.

[45] Novo CL, Londono-Vallejo JA. Telomeres and the nucleus. Seminars in Cancer Biology. 2013;23(2):116-24.

[46] Hou L, Zhang X, Gawron AJ, Liu J. Surrogate tissue telomere length and cancer risk: Shorter or longer? Cancer Letters. 2012;319(2):130-5.

[47] Prescott J, Wentzensen IM, Savage SA, De Vivo I. Epidemiologic evidence for a role of telomere dysfunction in cancer etiology. Mutation Research-Fundamental and Molecular Mechanisms of Mutagenesis. 2012;730(1-2):75-84.

[48] Thomas P, Callaghan NJO, Fenech M. Telomere length in white blood cells, buccal cells and brain tissue and its variation with ageing and Alzheimer's disease. Mechanisms of Ageing and Development. 2008;129(4):183-90.

[49] Tamura Y, Takubo K, Aida J, Araki A, Ito H. Telomere attrition and diabetes mellitus. Geriatrics & Gerontology International. 2016;16:66-74.

[50] Zhu X, Han W, Xue W, Zou Y, Xie C, Du J, et al. The association between telomere length and cancer risk in population studies. Scientific Reports. 2016;6:1–10. doi: 10.1038/srep22243.

[51] Forero DA, Gonzalez-Giraldo Y, Lopez-Quintero C, Castro-Vega LJ, Barreto GE, Perry G. Telomere length in Parkinson's disease: A meta-analysis. Experimental Gerontology. 2016;75:53-5.

[52] Hayashi MT, Cesare AJ, Fitzpatrick JAJ, Lazzerini-Denchi E, Karlseder J. A telomere-dependent DNA damage checkpoint induced by prolonged mitotic arrest. Nature Structural & Molecular Biology. 2012;19(4):387-94.

[53] Njajou OT, Cawthon RM, Blackburn EH, Harris TB, Li R, Sanders JL, et al. Shorter telomeres are associated with obesity and weight gain in the elderly. International Journal of Obesity. 2012;36(9):1176-9.

[54] Prigione A, Fauler B, Lurz R, Lehrach H, Adjaye J. The senescence-related mitochondrial/oxidative stress pathway is repressed in human induced pluripotent stem cells. Stem Cells. 2010;28(4):721-33.

[55] Zhou Y, Ning Z, Lee Y, Hambly BD, McLachlan CS. Shortened leukocyte telomere length in type 2 diabetes mellitus: Genetic polymorphisms in mitochondrial uncoupling proteins and telomeric pathways. Clinical and Translational Medicine. 2016;5:8.

[56] Burnett-Hartman AN, Fitzpatrick AL, Kronmal RA, Psaty BM, Jenny NS, Bis JC, et al. Telomere-associated polymorphisms correlate with cardiovascular disease mortality in Caucasian women: The Cardiovascular Health Study. Mechanisms of Ageing and Development. 2012;133(5):275-81.

[57] Fitzpatrick AL, Kronmal RA, Gardner JP, Psaty BM, Jenny NS, Tracy RP, et al. Leukocyte telomere length and cardiovascular disease in the cardiovascular health study. American Journal of Epidemiology. 2007;165(1):14-21.

[58] Armanios M. Syndromes of telomere shortening. Annual Review of Genomics and Human Genetics. 2009;10:45-61.

[59] Sanders JL, Newman AB. Telomere Length in Epidemiology: A Biomarker of Aging, Age-Related Disease, Both, or Neither? Epidemiologic Reviews. 2013;35:112-31.

[60] Scheinberg P. Prognostic value of telomere attrition in patients with aplastic anemia. International Journal of Hematology. 2013;97(5):553-7.

[61] Valdes AM, Richards JB, Gardner JP, Swaminathan R, Kimura M, Xiaobin L, et al. Telomere length in leukocytes correlates with bone mineral density and is shorter in women with osteoporosis. Osteoporosis International. 2007;18(9):1203-10.

[62] Tang NLS, Woo J, Suen EWC, Liao CD, Leung JCS, Leung PC. The effect of telomere length, a marker of biological aging, on bone mineral density in elderly population. Osteoporosis International. 2010;21(1):89-97.

[63] Nielsen BR, Linneberg A, Bendix L, Harboe M, Christensen K, Schwarz P. Association between leukocyte telomere length and bone mineral density in women 25-93 years of age. Experimental Gerontology. 2015;66:25-31.

[64] Sanders JL, Cauley JA, Boudreau RM, Zmuda JM, Strotmeyer ES, Opresko PL, et al. Leukocyte telomere length is not associated with BMD, osteoporosis, or fracture in older adults: Results from the Health, Aging and Body Composition Study. Journal of Bone and Mineral Research. 2009;24(9):1531-6.

[65] Mirabello L, Yu K, Kraft P, De Vivo I, Hunter DJ, Prescott J, et al. The association of telomere length and genetic variation in telomere biology genes. Human Mutation. 2010;31(9):1050-8.

[66] Vasa-Nicotera M, Brouilette S, Mangino M, Thompson JR, Braund P, Clemitson JR, et al. Mapping of a major locus that determines telomere length in humans. American Journal of Human Genetics. 2005;76(1):147-51.

[67] Kim S, Parks CG, Xu Z, Carswell G, DeRoo LA, Sandler DP, et al. Association between genetic variants in DNA and histone methylation and telomere length. PLoS One. 2012;7(7):1–7. doi: 10.371/journal.pone.0040504.

[68] Andrew T, Aviv A, Falchi M, Surdulescu GL, Gardner JP, Lu XB, et al. Mapping genetic loci that determine leukocyte telomere length in a large sample of unselected female sibling pairs. American Journal of Human Genetics. 2006;78(3):480-6.

[69] Matsubara Y, Murata M, Watanabe K, Saito I, Miyaki K, Omae K, et al. Coronary artery disease and a functional polymorphism of hTERT. Biochemical and Biophysical Research Communications. 2006;348(2):669-72.

[70] Hochstrasser T, Marksteiner J, Humpel C. Telomere length is age-dependent and reduced in monocytes of Alzheimer patients. Experimental Gerontology. 2012;47(2): 160-3.

[71] Takata Y, Kikukawa M, Hanyu H, Koyama S, Shimizu S, Umahara T, et al. Association between ApoE phenotypes and telomere erosion in Alzheimer's disease. Journals of Gerontology Series a-Biological Sciences and Medical Sciences. 2012;67(4):330-5.

[72] Kananen L, Surakka I, Pirkola S, Suvisaari J, Lonnqvist J, Peltonen L, et al. Childhood adversities are associated with shorter telomere length at adult age both in individuals with an anxiety disorder and controls. PLoS One. 2010;5(5).

[73] Theall KP, Brett ZH, Shirtcliff EA, Dunn EC, Drury SS. Neighborhood disorder and telomeres: Connecting children's exposure to community level stress and cellular response. Social Science & Medicine. 2013;85:50-8.

[74] Deng W, Cheung ST, Tsao SW, Wang XM, Tiwari AFY. Telomerase activity and its association with psychological stress, mental disorders, lifestyle factors and interventions: A systematic review. Psychoneuroendocrinology. 2016;64:150–163.

[75] Jones CH, Pepper C, Baird DM. Telomere dysfunction and its role in haematological cancer. British Journal of Haematology. 2012;156(5):573-87.

[76] Bonassi S, Au WW. Biomarkers in molecular epidemiology studies for health risk prediction. Mutation Research-Reviews in Mutation Research. 2002;511(1):73-86.

[77] Angerer J, Ewers U, Wilhelm M. Human biomonitoring: State of the art. International Journal of Hygiene and Environmental Health. 2007;210(3-4):201-28.

[78] Manno M, Viau C, Cocker J, Colosio C, Lowry L, Mutti A, et al. Biomonitoring for occupational health risk assessment (BOHRA) introduction. Toxicology Letters. 2010;192(1):3-16.

[79] Hou L, Andreotti G, Baccarelli AA, Savage S, Hoppin JA, Sandler DP, et al. Lifetime pesticide use and telomere shortening among male pesticide applicators in the agricultural health study. Environmental Health Perspectives. 2013;121(8):919-24.

[80] Li H, Åkerman G, Lidén C, Alhamdow A, Wojdacz TK, Broberg K, et al. Alterations of telomere length and DNA methylation in hairdressers: A cross-sectional study. Environmental and Molecular Mutagenesis. 2016;57:159-67.

[81] Da Silva FR, Da Silva J, Allgayer MdC, Simon CF, Dias JF, dos Santos CEI, et al. Genotoxic biomonitoring of tobacco farmers: Biomarkers of exposure, of early biological effects and of susceptibility. Journal of Hazardous Materials. 2012;225:81-90.

[82] Da Silva FR, Kvitko K, Rohr P, Abreu MB, Thiesen FV, Da Silva J. Genotoxic assessment in tobacco farmers at different crop times. Science of the Total Environment. 2014;490:334-41.

[83] Da Silva FR, Da Silva J, Nunes E, Benedetti D, Kahl V, Rohr P, et al. Application of the buccal micronucleus cytome assay and analysis of PON1Gln192Arg and CYP2A6*9(-48T> G) polymorphisms in tobacco farmers. Environmental and Molecular Mutagenesis. 2012;53(7):525-34.

[84] Alves JS, Da Silva FR, Silva GF, Salvador M, Kvitko K, Rohr P, et al. Investigation of potential biomarkers for the early diagnosis of cellular stability after the exposure of agricultural workers to pesticides. Annals of the Brazilian Academy of Science. 2016;88(1):349-60.

[85] Muniz JF, McCauley L, Scherer J, Lasarev M, Koshy M, Kow YW, et al. Biomarkers of oxidative stress and DNA damage in agricultural workers: A pilot study. Toxicology and Applied Pharmacology. 2008;227(1):97-107.

[86] Bolognesi C. Genotoxicity of pesticides: A review of human biomonitoring studies. Mutation Research-Reviews in Mutation Research. 2003;543(3):251-72.

[87] Benedetti D, Nunes E, Sarmento M, Porto C, Iochims dos Santos CE, Dias JF, et al. Genetic damage in soybean workers exposed to pesticides: Evaluation with the comet and buccal micronucleus cytome assays. Mutation Research-Genetic Toxicology and Environmental Mutagenesis. 2013;752(1-2):28-33.

[88] Mostafalou S, Abdollahi M. Pesticides and human chronic diseases: Evidences, mechanisms, and perspectives. Toxicology and Applied Pharmacology. 2013;268(2): 157-77.

[89] von Zglinicki T, Martin-Ruiz CM, Saretzki G. Telomeres, cell senescence and human aging. Journal of Signal Transduction. 2005;5(3):103-14.

[90] Kahl VFS, Da Silva J, Da Silva FR. Influence of exposure to pesticides on telomere length maintenance in tobacco farmers: A biology system approach. *in prep*.

[91] Vabulas RM. Proteasome function and protein biosynthesis. Current Opinion in Clinical Nutrition and Metabolic Care. 2007;10(1):24-31.

[92] Andreotti G, Hoppin JA, Hou L, Koutros S, Gadalla SM, Savage SA, et al. Pesticide use and relative leukocyte telomere length in the agricultural health study. PLoS One. 2015;10(7):1–10. doi: 10.371/journal.pone.0133382..

[93] Reste J, Zvigule G, Zvagule T, Kurjane N, Eglite M, Gabruseva N, Telomere length in Chernobyl accident recovery workers in the late period after the disaster. Journal of Radiation Research. 2014;55:1089-100.

[94] Collotta M, Bertazzi PA, Bollati V. Epigenetics and pesticides. Toxicology. 2013;307:35-41.

[95] Gadalla SM, Katki HA, Shebl FM, Giri N, Alter BP, Savage SA. The relationship between DNA methylation and telomere length in dyskeratosis congenita. Aging Cell. 2012;11(1):24-8.

[96] Hou L, Zhang X, Wang D, Baccarelli A. Environmental chemical exposures and human epigenetics. International Journal of Epidemiology. 2012;41(1):79-105.

[97] Cortessis VK, Thomas DC, Levine AJ, Breton CV, Mack TM, Siegmund KD, et al. Environmental epigenetics: Prospects for studying epigenetic mediation of exposure-response relationships. Human Genetics. 2012;131(10):1565-89.

[98] Pawlas N, Plachetka A, Kozlowska A, Broberg K, Kasperczyk S. Telomere length in children environmentally exposed to low-to-moderate levels of lead. Toxicology and Applied Pharmacology. 2015;287:111-8.

[99] Salihu HM, Pradhan A, King L, Paothong A, Nwoga C, Marty PJ, et al. Impact of intrauterine tobacco exposure on fetal telomere length. American Journal of Obstetrics and Gynecology. 2015;212(2):205.e1–8. doi: 10.1016/j.ajog.2014.08.026.

[100] Das B, Saini D, Seshadri M. No evidence of telomere length attrition in newborns from high level background radiation ares in Kerala coast, south west India. International Journal of Radiation Biology. 2012;88(9):642-7.

[101] Bijnens E, Zeegers MP, Gielen M, Kicinski M, Hageman GJ, Pachen D, et al. Lower placental telomere length may be attributed to maternal residential traffic exposure; a twin study. Environment International. 2015;79:1-7.

[102] De Felice B, Nappi C, Zizolfi B, Guida M, Di Spiezio Sardo A, Bifulco G, et al. Telomere shortening in women resident close to waste landfill sites. Gene. 2012;500(1):101-6.

[103] Fillman T, Shimizu-Furusawa H, Ng CF, Parajuli RP, Watanabe C. Association of cadmium and arsenic exposure with salivary telomere length in adolescents in Terai, Nepal. Environment Research. 2016;149:8-14.

[104] Chatterjee D, Bhattacharjee P, Sau TJ, Das JK, Sarma N, Bandyopadhyay AK, et al. Arsenic exposure through drinking water leads to senescence and alteration of telomere length in humans: A case-control in West Bengal, India. Molecular Carcinogenesis. 2015;54(9):800-9.

[105] Cheng T-F, Choudhuri S, Muldoon-Jacobs K. Epigenetic targets of some toxicologically relevant metals: A review of the literature. Journal of Applied Toxicology. 2012;32(9): 643-53.

[106] Østhus IBØ, Sgura A, Berardinelli F, Alsnes IV, Brønstad E, Rehn T, et al. Telomere length and long-term endurance exercise: Does exercise training affect biological age? A pilot study. PLoS One. 2012;7(12):e52769.

[107] Bull CF, Mayrhofer G, O'Callaghan NJ, Au AY, Pickett HA, Low GK, et al. Folate deficiency induces dysfunctional long and short telomeres; both states are associated with hypomethylation and DNA damage in human WIL2-NS cells. Cancer Prevention Research. 2014;7(1):128-38.

[108] Bull C, Fenech M. Genome-health nutrigenomics and nutrigenetics: Nutritional requirements or 'nutriomes' for chromosomal stability and telomere maintenance at the individual level. Proceedings of the Nutrition Society. 2008;67(2):146-56.

[109] Moores CJ, Fenech M, O'Callaghan NJ. Telomere dynamics: The influence of folate and DNA methylation. Nutrition and Physical Activity in Aging, Obesity, and Cancer. 2011;1229:76-88.

[110] Paul L, Cattaneo M, D'Angelo A, Sampietro F, Fermo I, Razzari C, et al. Telomere length in peripheral blood mononuclear cells is associated with folate status in men. Journal of Nutrition. 2009;139(7):1273-8.

[111] Fenech M. Folate (vitamin B9) and vitamin B12 and their function in the maintenance of nuclear and mitochondrial genome integrity. Mutation Research-Fundamental and Molecular Mechanisms of Mutagenesis. 2012;733(1-2):21-33.

[112] Milne E, O'Callaghan N, Ramankutty P, de Klerk NH, Greenop KR, Armstrong BK, et al. Plasma micronutrient levels and telomere length in children. Nutrition. 2015;31(2): 331-6.

[113] Sharif R, Thomas P, Zalewski P, Fenech M. The role of zinc in genomic stability. Mutation Research. 2012;733(1-2):111-21.

[114] Liu JJ, Prescott J, Giovannucci E, Hankinson SE, Rosner B, Han J, et al. Plasma vitamin D biomarkers and leukocyte telomere length. American Journal of Epidemiology. 2013;177(12):1411-7.

[115] Xu Q, Parks CG, DeRoo LA, Cawthon RM, Sandler DP, Chen H. Multivitamin use and telomere length in women. American Journal of Clinical Nutrition. 2009;89(6):1857-63.

[116] Kahl VFS, Reyes JM, Sarmento MS, da Silva J. Mitigation by vitamin C of the genotoxic effects of nicotine in mice, assessed by the comet assay and micronucleus induction. Mutation Research-Genetic Toxicology and Environmental Mutagenesis. 2012;744(2): 140-4.

[117] Franke SIR, Pra D, Da Silva J, Erdtmann B, Henriques JAP. Possible repair action of vitamin C on DNA damage induced by methyl methanesulfonate, cyclophosphamide, $FeSO_4$ and $CuSO_4$ in mouse blood cells in vivo. Mutation Research. 2005;583:75-84.

[118] Cooke MS, Evans MD, Podmore ID, Herbert KE, Mistry P, Hickenbotham PT, et al. Novel repair action of vitamin C upon in vivo oxidative DNA damage. FEBS Letters. 1998;439(3):363-7.

[119] Eroglu S, Pandir D, Uzun FG, Bas H. Protective role of vitamins C and E in diclorvos-induced oxidative stress in human erythrocytes *in vitro*. Biological Research. 2013;46:33-8.

[120] Guan JZ, Guan WP, Maeda T, Makino N. Effect of vitamin E administration on the elevated oxygen stress and the telomeric and subtelomeric status in Alzheimer's disease. Gerontology. 2012;58(1):62-9.

[121] Galaris D, Pantopoulos K. Oxidative stress and iron homeostasis: Mechanistic and health aspects. Critical Reviews in Clinical Laboratory Sciences. 2008;45(1):1-23.

[122] Prá D, Franke SIR, Henriques JA, Fenech M. Iron and genome stability: An update. Mutation Research. 2012;733(1-2):92-9.

[123] Kepinska M, Szyller J, Milnerowicz H. The influence of oxidative stress induced by iron on telomere length. Environmental Toxicology and Pharmacology. 2015;40(3):931-5.

[124] Orenish D, Lin J, Daubenmier J, Weidner G, Epel E, Kemp C, et al. Increased telomerase activity and comprehensive lifestyle changes: A pilot study. The Lancet. Oncology. 2008;9(11):1048-57.

[125] Cassidy A, De Vivo I, Liu Y, Han J, Prescott J, Hunter DJ, et al. Associations between diet, lifestyle factors, and telomere length in women. American Journal of Clinical Nutrition. 2010;91(5):1273-80.

[126] Puterman E, Lin J, Blackburn E, O'Donovan A, Alder N, Epel E. The power of exercise: Buffering the effect of chronic stress on telomere length. PLoS One. 2010;5(5):e10837.

Chapter 9

# On the Far Side of Telomeres: The Many Roles of Telomerase in the Acquisition and Retention of Cancer Stemness

Kerem Teralı and Açelya Yilmazer

Additional information is available at the end of the chapter

http://dx.doi.org/10.5772/65762

**Abstract**

It is well recognised that upregulation/reactivation of telomerase, the telomere-lengthening enzyme, is the *sine qua non* of cellular immortalisation and malignant transformation. But there is also convincing evidence that telomerase stands at a crossroads where several developmental signalling pathways meet and that its upregulation/reactivation has effects beyond maintaining telomere length, such as altering energy metabolism and modulating gene expression. We believe that it is important to realise that, in a pathological context, such extratelomeric effects of telomerase are related to the emergence and persistence of the cancer stem cell (CSC) phenotype. Given the common conception of cancer stemness as a major contributor to therapy resistance and tumour relapse, a more complete annotation of biological mechanisms for its regulation by telomerase will provide the opportunity to develop telomerase-targeted anticancer therapies which kill or differentiate CSCs effectively.

**Keywords:** telomeres, telomerase, TERT, cancer stemness, CSCs, targeted anticancer therapy

## 1. Introduction

Telomeres are specialised structures that define the very ends of linear eukaryotic chromosomes and provide for their stability by protecting against degradation or end-to-end fusion. In mammals, telomeres are localised throughout the nucleus and associated with the nuclear matrix. Telomeric DNA of human cells is composed of a long (5 to 15 kb) stretch of the repeating hexanucleotide sequence 5'–TTAGGG–3' on one strand (the G-rich strand) and the complementary 5'–CCCTAA–3' on the other (the C-rich strand). The G-rich strand has a short (35 to

600 nt) single-stranded overhang at its 3' end (the G-overhang) which folds back and base pairs with the C-rich strand, forming a T-loop [1]. In humans, hexameric telomere repeats act as binding sites for various telomere-binding proteins collectively termed the shelterin complex, a dynamic ensemble of interactions that allows the cell to distinguish between natural chromosome ends and DNA double-strand breaks, preventing the cell's DNA damage response (DDR) from improper activation [2]. Telomeres undergo progressive shortening with each cell division as a result of incomplete lagging strand synthesis, less widely known end-processing events, and oxidative damage [3, 4]. This so-called telomere erosion operates as a kind of mitotic clock that determines ageing of the whole organism and suppresses malignant transformation of its constituent cells. The biological function of telomeres is heavily regulated and relies on both a minimal length of telomeric DNA and the proper functioning of the associated shelterin complex. A unique enzyme termed telomerase assists in replicating linear chromosomes through *de novo* synthesis of telomeric repeats, thereby counteracting the progressive telomere erosion that would otherwise occur in its partial or complete absence. In addition to its role in telomere length homeostasis, telomerase also performs telomere length-independent functions such as modulation of gene expression. In a pathological context, telomerase's new talents are intimately related to tumour development and progression to metastatic disease. This chapter summarises the newly discovered extracurricular activities of telomerase and describe how these are involved in regulating cancer stemness, the stem-like component of human tumours.

## 2. Telomerase and the cancer connection

Telomerase is a conserved RNA-dependent DNA polymerase canonically responsible for the maintenance of telomere length above a critical threshold. Human telomerase is primarily localised in the nucleus, as deducible from its role in telomere biology, but it can also be found in other cellular compartments such as the cytosol and mitochondria [5]. Telomerase is ribonucleoprotein in nature and consists minimally and essentially of a protein catalytic subunit (telomerase reverse transcriptase, TERT) and a large RNA subunit (telomerase RNA, TER). Active human telomerase has a bilobal architecture where one TERT subunit and one TER subunit participate in the formation of each lobe and a hinge region connects the two lobes [6]. This conformationally flexible, dimeric structure of the human enzyme undoubtedly has profound functional implications with respect to the catalytic cycle. Firstly, during the synthesis of telomeric DNA by telomerase, the 3′ end of the G-overhang is positioned in the active site of TERT and aligned by base pairing with the 3' end of the RNA template in TER. Secondly, TERT catalyses the addition of deoxyribonucleotides to the chromosome substrate through reverse transcribing TER into hexameric telomere repeats until the 5' end of the RNA template is reached. Lastly, telomerase translocates and realigns with the newly synthesised 3' end of the chromosome substrate to restart the catalytic cycle [7, 8]. In spite of the fact that TERT and TER are the two subunits that provide the catalytic core of telomerase, there are several other molecules that associate with telomerase and are involved in its biogenesis, trafficking, recruitment, and activation. Some of the most well-known telomerase-associated proteins include the nucleolar protein dyskerin [9], the three other nucleolar proteins NOP10, NHP2 and GAR1 [10], the two AAA+ ATPases pontin and reptin [11], and the WD40-repeat protein TCAB1 [12]. It should be noted that not all cells necessarily rely upon telomerase to maintain telomere length. Some telomerase-negative immortalised cell lines and tumours are able to elongate their telomeres by the much rarer alternative lengthening of telomeres (ALT) pathway. In contrast to telomerase, which utilises an RNA template to *de novo* synthesise telomeric repeats, the ALT pathway utilises a DNA template for DNA copying in an inter- or intramolecular recombination event [13].

Cancer is usually an age-related genetic disease, manifesting only when normal cells develop genomic instability over a reasonable period of time and acquire unlimited replicative potential that leads to the generation of macroscopic tumours. Telomerase upregulation/reactivation is observed in at least 85% of advanced human tumours, strongly suggesting a crucial role during human tumour pathogenesis [14, 15]. The most widely accepted multistep model of general tumourigenesis for explaining the part played by telomerase in telomere maintenance and cellular immortalisation is provided in section 3.2. Besides being found in primary tumours, telomerase activity is also detected in circulating tumour cells in, for instance, breast [16], ovarian [17] and prostate [18] cancers. Telomerase is upregulated/reactivated in premalignant cells by five common mechanisms: (i) increased transcriptional activation of *TERT* and/or *TER*; (ii) loss of transcriptional repressors of *TERT*; (iii) mutations in the *TERT* gene promoter/enhancer region (which result in the transactivation of this gene); (iv) several kinases (which phosphorylate and thus enhance the activity of TERT); and (v) gain of copy number of *TERT* and/or *TER* [13]. Somatic mutations in the *TERT* gene promoter region are frequent events in cancers of the bladder, central nervous system, skin (melanoma) and thyroid (follicular cell-derived) [19]. Two mutually exclusive and highly recurrent *TERT* promoter mutations are C250T and C228T [20, 21]. Although both mutations create a similar binding motif for E-twenty-six (ETS) transcription factors, they are functionally distinct in such a way that the the C250T *TERT* promoter but not the C228T *TERT* promoter additionally requires non-canonical NF-κB signalling in order to be transcriptionally driven [22]. Collectively, these findings highlight the contribution of *TERT* promoter mutations and non-canonical NF-κB signalling to tumourigenesis and decipher a fundamental mechanism for the reactivation of TERT in various tumours.

## 3. Cancer stemness

Cancer cells within a single tumour often exist in distinct phenotypic states which differ in functional attributes. This so-called intratumoural heterogeneity originates from a myriad of cell types recruited to the tumour as well as from genetic, epigenetic and metabolic differences amongst the cancer cells themselves and may result in variable or unpredictable responses to treatment [23]. Postulated to be the driving force behind tumour maintenance, hypermalignant stem-like cells called cancer stem cells (CSCs) represent a unique dimension of intratumoural heterogeneity. This often-small subpopulation of cancer cells is thought to play pivotal roles in tumour initiation and progression, spreading, therapy resistance, and recurrence, all of which lead to poor prognosis.

### 3.1. Definitions and measurements

CSCs have critical implications for nearly, if not quite, all types of cancers, including leukaemias [24–26], lymphomas [27], melanomas [28, 29], sarcomas [30], and various carcinomas such as brain [31], skin [32], head and neck [33], lung [34, 35], liver [36], gastric [37], colorectal [38, 39], bladder [40], pancreatic [41, 42], prostate [43], breast [44] and ovarian [45] cancers. The functions assumed by CSCs in human cancers are diverse, ranging from sustaining tumour growth and dissemination to treatment failure and tumour relapse. The three clear-cut features that contribute to the aforementioned functions of CSCs, aka cancer stemness traits, are: (i) their unrestricted ability to self-renew; (ii) their aberrant ability to differentiate into mixed populations of tumour cells; and (iii) their high ability to transition from a proliferative to a quiescent state. In spite of the fact that these operational characteristics are, to a large extent, shared by both CSCs and physiological stem cells, CSCs are the ones that are known to be related to several malignant phenotypes, including induction of invasion and metastasis and resistance to apoptosis. In addition, CSCs are distinguished from bulk tumour cells by their capacity to form nonadherent spheres when cultured in stem cell media, their propensity to found fresh tumours when transplanted into severe combined immunodeficient mice and their expression of a selected repertoire of stem cell-surface markers [46]. Therefore, it is important here to realise that cancer stemness, no matter how it is measured, stresses the ways in which CSCs differ from bulk cancer cells as well as from physiological stem cells. The cancer stemness phenomenon is of considerable clinical importance and significance because it prognosticates that successful anticancer therapy must involve strategies that will eradicate CSCs, as these cells are able to dominate any residual tumour cells that survive conventional anticancer therapies.

### 3.2. Determinants and signatures

In the past, the cancer stemness model was widely seen as a static one which suggested a stable CSC population and a hierarchical organisation of cell division and differentiation. In recent times, however, the cancer stemness model has evolved into a dynamic one where CSCs are rather accepted as a functional subpopulation of cancer cells and can also be formed by the process of dedifferentiation from mature cancer cells under proper environmental conditions [47]. Accumulating data have revealed that cancer stemness is governed by genetic changes (such as oncogene activation and oncosuppressor gene inactivation), epigenetic changes (such as miRNA targeting and promoter DNA hypomethylation/hypermethylation) and metabolic changes (such as the shift to aerobic glycolysis) concomitant with changes in the tumour microenvironment, especially the CSC niche (Figure 1). These changes are a prerequisite for the oncogenic transformation and cellular (nuclear and metabolic) reprogramming of non-CSCs to CSCs and precipitate a spectrum of drastic cellular consequences, including overproduction of certain oncoproteins, disruption of certain oncosuppressor proteins, upregulation/reactivation of telomerase, reactivation of the epithelial-to-mesenchymal transition (EMT)

http://dx.doi.org/10.5772/65762

programme, modulation of energy metabolism, stimulation of a number of embryonic/oncogenic signalling pathways, and differential expression of several microRNAs (miRNAs).

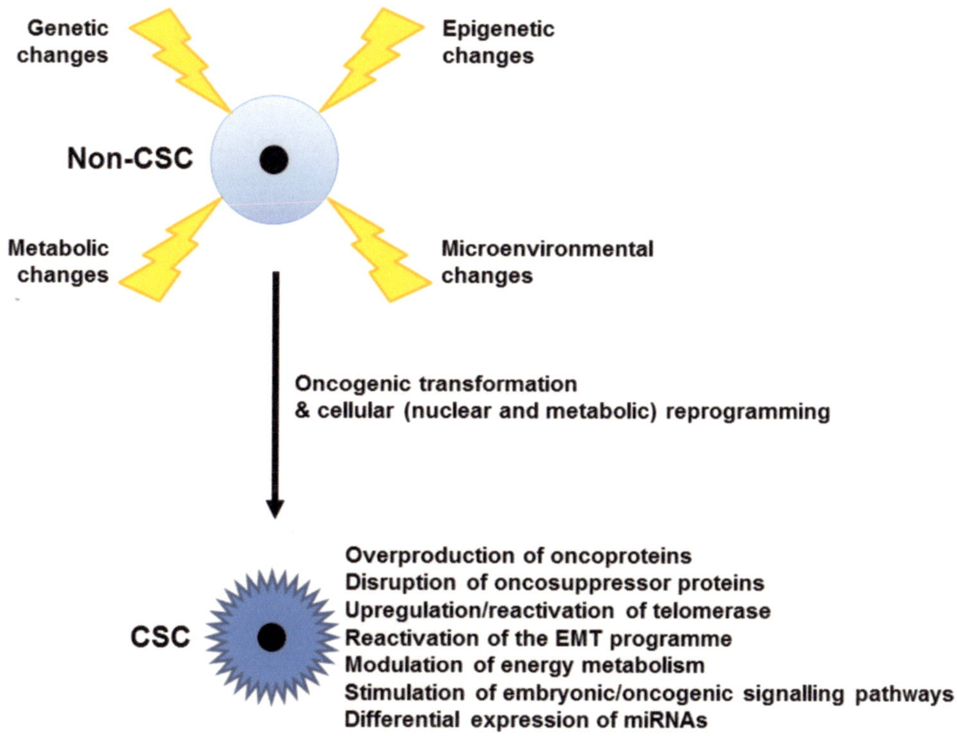


**Figure 1. How do CSCs arise?** The joint impact of genetic, epigenetic, metabolic and microenvironmental factors is believed to determine the conversion of non-CSCs (which could be normal stem cells, mature cancer cells, or others) to CSCs. This process somehow is a dynamic one and CSCs are a functional and not merely territorial subpopulation of cancer cells.

Disruption of diverse oncosuppressor proteins with antiproliferative, prodifferentiative and/or proapoptotic effects accounts for an early molecular event accompanying the emergence of cancer stemness traits. p53, pRB, PTEN, and $p16^{INK4A}$ are by far among the most commonly inactivated oncosuppressor proteins in advanced human tumours [48]. Their inactivation permits premalignant cells to avoid replicative senescence, apoptosis, or both, thereby continuing to divide and accumulating further tumourigenic alterations like genomic (chromosomal) instability that follows telomere erosion [49]. The subsequent upregulation/reactivation of telomerase compensates for telomere erosion (which would otherwise trigger entry of cells into a period of crisis with massive cell death), suppressing genomic (chromosomal) instability and allowing premalignant cells to proliferate for a virtually infinite number of cell divisions. Additionally, and surprisingly, there is accumulating evidence that telomerase upregulation/reactivation provides susceptible cells with cancer stemness traits. The many functions of telomerase in the development and maintenance of cancer stemness will be addressed in more detail in the next sections of this chapter.

A further means by which non-CSCs acquire cancer stemness traits is through the EMT process. Physiologically, EMT causes cells to change from a stationary epithelial to a motile mesenchymal morphology, thereby allowing for wound healing, tissue regeneration and organ fibrosis in adults and cell migration and tissue remodelling in developing embryos [50]. In the context of epithelium-derived carcinoma, however, the reactivation of the EMT programme contributes to the evolution of primary tumours towards increasingly aggressive phenotypes. The complex molecular, cellular and morphological alterations linked to pathological EMT are generally mediated by the joint action of the signals from the tumour microenvironment that induce the EMT programme (for example, TGF-β signalling, inflammatory cytokines, and hypoxia), the transcription factors that coordinate the EMT programme (for example, SNAI-1, SNAI-2, ZEB-1, ZEB-2, TWIST-1, and TWIST-2), and the effector proteins that execute the EMT programme (for example, low levels of E-cadherin and high levels of vimentin, N-cadherin, fibronectin, CD44, and MMPs) [51]. Such cooperation between the cell-extrinsic signals and the cell-intrinsic regulators is fully important and primarily responsible for endowing epithelial tumour cells with CSC-like properties, ranging from cell motility to invasiveness to cell survival, which are indispensable to metastatic dissemination from the primary tumour site, secondary tumour growth at a distant site, and resistance to therapy, respectively. Although CSCs originating from bulk tumour cells within epithelium-derived carcinomas achieve their final stemness state possibly *via* EMT, the degree to which they resemble or depart from CSCs originating from adult stem cells has yet to be fully explored.

Metabolic reprogramming is also an obvious mechanism of intervening and redirecting the cell fate of differentiated (normal or non-CSC tumour) cells. Traditionally, energy metabolism was widely accepted as a passive process that generated ATP and building blocks to meet the demands of the specialised cell types of the body in response to extra- and/or intracellular signals. Today, however, the modulation of energy metabolism and build-up of oncogenic metabolites are viewed as the harbingers of cancer stemness [52]. Typically, cancer cells are dependent more on glycolysis for energy production, even in the presence of sufficient oxygen to support oxidative phosphorylation. This phenomenon of aerobic glycolysis is commonly referred to as the Warburg effect and appears to fulfil the requirement of proliferating cancer cells to rapidly yield ATP and to provide anabolic substrates (such as amino acids, nucleotides, and phospholipids) for their daughter cells [53]. Besides, increased lactate generation during aerobic glycolysis provokes the acidification of the tumour microenvironment, ultimately giving rise to motile, invasive/metastatic and drug-resistant cells [54]. In agreement with this, a recent report confirmed and substantiated the need for a metabolic switch to glycolysis in the emergence of EMT-driven CSC-like characteristics in basal-like breast cancer cells [55]. Another report utilising nasopharyngeal carcinoma as a model system established that behaviourally-selected and accordingly-assayed CSCs, as distinct from their differentiated progenies, exhibit a metabolic shift from oxidative phosphorylation to glycolysis for ATP supply [56]. Nevertheless, contradictory evidence on the metabolic profile of CSCs has also been presented; two independent research groups reported that the bioenergetic and biosynthetic demands of quiescent/slow-cycling CSCs are likely to be met by oxidative phosphorylation, not by glycolysis [57, 58].

CSCs maintain their prolonged residence in the stemness state through diverting and co-opting elegant signalling pathways that are normally active during embryonic development. The embryonic/oncogenic signalling pathways operating in CSCs include Notch, Hedgehog (HH), Wnt/β-catenin, cytokine receptor-mediated JAK/STAT, TNF-α receptor-mediated NF-κB, growth factor receptor (receptor tyrosine kinase)-mediated PI3K/AKT/mTOR, TGF-β/BMP receptor-mediated SMAD, and Hippo-YAP/TAZ [59–61]. Sustained activation of and crosstalk between these cascades ultimately enhance the expression of cell-surface proteins (for example, CD133, CD44, integrins, and CXCR4), prosurvival proteins (for example, BCL-2, BCL-XL, MCL-1, survivin, and MIC-1), induced pluripotency-associated transcription factors (for example, BMI-1, OCT-3/4, SOX-2, MYC, and NANOG), EMT-associated proteins (for example, MMPs, vimentin, N-cadherin, SNAI, TWIST, and ZEB), glycolysis-associated proteins (for example, GLUTs and glycolytic enzymes), treatment resistance-associated proteins (for example, GSH, ALDH1, ABCB1, ABCC1, ABCG2, CHK-1, and CHK-2), proangiogenic factors (for example, VEGF and COX-2), and proinflammatory cytokines (for example, IL-6 and TNF-α) [60, 62, 63].

Lastly, several miRNAs have been observed to support the emergence of cancer stemness traits through targeting signalling elements and gene groups implicated in CSC biology. miRNAs are a fast-growing class of short (19 to 22 nt), noncoding, regulatory RNA molecules that customarily bind to the 3′-untranslated region (3′-UTR) of their target transcripts to induce translational repression, degradation, or destabilisation. Although miRNAs generally help regulate the transitions between different stages of development, they are also linked with tumourigenesis. As such, CSC-specific miRNA expression profiles may be useful for prognostic purposes. Those miRNAs that are highly expressed in CSCs of a specific tumour are termed oncomiRs; those that are excluded from CSCs of the same tumour are known as tumour-suppressor miRs. Breast CSCs were the first CSCs in which differential expression of miRNAs was demonstrated [64].

## 4. Regulation of cancer stemness by telomerase

Most adult somatic cells do not or only transiently express telomerase and undergo telomere shortening with every cell division until the cell eventually dies. Most tumour cells, including CSCs, however, display high levels of telomerase activity and possess the ability to continually regenerate their telomeres [65]. As a result, telomerase upregulation/reactivation serves as an important mechanism for CSCs to attain indefinite (or at least extremely long) replicative lifespans. In fact, in reality, telomerase undertakes roles that significantly diverge from its normal role in elongating telomeres, as suggested by contemporary research on manipulation of telomerase expression and/or function in cells representing potential targets for oncogenic transformation and cellular (nuclear and metabolic) reprogramming. Central to the extratelomeric roles of telomerase (particularly of TERT) is its interaction with key downstream components of the main embryonic/oncogenic signalling pathways or with other macromolecules (such as DNA and transcription factors) by which gene expression is regulated. The presence of a few to several hundred copies of TERT, which are not assembled into telomerase, in human immortalised cell lines reasonably provides a molecular basis for the formidable power of TERT as a transcriptional cofactor in oncogenic transformation and cellular (nuclear and metabolic) reprogramming, irrespectively of its TER-dependent DNA polymerase activity [66]. A very recent systemic review of the literature by us disclosed that most of the non-canonical responsibilities of telomerase identified so far strongly relate to the control of cancer stemness traits [67]. Telomerase/TERT-controlled aspects of the CSC phenotype involve proliferation, survival, therapy resistance, induced pluripotency, motility, glycolytic metabolism, and niche establishment and integrity (Figure 2). Equally strikingly, there seems to be a positive feedback loop between a number of gene products targeting TERT and TERT expression itself, plausibly amplifying the effects of central oncogenes and oncogenic pathways associated with the generation and/or maintenance of cancer stemness traits in a cell-autonomous manner. Although some of the observed cell-intrinsic/microenvironmental changes may require a catalytically active enzyme, there are several examples of oncogenic alterations brought about by catalytically inactive telomerase, as in the case of alternatively spliced (AS) TERT variants. To date, as many as twenty different AS TERT variants have been identified [68]. These variants tend to occur more frequently in cancer cells than in normal cells, indicating that they may be evolutionarily favoured in the context of pathology.

### 4.1. Stimulation of CSC proliferation

Given their role in the expansion of a tumour cell population, CSCs must display extensive proliferative capacity. Cell proliferation is both a matter of progression through the cell cycle and an issue necessitating cell growth (biosynthesis). There is a wealth of information in the literature on the promotive role of telomerase, independent of its telomere-elongating function, in cell proliferation. In an early study of the association between telomerase and cell proliferation, telomerase was shown to support the proliferation of human mammary epithelial cells through elevated EGFR signalling (even though it is quite ambiguous whether this effect is telomere length-independent or not) [69]. Moreover, TERT confers CSC characteristics to glioma cells by inducing EGFR expression, disconnectedly from its role in telomere biology [70]. Interestingly, telomerase upregulation was found to be closely linked to EGFR expression in actively proliferating normal human epithelial cells [71]. These observations imply the existence of a feed-forward loop that involves telomerase/TERT and EGFR. A plausible mechanism linking the EGFR–telomerase axis to cancer is that aberrant EGFR signalling may render CSCs less dependent on exogenous mitogens/growth factors and reinforce the persistent expression of telomerase in CSCs, thus playing a critical role in tumour development and progression.

Expanding these findings, one research group demonstrated that TERT promotes the proliferation of mammalian tissue progenitor cells *via* transcriptional control of a MYC- and Wnt-related developmental program [72]. To be more precise, TERT physically occupies the promoters of Wnt/β-catenin target genes, including those encoding cyclin D1 and MYC [73]. Cyclin D1 is a cell cycle control protein with oncogenic potential and has both enzymatic and nonenzymatic activities which are of great significance in tumour cells [74]. An additional molecular component involved in cyclin D1 expression in proliferating cells is nucleolar

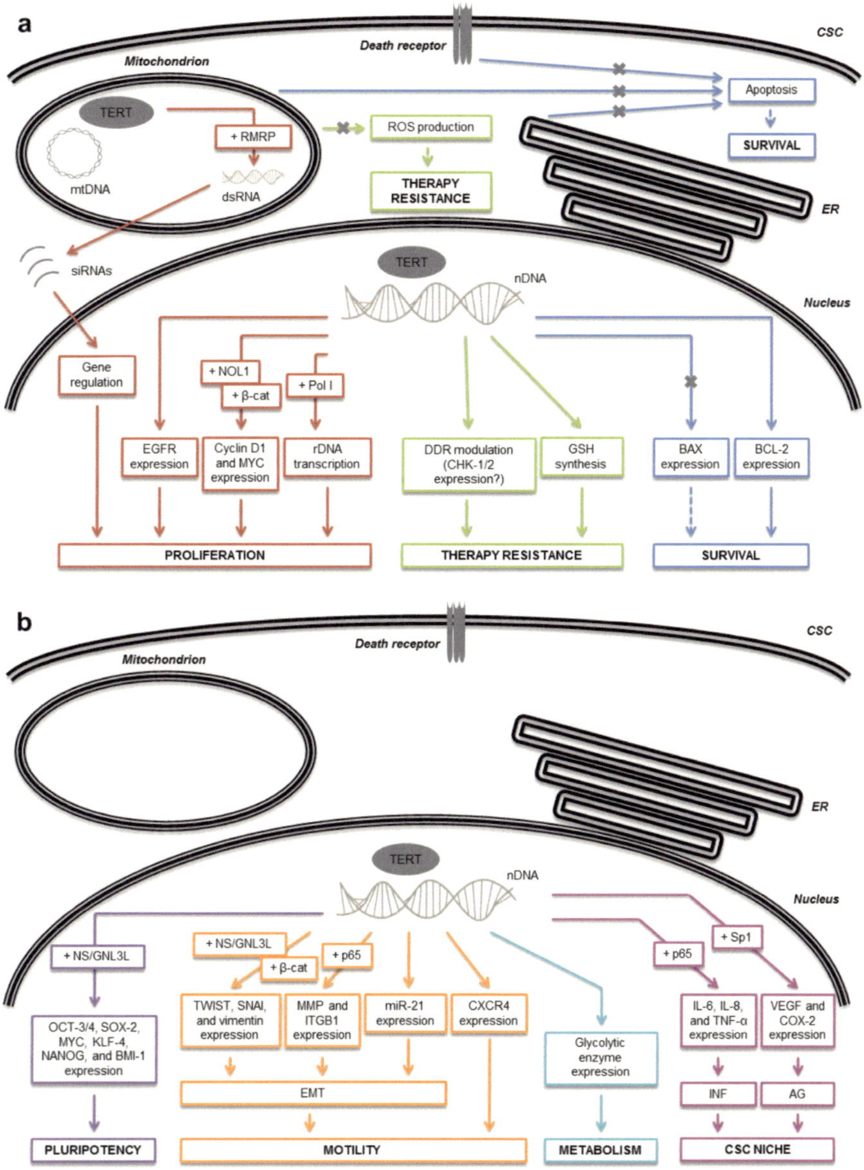


**Figure 2. Emergence and persistence of cancer stemness by telomerase/TERT (figure adapted from [67] with permission).** Clearly and unmistakably, telomerase/TERT is a powerful regulator of many aspects of the CSC phenotype, including: (a) proliferation, survival, therapy resistance; and (b) induced pluripotency, motility, glycolytic metabolism, niche establishment and integrity. This multifaceted ribonucleoprotein complex exerts its telomere-independent tumour-promoting effects partly by diverting and co-opting developmental signalling pathways and modulating gene expression. A cross symbol denotes an inhibition (blockage). A dashed arrow indicates that a given cancer stemness trait is not a direct consequence of the process shown in the preceding box, but of the inhibition of that process. AG, angiogenesis; DDR, DNA damage response; dsDNA, double-stranded DNA; dsRNA, double-stranded RNA; GSH, glutathione; INF, inflammation; mtDNA, mitochondrial DNA; nDNA, nuclear DNA; rDNA, ribosomal DNA; RMRP, RNA component of mitochondrial RNA-processing endoribonuclease; ROS, reactive oxygen species; siRNAs, small interfering RNAs

antigen p120 (NOL1), as suggested by the results of a very recent study [75]. In this study, telomerase was found to interact, in a TER-dependent fashion, with NOL1 and activate the transcription of the gene coding for cyclin D1. The relationship between TERT and cyclin D1 expression was corroborated also by other scientists [76–79]. Further support for TERT involvement in the stimulation of Wnt signalling-mediated cell proliferation was evidenced by an independent approach employing the Δ4–13 AS variant of human TERT that is devoid of reverse transcriptase activity [80]. In this approach, ectopic expression and small interfering RNA (siRNA)-mediated knockdown of the Δ4–13 AS variant in ALT cells, transformed telomerase-positive cell lines and telomerase-negative normal cells unquestionably proved that the proliferative effect of TERT is not coupled to telomerase activity. Because β-catenin is known to modulate TERT expression in stem cells and tumour cells [81], it is tempting to speculate that telomerase and Wnt/β-catenin signalling may act together in a positive feedback circuit to actively encourage the proliferation of CSCs.

Intriguingly, one group failed to find evidence that TERT promotes Wnt signalling in human breast cancer cells, indicating that TERT's effect on Wnt signalling is possibly context- and cell type-dependent [82]. Their findings are in the same direction as those from a former study on telomerase-null mouse models, where TERT loss-of-function in a physiological setting was reported to have no evident effects on Wnt signalling [83]. An alternative mechanism of action of telomerase on cell proliferation, as deduced by reverse genetics in human mammary epithelial cells, is that TERT-induced cell proliferation may result primarily from decreased levels of the RNA component of mitochondrial RNA-processing endoribonuclease (RMRP), not from increased Wnt signalling [78]. TERT and RMRP form a definite ribonucleoprotein complex that exhibits RNA-dependent RNA polymerase activity and, using RMRP as a template, produces double-stranded RNAs that can be later processed into siRNAs in a Dicer-dependent fashion [84]. siRNAs regulate gene expression at the posttranscriptional level as well as at the level of chromatin structure; therefore, it is reasonable to question whether their mutations or altered expression correlate with human cancers.

Aside from activating Wnt signalling and regulating gene expression (in the presence of RMRP), telomerase also stimulates ribosomal biogenesis through increased Pol I-directed ribosomal DNA transcription, exerting a positive influence on cell cycle and proliferation dynamics [85]. This may ultimately improve the protein synthesis capacity of CSCs for unrestrained growth. The molecular mechanism behind telomerase-induced ribosomal biogenesis was investigated in a very recent report where a MYC-driven oncogenesis model was proposed [79].

### 4.2. Promotion of CSC survival

Apoptosis is a form of cell death induced by miscellaneous stimuli and mediated by a subset of cysteine proteases termed caspases. A cancer cell's ability to evade death signals, thus preventing self-destruction by the activation of an apoptotic programme, is regarded as one of the hallmarks of cancer [86]. Several pieces of information suggest that telomerase exerts antiapoptotic effects in cancer cells through telomere-independent mechanisms. In the case of CSCs, telomerase-mediated inhibition of apoptosis may contribute to the enhanced and

http://dx.doi.org/10.5772/65762

continued survival of these cells in tumours. In keeping with its cytoprotective function, TERT was revealed to inhibit cell death by blocking the death receptor-initiated (or extrinsic) apoptotic pathway in acute promyelocytic cells [87]. Similarly, yet in a mechanistically different way, TERT was also shown to block the mitochondrion-initiated (or intrinsic) apoptotic pathway in colon and cervical carcinoma cell lines [88]. A more thorough probing of the molecular mechanism behind telomerase-mediated suppression of the intrinsic apoptotic pathway found that TERT overexpression upregulates the expression of the antiapoptotic mitochondrial protein BCL-2, downregulates the expression of some proapoptotic mitochondrial proteins (for example, BAX) and reduces the activation of some caspases (for example, caspase-9) in ovarian surface epithelial cells [89]. Given the capacity of BCL-2 to increase telomerase activity in human colorectal and cervical carcinoma cell lines [90], it is conceivable that telomerase and BCL-2 are engaged in a positive feedback loop that impedes apoptosis. In this connection, it is well to add that the introduction of a constitutively expressed TERT construct into colon carcinoma and Burkitt's lymphoma cell lines was, independently of telomerase activity, associated with the reversion of a transcriptional programme coordinated by p53, a potent and common activator of both the intrinsic and extrinsic apoptotic pathways [91].

Apart from suppressing mitochondrion-initiated cell death, overexpression of TERT was also found to suppress, in a telomere-independent manner, endoplasmic reticulum (ER) stress-induced cell death in murine primary neural cells and human cancer cell lines [92]. ER stress arises as a result of perturbations in ER function and elicits the unfolded protein response (UPR), a conserved signal transduction pathway for dealing with misfolded proteins. When the UPR-induced mechanisms fail to alleviate ER stress, both the intrinsic and extrinsic apoptotic pathways may become activated [93]. Reciprocally, specific activation of ER stress was demonstrated to upregulate TERT expression in a breast cancer cell line [94]. It therefore seems reasonable to suggest that TERT and ER stress are involved in a dynamic interplay supporting CSC survival in abnormal metabolic conditions such as glucose starvation.

### 4.3. Induction of pluripotency

Restoration of the molecular circuitry that forms the necessary base of pluripotency in embryonic stem cells (ESCs) strongly correlates with the gaining and retention of cancer stemness. In ESCs, this circuitry is made up of special transcription factors and function as a repressor of differentiation. Takahashi and Yamanaka were the first to demonstrate that a cocktail of four transcription factors (namely OCT-3/4, SOX-2, MYC, and KLF4) are necessary and sufficient for nuclear reprogramming into an ESC-like state [95]. In CSCs, the so-called Yamanaka factors, besides driving the induction of pluripotency, are additionally involved in inhibiting apoptosis [96]. A valued piece of work documented that TERT forms a ternary complex with the nucleolar GTP-binding protein NS/GNL3L and the chromatin remodelling factor BRG1 and that the resulting NS/GNL3L TERT BRG1 complex is required for NS/GNL3L-induced upregulation of the nuclear reprogramming factors OCT-3/4, MYC, and KLF-4 [97]. The likely part played by TERT/telomerase in contributing to the pluripotent character of CSCs is also congruous with the later finding that siRNA-mediated hTERT depletion in gastric CSCs downregulates the induced pluripotency-associated transcription factor OCT-4 [98].

### 4.4. Increase of CSC motility and invasiveness

Migrating CSCs and EMT-phenotypic cells have the ability to disseminate from their primary site and are thus present in the invasive front of tumours. The initial evidence for telomerase/TERT participation in cell migration came from experiments measuring the *in vitro* migration rate of telomerase-positive progenitor cells and cancer cell lines [99, 100]. Later experiments aiming at uncovering the molecular mechanism behind this positive trend showed that telomerase reconstitution boosts cell migration through the activation of Rho family members and the SDF-1–CXCR4 axis [101]. With respect to CSC motility, expression of the chemokine receptor CXCR4 may enable CSCs to migrate along a gradient of the ligand SDF-1 and thus help facilitate their spread. Therapeutic strategies intended to interfere with the SDF-1–CXCR4 axis can possibly have useful clinical relevance and application in the prevention of metastatic disease.

Differentiated epithelial cells that have undergone EMT may as well exhibit augmented motility and invasiveness leading to metastasis. The ternary complex containing TERT, BRG1, and NS or GNL3L (see section 4.3) acts in a telomere-independent mode to activate the EMT programme *via* NS/GNL3L-induced upregulation of vimentin, SNAI, and TWIST, three of the mesenchymal cell markers, in genetically defined cancer cells [97]. TERT additionally stimulates EMT in gastric cancer cells through directly regulating the expression of Wnt/β-catenin target genes like those coding for vimentin and SNAI-1 [98]. Equally important is the fact that TERT, in a telomere-independent manner, regulates the expression of several MMP family members, such as MMP-9, *via* the NF-κB pathway [102]. MMPs are the key mediators promoting extracellular matrix (ECM) degradation and remodelling, both of which pave the way for EMT and subsequent metastasis. The indirect involvement of TERT in dissemination was also highlighted by a separate set of data which documented that changes in the motility and invasiveness of malignant cells are likely to result from the TERT-induced upregulation of the metastasis-implicated proteins RhoC and MMP-9 [103]. Interestingly, MMP-9 silencing was shown to downregulate TERT expression *via* ITGB1-mediated FAK signalling in glioma xenograft cells [104]. It is worth mentioning here that a very recent report found that ITGB1 itself is regulated by TERT and that TERT may promote the invasion and metastasis of gastric cancer cells by enhancing ITGB1 protein levels [105]. Collectively, these findings reinforce the notion that there is an indirect, metastasis-favouring interaction between TERT, MMP-9 and ITGB1 in cancer cells. Another study discovered that TERT upregulates the levels of MAC2BP, a metastasis-related secreted ECM glycoprotein, in gastric cancer cells [106]. MAC2BP is believed to support metastasis through interacting with galectins and altering cell–cell and cell–matrix adhesion properties [107].

Another contribution to knowledge came from a very recent report in which TERT was found to stimulate the expression of oncomiRs, including miR-21, in human leukaemia and HeLa cell lines [108]. Extant research identifies miR-21 as being among the most frequently upregulated miRNAs in epithelial cell-derived solid tumours [109] and also as having a decisive role in the conservation of CSC phenotype *via* the AKT and ERK1/2 signalling pathways targeting PTEN [110]. The centrality of miR-21 to cancer stemness was confirmed in a recent study on the antisense oligonucleotide-mediated inhibition of miR-21 in two different anaplastic thyroid carcinoma (ATC) cell lines, where the knockdown of miR-21 disturbed the stemness state of ATC cells, as assessed by a decreased expression of the genes encoding OCT-4 and ABCG2 [111].

### 4.5. Modulation of energy metabolism

Apparently, genetic, epigenetic and microenvironmental changes that regulate the transition to a CSC-like state cannot occur without the presence of a favourable metabotype. In general, stimulation of aerobic glycolysis promotes metabolic reprogramming, whereas inhibition of glycolytic enzymes impairs metabolic reprogramming. In harmony with the concept that metabolism is involved in the control of cancer stemness, a microarray-based gene expression profiling study elucidated that ribozyme-mediated targeting of telomerase in murine melanoma cells downregulates the expression of more than a few glycolytic pathway genes such as those coding for phosphofructokinase and aldolase C [112]. Additionally, a very recent report showed that siRNA-mediated knockdown of TERT in human lymphoma cells lowers the expression of MYC-regulated target genes such as those coding for the glycolytic enzymes lactate dehydrogenase, hexokinase 2, and pyruvate kinase M2 isoform [79]. Due to the fact that MYC is a well-established oncogenic transcription factor activating TERT expression [113], a feed-forward mechanism for the rewiring of glucose metabolism in CSCs is likely to prevail between TERT and MYC.

### 4.6. Contribution to therapy resistance

CSCs are notorious for their resistance to existing cancer treatment regimens, including radiotherapy and chemotherapy. Both cell-intrinsic and microenvironmental factors appear to contribute to the emergence of therapy resistance in CSCs. Radiotherapy works by directing ionising radiation toward tumours to induce the generation of reactive oxygen species (ROS) which react with and cause damaging of DNA. By the same token, a number of chemotherapeutic agents such as platinum-based antitumour drugs are known to bind to and cause crosslinking of DNA. In this regard, implementation by CSCs of fast and efficient DNA repair mechanisms as well as potent antioxidant/scavenger systems may prove vital to circumvent the deleterious effects of irradiation and several classes of antitumour compounds.

Growing evidence points to a role for telomerase in modulating DDR and contributing to DNA repair. In a prior report, TERT was proposed to, independently of its effect on telomere length, set in motion a transcriptional programme leading to enlarged ribonucleotide (NTP) pools, enhanced DNA repair, and increased chromosomal stability [114]. A circumstantial investigation into the enhanced DNA repair capability of telomerase-expressing cells suggested that TERT/telomerase increases DNA end-joining repair and accelerates nucleotide excision repair through recruiting proteinaceous factors to sites where DNA damage is occurring [115]. The aforementioned findings are consistent with a newer report which showed that TERT expression affords a means of protecting human transformed cells against double-stranded DNA-damaging drugs and increases their endurance to chromosomal instability [116]. Specifically expressing TERT mutants lacking catalytic activity in ALT cells, the authors of the same report reached the conclusion that the observed cytoprotective effect of telomerase is distinct from its function in telomere biosynthesis. In a separate study providing evidence for an epigenetic component to telomerase-induced treatment resistance, stable short hairpin RNA (shRNA)-mediated suppression of TERT expression was demonstrated to, in a telomere length-independent way, diminish the response of human fibroblasts to DNA double strand breaks, most likely through a mechanism altering the overall state (that is to say, configuration) of chromatin [117].

Telomerase upregulation/reactivation also seems to be involved in counteracting oxidative stress-induced intracellular injury that often follows therapy, as evident from several experimental studies. The initial study examining the extratelomeric function of telomerase under oxidative stress found that mitochondrially-localised TERT decreases cellular peroxide levels and mitochondrial superoxide production, increases mitochondrial membrane potential and protects mitochondrial DNA from oxidative damage in human lung fibroblasts [118]. The observation that telomerase provides resistance to oxidative stress was validated and extended in an ensuing study where TERT was shown to bind to mitochondrial DNA and accordingly protect it and its function against damage [119]. An alternative explanation for telomerase-induced resistance to oxidative stress came from a more recent study in which TERT overexpression in cancer cells was demonstrated to alleviate basal ROS levels and intracellular ROS production through potentiating the effects of endogenous antioxidants or free radical scavengers such that the proportion of reduced to oxidised glutathione (GSH/GSSG) is increased and peroxiredoxin is replenished in the interior of the cell [120]. Apart from serving to keep mitochondrial DNA damage-free, mitochondrially-localised telomerase also guards nuclear DNA against oxidative attack through decreasing mitochondrial ROS production [121]. Finally, it is appropriate to mention that the β-deletion variant, a catalytically defective AS variant of TERT, localises to both mitochondria and the nucleus and, distinct from the canonical role of TERT in telomere extension, protects three basal breast cancer cell lines from cisplatin-induced apoptosis, endowing breast tumours with chemotherapy resistance [122].

### 4.7. Establishment and integrity of the CSC niche

The tumour microenvironment (TME) is an umbrella term that encompasses all cellular and non-cellular components surrounding a tumour. These components include tumour-adjacent stromal cells (for example, endothelial cells and fibroblasts), diverse effectors of the immune system (for example, lymphocytes and mesenchymal stem cells), ECM elements, proteases, and networks of cytokines, growth factors and other soluble factors. Specifically, both the immediate TME (cell–cell and cell–matrix connections) and the extended TME (for example, vascular bed) are thought to be implicated in tumour progression. The TME is also capable of creating a niche for CSCs, in which they remain in an undifferentiated state until stimulated to differentiate into non-CSC tumour cells and form tumour bulk. Modulation of gene expression and metabolism by telomerase in CSCs may recondition the CSC niche in favour of the hypermalignant (that is to say, highly metastatic, therapy-resistant) nature of these cells.

It is in this regard that a recent study demonstrated that telomerase binds to p65 and localises to promoters of NF-κB target genes, such as those encoding IL-6, TNF-$\alpha$, and IL-8, proinflammatory cytokines that are the critical triggers of inflammatory responses [123]. Inflammation is considered an enabling characteristic of cancer for the reason that it supplies bioactive molecules (for example, growth factors and EMT-inducing ligands) to the TME and primes cells to release ROS and other chemicals that drive the mutagenesis, and hence genetic evolution, of nearby tumour cells toward hypermalignancy [86]. Since NF-κB is known to transcriptionally upregulate telomerase levels [124], this finding implies that a positive feedback loop between telomerase and NF-κB may explain the grounds for the coexistence of chronic inflammation and sustained telomerase activity in neoplastic lesions.

Furthermore, it was reported that TERT activates the transcription of VEGF, an endothelial mitogen and master orchestrator of angiogenesis, independently of telomerase activity in HeLa cells [125]. Further dissection of the underlying regulatory mechanism led to the conclusion that TERT upregulates VEGF expression through its interaction with the specificity protein 1 (Sp1) transcription factor [126]. Angiogenesis is the process of growth or formation of fresh blood vessels from the pre-existing vasculature, and its induction is widely considered an essential attribute of tumour growth as well as metastasis as solid tumours larger than 1 $cm^3$ have to develop their own blood supply to circumvent necrotic cell death. Given the prior discovery that VEGF stimulates the production of TERT [127], it may be that there is a positive feedback circuit between TERT and VEGF. This regulation may account for the combined and continuing contribution of these two proteins to the maintenance of CSCs in solid tumours. Moreover, siRNA-mediated knockdown of TERT was shown to downregulate the prostaglandin-synthesising enzyme COX-2 in pancreatic cancer cells [128]. COX-2, like VEGF, is a proangiogenic factor that has the potential to establish a selective niche favourable to the preservation of CSCs. Subsequent studies showed that COX-2 stimulates the expression of TERT in cervical cancer cells [129]. Collectively, these data indicate that a feed-forward regulation, which could be important in carcinoma growth and progression, occurs between TERT and COX-2.

## 5. Prospects for telomerase-targeted anticancer therapies

There is little doubt that telomerase is not only an effector in human tumour pathogenesis but also a regulator of essentially all aspects of malignant behaviour, including spreading to secondary sites. This being the case, specifically and sensitively measuring telomerase activity in clinical samples represents both an early diagnostic marker and a negative prognostic factor for patients with malignant disease. The obvious capacity of telomerase to directly regulate an ever-expanding number of tumour-promoting genes and pathways renders this gifted ribonucleoprotein particle an attractive and almost universal target for human cancers. Given the integral role played by cancer stemness in disease recurrence, selectively targeting and eradicating CSCs with low toxicity to somatic cells and with minimal side effects holds the promise of a full cure for cancer. Besides being pursued with vigour in the hope of improving patient outcomes, successfully suppressing cancer stemness may also provide the ultimate evidence for the CSC concept. As summarised in this chapter, telomerase contributes to carcinogenesis most likely through the emergence and persistence of conspicuous CSC qualities. Accordingly, telomerase inhibition in CSCs is predicted to: (i) shrink telomeres; (ii) restrain anchorage-independent growth and inhibit proliferation by cell cycle arrest; (iii) induce CSC death; (iv) induce CSC differentiation; (v) inhibit CSC migration and reverse the EMT programme; (vi) deteriorate glucose metabolism; (vii) enhance radio- and chemosensitivity; and (viii) disrupt the CSC niche. Serious telomere shrinkage is assumed to be a long-term effect of telomerase inhibition in CSCs so the tumour mass will continue to expand for a time after treatment until its constituent cells enter crisis and begin to die in large numbers. The rest of the aforementioned effects, however, are likely to occur after short-term exposure of CSCs to telomerase inhibitors, inducing relatively rapid initial responses to treatment. Natural telomerase inhibitors (phytochemicals) and small-molecule telomerase inhibitors, antisense oligonucleotides and chemically modified nucleic acids, immunotherapeutic agents, and telomerase-directed gene therapy are promising treatment options and may play a larger role in the near future [130]. Imetelstat (GRN163L), which was designed by Geron Corporation in 2003, is the first telomerase inhibitor to advance to clinical development. It is a lipid-conjugated 13-mer (5'–TAGGGTTAGACAA–3') antisense oligonucleotide that is complementary to and binds with high affinity to TER, thereby directly inhibiting telomerase activity and interfering with telomere length homeostasis. It is perhaps safe here to assume that Imetelstat impairs the regulatory role of telomerase in CSC biology not only through telomere shortening but also through negatively influencing its telomere length-independent tumour-promoting functions. In support of this, short-term (72-hour) Imetelstat exposure was shown to promote the differentiation and inhibit the colony-forming ability of multiple myeloma CSCs through a telomere length-independent mechanism [131]. Similarly, *in vitro* Imetelstat treatment was found to deplete breast and pancreatic CSCs, as measured by the reduced proportion of ALDH-positive and CSC-surface marker-expressing cells, through a mechanism of action independent of telomere shortening [132]. Although Imetelstat is known to form thermodynamically stable and sequence-specific duplexes with TER, the possibility that even less thermodynamically stable tetraplexes of Imetelstat may bind to and interfere with some other, yet to be identified, proteins (particularly those that interact with telomerase) should not be excluded [133]. There also exists a possibility that telomerase inhibitors like Imetelstat may be coupled with conventional therapies such as surgical (debulking) therapy, radiotherapy, and chemotherapy, all of which have their own weaknesses and inadequacies. Such combination therapy is predicted to result in rapid and durable clinical responses in broad tumour types (Figure 3). As shown by the sources provided earlier in this chapter and elsewhere in the literature, the principal signalling pathways governing CSC biology operate in physiological stem cells as well. This complicates telomerase inhibition therapy because of the risk of telomerase inhibitors exerting an adverse influence on the size of the physiological stem cell pool and/or on the integrity of the physiological stem cell niche. The notion that physiological stem cells only transiently express telomerase and have relatively long telomeres [65], however, means that there is likely to be a narrow but safe therapeutic window where only CSCs will be depleted by telomerase inhibitors and normal stem cells will remain unaffected. Furthermore, rational approaches that disrupt the interactions of telomerase with important downstream components of embryonic/oncogenic signalling pathways (Wnt/β-catenin and NF-κB being the most prominent of all so far) may be conceived and executed as therapeutic tactics to specifically target and eliminate CSCs. As far as targeting protein–protein interactions is concerned, a future challenge is to add to existing pathways or identify new ones where telomerase, independently of its role in preventing telomere loss, intervenes and contributes to CSC phenotype. The essential nature of telomerase in the promotion and maintenance of cancer stemness provides a logical basis for believing that CSCs will not develop resistance to any of the aforementioned telomerase-focused therapeutics, in contrast to other targeted anticancer therapies whose targets are likely to be compensated for by functionally equivalent gene products and signalling pathways.

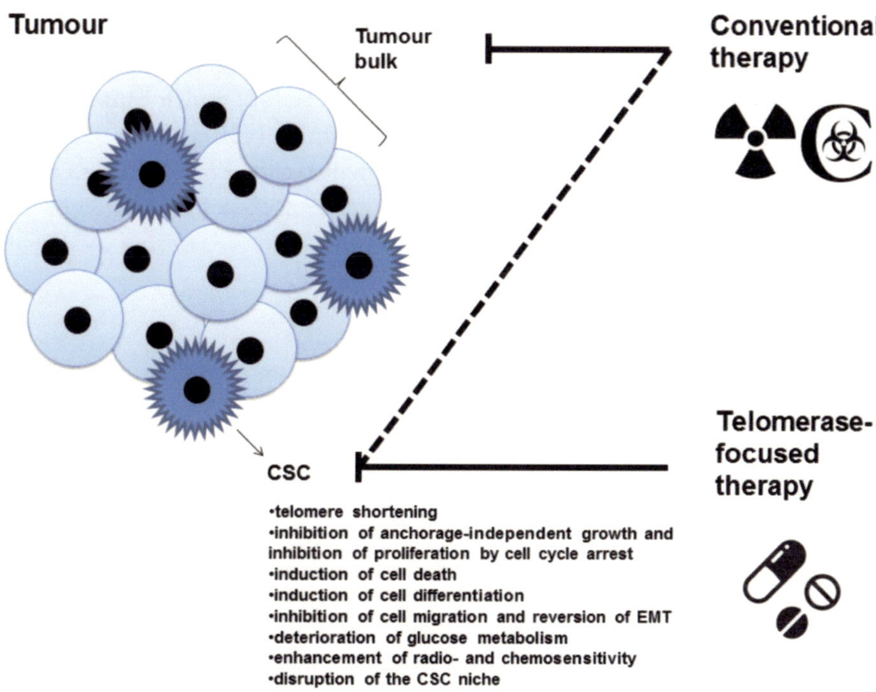


**Figure 3. Combination therapy for predicting rapid and durable clinical responses in broad tumours.** Here, telomerase-focused therapy is proposed as a strategy to effectively target CSCs. Combining telomerase-focused therapy with conventional therapy may provide scope for the elimination of bulk tumour cells while preventing recurrence by simultaneously eradicating the stem-like component of the tumour. Combination therapy may also prevent non-CSC tumour cells from acquiring cancer stemness traits *via*, for example, EMT. A bar-headed solid line denotes a strong inhibitory (negative) effect. A bar-headed dashed line denotes a weak inhibitory (negative) effect.

## 6. Abbreviations

ABC, ATP-binding cassette; Akt, protein kinase B; ALDH1, aldehyde dehydrogenase 1; BAX, BCL-2-associated protein X; BCL, B-cell lymphoma family protein; BMI-1, B lymphoma Mo-MLV insertion region 1 homolog; BMP, bone morphogenetic protein; BRG1, Brahma-related gene 1; CD, cluster of differentiation; CHK, checkpoint kinase; COX-2, cyclooxygenase-2;

CXCR4, C–X–C chemokine receptor type 4; EGFR, epidermal growth factor receptor; ERK1/2, extracellular signal-related kinase 1/2; FAK, focal adhesion kinase; GLUTs, glucose transporters; GNL3L, guanine nucleotide-binding protein-like 3-like; IL, interleukin; ITGB1, integrin beta-1; JAK, Janus kinase; KLF-4, Kruppel-like factor-4; MAC2BP, Mac-2-binding protein; MCL-1, myeloid cell leukaemia-1; MIC-1, macrophage inhibitory cytokine-1; MMPs, matrix metalloproteinases; MYC, v-myc avian myelocytomatosis viral oncoprotein homolog; mTOR, mammalian target of rapamycin; NANOG, Nanog homeobox transcription factor; NF-κB, nuclear factor-κB; NS, nucleostemin; OCT-3/4, octamer-binding transcription factor-3/4; PI3K, phosphoinositide 3-kinase; PTEN, phosphatase and tensin homolog; SDF-1, stromal cell-derived factor-1; SMAD, small mother against decapentaplegic homolog; SNAI, snail family zinc-finger transcription factor; SOX-2, SRY (sex determining region Y)-box 2; STAT, signal transducer and activator of transcription; TAZ, Tafazzin; TGF-β, transforming growth factor-β; TNF-α, tumour necrosis factor-α; TWIST, twist family bHLH (basic helix-loop-helix) transcription factor; VEGF, vascular endothelial growth factor; Wnt, Wingless ligand; YAP, Yes-associated protein; ZEB, zinc-finger E-box-binding homeobox family protein

## Author details

Kerem Teralı[1*] and Açelya Yilmazer[2]

*Address all correspondence to: kerem.terali@neu.edu.tr

1 Department of Medical Biochemistry, Faculty of Medicine, Near East University, Nicosia, North Cyprus, via Mersin, Turkey

2 Department of Biomedical Engineering, Faculty of Engineering, Ankara University, Tandogan, Ankara, Turkey

## References

[1] Samassekou O, Gadji M, Drouin R, Yan J. Sizing the ends: normal length of human telomeres. Ann Anat. 2010;192:284–91.

[2] Palm W, de Lange T. How shelterin protects mammalian telomeres. Annu Rev Genet. 2008;42:301–34.

[3] de Lange T. Mammalian telomeres. In: de Lange T, Lundblad V, Blackburn E, editors. Telomeres. 2nd ed. NY: Cold Spring Harbor Laboratory Press; 2006.

[4] von Zglinicki T. Oxidative stress shortens telomeres. Trends Biochem Sci. 2002;27:339–44.

[5] Saretzki G. Extra-telomeric functions of human telomerase: cancer, mitochondria and oxidative stress. Curr Pharm Des. 2014;20:6386–403.

[6] Sauerwald A, Sandin S, Cristofari G, Scheres SHW, Lingner J, Rhodes D. Structure of active dimeric human telomerase. Nat Struct Mol Biol. 2013;20:454–60.

[7] Blackburn EH, Collins K. Telomerase: an RNP enzyme synthesizes DNA. Cold Spring Harb Perspect Biol. 2011;3:a003558.

[8] Pfeiffer V, Lingner J. Replication of telomeres and the regulation of telomerase. Cold Spring Harb Perspect Biol. 2013;5:a010405.

[9] Mitchell JR, Wood E, Collins K. A telomerase component is defective in the human disease dyskeratosis congenita. Nature. 1999;402:551–5.

[10] Fu D, Collins K. Purification of human telomerase complexes identifies factors involved in telomerase biogenesis and telomere length regulation. Mol Cell. 2007;28:773–85.

[11] Venteicher AS, Meng Z, Mason PJ, Veenstra TD, Artandi SE. Identification of ATPases pontin and reptin as telomerase components essential for holoenzyme assembly. Cell. 2008;132:945–57.

[12] Venteicher AS, Abreu EB, Meng Z, McCann KE, Terns RM, Veenstra TD, Terns MP, Artandi SE. A human telomerase holoenzyme protein required for Cajal body localization and telomere synthesis. Science. 2009;323:644–648.

[13] Reddel RR. Telomere maintenance mechanisms in human cancer: clinical implications. Curr Pharm Des. 2014;20:6361–74.

[14] Kim NW, Piatyszek MA, Prowse KR, Harley CB, West MD, Ho PL, Coviello GM, Wright WE, Weinrich SL, Shay JW. Specific association of human telomerase activity with immortal cells and cancer. Science. 1994;266:2011–5.

[15] Shay JW, Bacchetti S. A survey of telomerase activity in human cancer. Eur J Cancer. 1997;33:787–91.

[16] Soria JC, Gauthier LR, Raymond E, Granotier C, Morat L, Armand JP, Boussin FD, Sabatier L. Molecular detection of telomerase-positive circulating epithelial cells in metastatic breast cancer patients. Clin Cancer Res. 1999;5:971–5.

[17] Sapi E, Okpokwasili NI, Rutherford T. Detection of telomerase-positive circulating epithelial cells in ovarian cancer patients. Cancer Detect Prev. 2002;26:158–67.

[18] Goldkorn A, Ely B, Tangen CM, Tai YC, Xu T, Li H, Twardowski P, Veldhuizen PJ, Agarwal N, Carducci MA, et al. Circulating tumor cell telomerase activity as a prognostic marker for overall survival in SWOG 0421: A phase III metastatic castration resistant prostate cancer trial. Int J Cancer. 2015;136:1856–62.

[19] Vinagre J, Almeida A, Pópulo H, Batista R, Lyra J, Pinto V, Coelho R, Celestino R, Prazeres H, Lima L, et al. Frequency of TERT promoter mutations in human cancers. Nat Commun. 2013;4:2185.

[20] Huang FW, Hodis E, Xu MJ, Kryukov GV, Chin L, Garraway LA. Highly recurrent TERT promoter mutations in human melanoma. Science. 2013;339:957–9.

[21] Horn S, Figl A, Rachakonda PS, Fischer C, Sucker A, Gast A, Kadel S, Moll I, Nagore E, Hemminki K, et al. TERT promoter mutations in familial and sporadic melanoma. Science. 2013;339:959–61.

[22] Li Y, Zhou QL, Sun W, Chandrasekharan P, Cheng HS, Ying Z, Lakshmanan M, Raju A, Tenen DG, Cheng SY, et al. Non-canonical NF-kappaB signalling and ETS1/2 cooperatively drive C250T mutant TERT promoter activation. Nat Cell Biol. 2015;17:1327–38.

[23] Kreso A, Dick JE. Evolution of the cancer stem cell model. Cell Stem Cell, 2014;14:275–91.

[24] Lapidot T, Sirard C, Vormoor J, Murdoch B, Hoang T, Caceres-Cortes J, Minden M, Paterson B, Callgiuri MA, Dick JE. A cell initiating human acute leukaemia after transplantation into SCID mice. Nature. 1994;367:645–8.

[25] Bonnet D, Dick JE. Human acute myeloid leukemia is organized as a hierarchy that originates from a primitive hematopoietic cell. Nat Med. 1997;3:730–7.

[26] Graham SM, Jørgensen HG, Allan E, Pearson C, Alcorn MJ, Richmond L, Holyoake TL. Primitive, quiescent, Philadelphia-positive stem cells from patients with chronic myeloid leukemia are insensitive to STI571 in vitro. Blood. 2002;99:319–25.

[27] Chen Z, Ayala P, Wang M, Fayad L, Katz RL, Romaguera J, Caraway N, Neelapu SS, Kwak LW, Simmons PJ, McCarty N. Prospective isolation of clonogenic mantle cell lymphoma-initiating cells. Stem Cell Res. 2010;5:212–25.

[28] Fang D, Nguyen TK, Leishear K, Finko R, Kulp AN, Hotz S, Van Belle PA, Xu X, Elder DE, Herlyn M. A tumorigenic subpopulation with stem cell properties in melanomas. Cancer Res. 2005;65:9328–37.

[29] Schatton T, Murphy GF, Frank NY, Yamaura K, Waaga-Gasser AM, Gasser M, Zhan Q, Jordan S, Duncan LM, Weishaupt C, Fuhlbrigge RC, Kupper TS, Sayegh MH, Frank MH. Identification of cells initiating human melanomas. Nature. 2008;451:345–9.

[30] Suvà ML, Riggi N, Stehle JC, Baumer K, Tercier S, Joseph JM, Suvà D, Clément V, Provero P, Cironi L, Osterheld MC, Guillou L, Stamenkovic I. Identification of cancer stem cells in Ewing's sarcoma. Cancer Res. 2009;69:1776–81.

[31] Singh SK, Hawkins C, Clarke ID, Squire JA, Bayani J, Hide T, Henkelman RM, Cusimano MD, Dirks PB. Identification of human brain tumour initiating cells. Nature. 2004;432:396–401.

[32] Malanchi I, Peinado H, Kassen D, Hussenet T, Metzger D, Chambon P, Huber M, Hohl D, Cano A, Birchmeier W, Huelsken J. Cutaneous cancer stem cell maintenance is dependent on beta-catenin signalling. Nature. 2008;452:650–3.

[33] Prince ME, Sivanandan R, Kaczorowski A, Wolf GT, Kaplan MJ, Dalerba P, Weissman IL, Clarke MF, Ailles LE. Identification of a subpopulation of cells with cancer stem cell properties in head and neck squamous cell carcinoma. Proc Natl Acad Sci USA. 2007;104:973–8.

[34] Kim CF, Jackson EL, Woolfenden AE, Lawrence S, Babar I, Vogel S, Crowley D, Bronson RT, Jacks T. Identification of bronchioalveolar stem cells in normal lung and lung cancer. Cell. 2005;121:823–35.

[35] Eramo A, Lotti F, Sette G, Pilozzi E, Biffoni M, Di Virgilio A, Conticello C, Ruco L, Peschle C, De Maria R. Identification and expansion of the tumorigenic lung cancer stem cell population. Cell Death Differ. 2008;15:504–14.

[36] Ma S, Chan KW, Hu L, Lee TK, Wo JY, Ng IO, Zheng BJ, Guan XY. Identification and characterization of tumorigenic liver cancer stem/progenitor cells. Gastroenterology. 2007;132:2542–56.

[37] Takaishi S, Okumura T, Tu S, Wang SS, Shibata W, Vigneshwaran R, Gordon SA, Shimada Y, Wang TC. Identification of gastric cancer stem cells using the cell surface marker CD44. Stem Cells. 2009;27:1006–20.

[38] O'Brien CA, Pollett A, Gallinger S, Dick JE. A human colon cancer cell capable of initiating tumour growth in immunodeficient mice. Nature. 2007;445:106–10.

[39] Ricci-Vitiani L, Lombardi DG, Pilozzi E, Biffoni M, Todaro M, Peschle C, De Maria R. Identification and expansion of human colon-cancer-initiating cells. Nature. 2007;445:111–5.

[40] Chan KS, Espinosa I, Chao M, Wong D, Ailles L, Diehn M, Gill H, Presti J Jr, Chang HY, van de Rijn M, Shortliffe L, Weissman IL. Identification, molecular characterization, clinical prognosis, and therapeutic targeting of human bladder tumor-initiating cells. Proc Natl Acad Sci USA 2009;106:14016–21.

[41] Li C, Heidt DG, Dalerba P, Burant CF, Zhang L, Adsay V, Wicha M, Clarke MF, Simeone DM. Identification of pancreatic cancer stem cells. Cancer Res. 2007;67:1030–7.

[42] Hermann PC, Huber SL, Herrler T, Aicher A, Ellwart JW, Guba M, Bruns CJ, Heeschen C. Distinct populations of cancer stem cells determine tumor growth and metastatic activity in human pancreatic cancer. Cell Stem Cell. 2007;1:313–23.

[43] Collins AT, Berry PA, Hyde C, Stower MJ, Maitland NJ. Prospective identification of tumorigenic prostate cancer stem cells. Cancer Res. 2005;65:10946–51.

[44] Al-Hajj M, Wicha MS, Benito-Hernandez A, Morrison SJ, Clarke MF. Prospective identification of tumorigenic breast cancer cells. Proc Natl Acad Sci USA. 2003;100:3983–8.

[45] Zhang S, Balch C, Chan MW, Lai HC, Matei D, Schilder JM, Yan PS, Huang TH, Nephew KP. Identification and characterization of ovarian cancer-initiating cells from primary human tumors. Cancer Res. 2008;68:4311–20.

[46] Valent P, Bonnet D, De MR, Lapidot T, Copland M, Melo JV, Chomienne C, Ishikawa F, Schuringa JJ, Stassi G, Huntly B, Herrmann H, Soulier J, Roesch A, Schuurhuis GJ, Wohrer S, Arock M, Zuber J, Cerny-Reiterer S, Johnsen HE, Andreeff M, Eaves C. Cancer stem cell definitions and terminology: the devil is in the details. Nat Rev Cancer. 2012;11:767–75.

[47] Islam F, Qiao B, Smith RA, Gopalan V, Lam AK. Cancer stem cell: fundamental experimental pathological concepts and updates. Exp Mol Pathol. 2015;98:184–91.

[48] Mimeault M, Batra SK. Recent insights into the molecular mechanisms involved in aging and the malignant transformation of adult stem/progenitor cells and their therapeutic implications. Ageing Res Rev. 2009;8:94–112.

[49] Feldser DM, Hackett JA, Greider CW. Telomere dysfunction and the initiation of genome instability. Nat Rev Cancer. 2003;3:623–7.

[50] Thiery JP, Acloque H, Huang RY, Nieto MA. Epithelial-mesenchymal transitions in development and disease. Cell. 2009;139:871–890.

[51] Tsai JH, Yang J. Epithelial–mesenchymal plasticity in carcinoma metastasis. Genes Dev. 2013;27:2192–206.

[52] Menendez JA, Alarcón T. Metabostemness: a new cancer hallmark. Front Oncol. 2014;4:262.

[53] Lunt SY, Vander Heiden MG. Aerobic glycolysis: meeting the metabolic requirements of cell proliferation. Annu Rev Cell Dev Biol. 2011;27:441–64.

[54] Abaza M, Luqmani YA. The influence of pH and hypoxia on tumor metastasis. Expert Rev Anticancer Ther. 2013;13:1229–42.

[55] Dong C, Yuan T, Wu Y, Wang Y, Fan TW, Miriyala S, Lin Y, Yao J, Shi J, Kang T, Lorkiewicz P, St Clair D, Hung MC, Evers BM, Zhou BP. Loss of FBP1 by Snail-mediated repression provides metabolic advantages in basal-like breast cancer. Cancer Cell. 2013;23:316–31.

[56] Shen YA, Wang CY, Hsieh YT, Chen YJ, Wei YH. Metabolic reprogramming orchestrates cancer stem cell properties in nasopharyngeal carcinoma. Cell Cycle. 2015;14:86–98.

[57] Vlashi E, Lagadec C, Vergnes L, Matsutani T, Masui K, Poulou M. Metabolic state of glioma stem cells and nontumorigenic cells. Proc Natl Acad Sci USA. 2011;108:16062–7.

[58] Lagadinou ED, Sach A, Callahan K, Rossi RM, Neering SJ, Minhajuddin M, Ashton JM, Pei S, Grose V, O'Dwyer KM, Liesveld JL, Brookes PS, Becker MW, Jordan CT. BCL-2 inhibition targets oxidative phosphorylation and selectively eradicates quiescent human leukemia stem cells. Cell Stem Cell. 2013;12:329–41.

[59] Pattabiraman DR, Weinberg RA. Tackling the cancer stem cells—what challenges do they pose? Nat Rev Drug Discov. 2014;13:497–512.

[60] Mimeault M, Batra SK. Altered gene products involved in the malignant reprogramming of cancer stem/progenitor cells and multitargeted therapies. Mol Aspects Med. 2014;39:3–32.

[61] Ajani JA, Song S, Hochster HS, Steinberg IB. Cancer stem cells: the promise and the potential. Semin Oncol. 2015;42(Suppl 1):S3–17.

[62] Mimeault M, Batra SK. Molecular biomarkers of cancer stem/progenitor cells associated with progression, metastases, and treatment resistance of aggressive cancers. Cancer Epidemiol Biomarkers Prev. 2014;23:234–54.

[63] Kim JK, Jeon HY, Kim H. The molecular mechanisms underlying the therapeutic resistance of cancer stem cells. Arch Pharm Res. 2015;38:389–401.

[64] Yu F, Yao H, Zhu P, Zhang X, Pan Q, Gong C, Huang Y, Hu X, Su F, Lieberman J, et al. let-7 regulates self renewal and tumorigenicity of breast cancer cells. Cell. 2007;131:1109–23.

[65] Shay JW, Wright WE. Telomeres and telomerase in normal and cancer stem cells. FEBS Lett. 2010;584:3819–25.

[66] Xi L, Cech TR. Inventory of telomerase components in human cells reveals multiple subpopulations of hTR and hTERT. Nucleic Acids Res. 2014;42:8565–77.

[67] Teralı K, Yilmazer A. New surprises from an old favourite: the emergence of telomerase as a key player in the regulation of cancer stemness. Biochimie. 2016;121:170–78.

[68] Bollmann FM. Physiological and pathological significance of human telomerase reverse transcriptase splice variants. Biochimie. 2013;95:1965–70.

[69] Smith LL, Coller HA, Roberts JM. Telomerase modulates expression of growth-controlling genes and enhances cell proliferation. Nat Cell Biol. 2003;5:474–9.

[70] Beck S, Jin X, Sohn YW, Kim JK, Kim SH, Yin J, Pian X, Kim SC, Nam DH, Choi YJ, Kim H. Telomerase activity-independent function of TERT allows glioma cells to attain cancer stem cell characteristics by inducing EGFR expression. Mol Cells. 2011;31:9–15.

[71] Kunimura C, Kikuchi K, Ahmed N, Shimizu A, Yasumoto S. Telomerase activity in a specific cell subset co-expressing integrin beta1/EGFR but not p75NGFR/bcl2/integrin beta4 in normal human epithelial cells. Oncogene. 1998;17:187–97.

[72] Choi J, Southworth LK, Sarin KY, Venteicher AS, Ma W, Chang W, Cheung P, Jun S, Artandi MK, Shah N, Kim SK, Artandi SE. TERT promotes epithelial proliferation through transcriptional control of a Myc- and Wnt-related developmental program. PLoS Genet. 2008;4:e10.

[73] Park JI, Venteicher AS, Hong JY, Choi J, Jun S, Shkreli M, Chang W, Meng Z, Cheung P, Ji H, McLaughlin M, Veenstra TD, Nusse R, McCrea PD, Artandi SE. Telomerase

modulates Wnt signalling by association with target gene chromatin. Nature. 2009;460:66–72.

[74] Musgrove EA, Caldon CE, Barraclough J, Stone A, Sutherland RL. Cyclin D as a therapeutic target in cancer. Nat Rev Cancer. 2011;11:558–72.

[75] Hong J, Lee JH, Chung IK. Telomerase activates transcription of cyclin D1 gene through an interaction with NOL1. J Cell Sci. 2016;129:1566–79.

[76] Jagadeesh S, Banerjee PP. Telomerase reverse transcriptase regulates the expression of a key cell cycle regulator, cyclin D1. Biochem Biophys Res Commun. 2006;347:774–80.

[77] Li J, Huang X, Xie X, Wang J, Duan M. Human telomerase reverse transcriptase regulates cyclin D1 and G1/S phase transition in laryngeal squamous carcinoma. Acta Otolaryngol. 2011;131:546–51.

[78] Mukherjee S, Firpo EJ, Wang Y, Roberts JM. Separation of telomerase functions by reverse genetics. Proc Natl Acad Sci USA. 2011;108:E1363–71.

[79] Koh CM, Khattar E, Leow SC, Liu CY, Muller J, Ang WX, Li Y, Franzoso G, Li S, Guccione E, Tergaonkar V. Telomerase regulates MYC-driven oncogenesis independent of its reverse transcriptase activity. J Clin Invest. 2015;125:2109–22.

[80] Hrdličková R, Nehyba J, Bose HR Jr. Alternatively spliced telomerase reverse transcriptase variants lacking telomerase activity stimulate cell proliferation. Mol Cell Biol. 2012;32:4283–96.

[81] Hoffmeyer K, Raggioli A, Rudloff S, Anton R, Hierholzer A, Del Valle I, Hein K, Vogt R, Kemler R. Wnt/beta-catenin signaling regulates telomerase in stem cells and cancer cells. Science. 2012;336:1549–54.

[82] Listerman I, Gazzaniga FS, Blackburn EH. An investigation of the effects of the core protein telomerase reverse transcriptase on Wnt signaling in breast cancer cells. Mol Cell Biol. 2014; 34:280–9.

[83] Strong MA, Vidal-Cardenas SL, Karim B, Yu H, Guo N, Greider CW. Phenotypes in mTERT+/- and mTERT-/- mice are due to short telomeres, not telomere-independent functions of telomerase reverse transcriptase. Mol. Cell Biol. 2011;31:2369–79.

[84] Maida Y, Yasukawa M, Furuuchi M, Lassmann T, Possemato R, Okamoto N, Kasim V, Hayashizaki Y, Hahn WC, Masutomi K. An RNA-dependent RNA polymerase formed by TERT and the RMRP RNA. Nature. 2009;461:230–5.

[85] Gonzalez OG, Assfalg R, Koch S, Schelling A, Meena JK, Kraus J, Lechel A, Katz SF, Benes V, Scharffetter-Kochanek K, Kestler HA, Gunes C, Iben S. Telomerase stimulates ribosomal DNA transcription under hyperproliferative conditions. Nat Commun. 2014;5:4599.

[86] Hanahan D, Weinberg RA. Hallmarks of cancer: the next generation. Cell. 2011;144:646–74.

[87] Dudognon C, Pendino F, Hillion J, Saumet A, Lanotte M, Segal-Bendirdjian E. Death receptor signaling regulatory function for telomerase: hTERT abolishes TRAIL-induced apoptosis, independently of telomere maintenance. Oncogene. 2004;23:7469–74.

[88] Del Bufalo D, Rizzo A, Trisciuoglio D, Cardinali G, Torrisi MR, Zangemeister-Wittke U, Zupi G, Biroccio A. Involvement of hTERT in apoptosis induced by interference with Bcl-2 expression and function. Cell Death Differ. 2005;12:1429–38.

[89] Bermudez Y, Erasso D, Johnson N, Matte AD, Lowell N, Kruk P. Telomerase confers resistance to caspase-mediated apoptosis. Clin Intervent Aging. 2006;1:155–67.

[90] Mandal M, Kumar R. Bcl-2 modulates telomerase activity. J Biol Chem. 1997;272:14183–7.

[91] Rahman R, Latonen L, Wiman KG. hTERT antagonizes p53-induced apoptosis independently of telomerase activity. Oncogene. 2005;24:1320–7.

[92] Zhou J, Mao B, Zhou Q, Ding D, Wang M, Guo P, Gao Y, Shay JW, Yuan Z, Cong YS. Endoplasmic reticulum stress activates telomerase. Aging Cell. 2014;13:197–200.

[93] Sano R, Reed JC. ER stress-induced cell death mechanisms. Biochim Biophys Acta. 2013;1833:3460–70.

[94] Hosoi T, Inoue Y, Nakatsu K, Matsushima N, Kiyose N, Shimamoto A, Tahara H, Ozawa K. TERT attenuated ER stress-induced cell death. Biochem Biophys Res Commun. 2014;447:378–82.

[95] Takahashi K, Yamanaka S. Induction of pluripotent stem cells from mouse embryonic and adult fibroblast cultures by defined factors. Cell. 2006;126:663–76.

[96] Liu A, Yu X, Liu S. Pluripotency transcription factors and cancer stem cells: small genes make a big difference. Chin J Cancer. 2013;32;483–487.

[97] Okamoto N, Yasukawa M, Nguyen C, Kasim V, Maida Y, Possemato R, Shibata T, Ligon KL, Fukami K, Hahn WC, Masutomi K. Maintenance of tumor initiating cells of defined genetic composition by nucleostemin. Proc Natl Acad Sci USA. 2011;108:20388–93.

[98] Liu Z, Li Q, Li K, Chen L, Li W, Hou M, Liu T, Yang J, Lindvall C, Bjorkholm M, Jia J, Xu D. Telomerase reverse transcriptase promotes epithelial-mesenchymal transition and stem cell-like traits in cancer cells. Oncogene. 2013;32:4203–13.

[99] Sato N, Maehara N, Mizumoto K, Nagai E, Yasoshima T, Hirata K, Tanaka M. Telomerase activity of cultured human pancreatic carcinoma cell lines correlates with their potential for migration and invasion. Cancer. 2001;91:496–504.

[100] Murasawa S, Uevadot J, Silver M, Isner JM, Losordo DW, Asahara T. Constitutive human telomerase reverse transcriptase expression enhances regenerative properties of endothelial progenitor cells. Circulation. 2002;106:1133–9.

[101] Qu Y, Mao M, Li X, Zhang L, Huang X, Yang C, Zhao F, Xiong Y, Mu D. Enhanced migration and CXCR4 over-expression in fibroblasts with telomerase reconstitution. Mol Cell Biochem. 2008;313:45–52.

[102] Ding D, Xi P, Zhou J, Wang M, Cong YS. Human telomerase reverse transcriptase regulates MMP expression independently of telomerase activity via NF-kappaB-dependent transcription. FASEB J. 2013;27:4375–83.

[103] Chen P, Peng J, Huang L, Li W, Wang W, Cui Z, Han H, Gong L, Xiang D, Qiao S, Yu X, Wei Y, Ma L, Li N, Zhu J, Leng X. Overexpression of human telomerase reverse transcriptase promotes the motility and invasiveness of HepG2 cells in vitro. Oncology Reports. 2013;30:1157–64.

[104] Ponnala S, Chetty C, Veeravalli KK, Dinh DH, Klopfenstein JD, Rao JS. MMP-9 silencing regulates hTERT expression via beta1 integrin-mediated FAK signaling and induces senescence in glioma xenograft cells. Cell Signal. 2011;23:2065–75.

[105] He B, Xiao YF, Tang B, Wu YY, Hu CJ, Xie R, Yang X, Yu ST, Dong H, Zhao XY, Li JL, Yang SM. hTERT mediates gastric cancer metastasis partially through the indirect targeting of ITGB1 by microRNA-29a. Sci Rep. 2016;6:21955.

[106] Park YP, Choi SC, Kim JH, Song EY, Kim JW, Yoon DY, Yeom YI, Lim JS, Kim JW, Paik SG, Lee HG. Up-regulation of Mac-2 binding protein by hTERT in gastric cancer. Int J Cancer. 2007;120:813–20.

[107] Grassadonia A, Tinari N, Iurisci I, Piccolo E, Cumashi A, Innominato P, D'Egidio M, Natoli C, Piantelli M, Iacobelli S. 90K (Mac-2 BP) and galectins in tumor progression and metastasis. Glycoconj J. 2004;19:551–6.

[108] Lassmann T, Maida Y, Tomaru Y, Yasukawa M, Ando Y, Kojima M, Kasim V, Simon C, Daub CO, Carninci P, Hayashizaki Y, Masutomi K. Telomerase reverse transcriptase regulates microRNAs. Int J Mol Sci. 2015;16:1192–208.

[109] Volinia S, Calin GA, Liu CG, Ambs S, Cimmino A, Petrocca F, Visone R, Iorio M, Roldo C, Ferracin M, Prueitt RL, Yanaihara N, Lanza G, Scarpa A, Vecchione A, Negrini M, Harris CC, Croce CM. A microRNA expression signature of human solid tumors defines cancer gene targets. Proc Nat Acad Sci USA. 2006;103:2257–61.

[110] Han M, Liu M, Wang Y, Chen X, Xu J, Sun Y, Zhao L, Qu H, Fan Y, Wu C. Antagonism of miR-21 reverses epithelial–mesenchymal transition and cancer stem cell phenotype through AKT/ERK1/2 inactivation by targeting PTEN. PLoS One. 2012;7:e39520.

[111] Haghpanah V, Fallah P, Tavakoli R, Naderi M, Samimi H, Soleimani M, Larijani B. Antisense-miR-21 enhances differentiation/apoptosis and reduces cancer stemness state on anaplastic thyroid cancer. Tumor Biol. 2016;37:1299–308.

[112] Bagheri S, Nosrati M, Li S, Fong S, Torabian S, Rangel J, Moore DH, Federman S, Laposa RR, Baehner FL, Sagebiel RW, Cleaver JE, Haqq C, Debs RJ, Blackburn EH, Kashani-Sabet M. Genes and pathways downstream of telomerase in melanoma metastasis. Proc Natl Acad Sci USA. 2006;103;11306–11.

[113] Wu KJ, Grandori C, Amacker M, Simon-Vermot N, Polack A, Lingner J, Dalla-Favera R. Direct activation of TERT transcription by c-MYC. Nat Genet. 1999;21:220–4.

[114] Sharma GG, Gupta A, Wang H, Scherthan H, Dhar S, Gandhi V, Iliakis G, Shay JW, Young CSH, Pandita TK. hTERT associates with human telomeres and enhances genomic stability and DNA repair. Oncogene. 2003;22:131–46.

[115] Shin KH, Kang MK, Dicterow E, Kameta A, Baluda MA, Park NH. Introduction of human telomerase reverse transcriptase to normal human fibroblasts enhances DNA repair capacity. Clin Cancer Res. 2004;10:2551–60.

[116] Fleisig HB, Hukezalie KR, Thompson CAH, Au-Yeung TTT, Ludlow AT, Xhao CR, Wong JMY. Telomerase reverse transcriptase expression protects transformed human cells against DNA-damaging agents, and increases tolerance to chromosomal instability. Oncogene. 2015;doi:10.1038/onc.2015.75.

[117] Masutomi K, Possemato R, Wong JM, Currier JL, Tothova Z, Manola JB, Ganesan S, Lansdorp PM, Collins K, Hahn WC. The telomerase reverse transcriptase regulates chromatin state and DNA damage responses. Proc Natl Acad Sci USA. 2005;102:8222–27.

[118] Ahmed S, Passos JF, Birket MJ, Beckmann T, Brings S, Peters H, Birch-Machin MA, von Zglinicki T, Saretzki G. Telomerase does not counteract telomere shortening but protects mitochondrial function under oxidative stress. J Cell Sci. 2008;121:1046–53.

[119] Haendeler J, Dröse S, Büchner N, Jakob S, Altschmied J, Goy C, Spyridopoulos I, Zeiher AM, Brandt U, Dimmeler S. Mitochondrial telomerase reverse transcriptase binds to and protects mitochondrial DNA and function from damage. Arterioscler Thromb Vasc Biol. 2009;29:929–35.

[120] Indran I, Hande P, Pervaiz S. hTERT overexpression alleviates intracellular ROS production, improves mitochondrial function, and inhibits ROS-mediated apoptosis in cancer cells. Cancer Res. 2011;71:266–76.

[121] Singhapol C, Pal D, Czapiewski R, Porika M, Nelson G, Saretzki GC. Mitochondrial telomerase protects cancer cells from nuclear DNA damage and apoptosis. PLoS One. 2013;8:e52989.

[122] Listerman I, Sun J, Gazzaniga FS, Lukas JL, Blackburn EH. The major reverse transcriptase-incompetent splice variant of the human telomerase protein inhibits telomerase activity but protects from apoptosis. Cancer Res. 2013;73:2817–28.

[123] Ghosh A, Saginc G, Leow SC, Khattar E, Shin EM, Yan TD, Wong M, Zhang Z, Li G, Sung WK, Zhou J, Chng WJ, Li S, Liu E, Tergaonkar V. Telomerase directly regulates NF-kappaB-dependent transcription. Nat Cell Biol. 2012;14:1270–81.

[124] Yin L, Hubbard AK, Giardina C. NF-kappa B regulates transcription of the mouse telomerase catalytic subunit. J Biol Chem. 2000;275:36,671–5.

[125] Zhou L, Zheng D, Wang M, Cong YS. Telomerase reverse transcriptase activates the expression of vascular endothelial growth factor independent of telomerase activity. Biochem Biophys Res Commun. 2009;386:739–43.

[126] Liu N, Ding D, Hao W, Yang F, Wu X, Wang M, Xu X, Ju Z, Liu JP, Song Z, Shay JW, Guo Y, Cong YS. hTERT promotes tumor angiogenesis by activating VEGF via interactions with the Sp1 transcription factor. Nuc Acids Res. 2016 (in press)

[127] Bermudez Y, Yang H, Saunders BO, Cheng JQ, Nicosia SV, Kruk PA. VEGF- and LPA-induced telomerase in human ovarian cancer cells is Sp1-dependent. Gynecol Oncol. 2007;106:526–37.

[128] Zhong YQ, Xia ZS, Fu YR, Zhu ZH. Knockdown of hTERT by siRNA suppresses growth of Capan-2 human pancreatic cancer cell via the inhibition of expressions of Bcl-2 and COX-2. J Dig Dis. 2010;11:176–84.

[129] Liu L, Liu C, Lou F, Zhang G, Wang X, Fan Y, Yan K, Wang K, Xu Z, Hu S, Björkholm M, Xu D. Activation of telomerase by seminal plasma in malignant and normal cervical epithelial cells. J Pathol. 2011;225:203–11.

[130] Jäger K, Walter M. Therapeutic targeting of telomerase. Genes. 2016;7:39.

[131] Brennan SK, Wang Q, Tressler R, Harley C, Go N, Bassett E, Huff CA, Jones RJ, Matsui W. Telomerase inhibition targets clonogenic multiple myeloma cells through telomere length-dependent and independent mechanisms. PLoS One. 2010;5:e12487.

[132] Joseph I, Tressler R, Bassett E, Harley C, Buseman CM, Pattamatta P, Wright WE, Shay JW, Go NF. The telomerase inhibitor imetelstat depletes cancer stem cells in breast and pancreatic cancer cell lines. Cancer Res. 2010;70:9494–504.

[133] Gryaznov SM. Oligonucleotide n3′–>p5′ phosphoramidates and thio-phoshoramidates as potential therapeutic agents. Chem Biodivers. 2010;7:477–93.